The Neurobiology of Addiction

The Neurobiology of Addiction:
New Vistas

Edited by

Trevor W. Robbins
Behavioural and Clinical Neuroscience Institute
Department of Experimental Psychology
University of Cambridge
Cambridge, UK

Barry J. Everitt
Behavioural and Clinical Neuroscience Institute
Department of Experimental Psychology
University of Cambridge
Cambridge, UK

David J. Nutt
Head of Department of Neuropsychopharmacology and Molecular Imaging
Division of Neuroscience & Mental Health
Imperial College London
London, UK

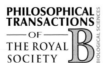

PHILOSOPHICAL TRANSACTIONS
— OF —
THE ROYAL SOCIETY B BIOLOGICAL SCIENCES

Originating from a Theme Issue first published in Philosophical
Transactions of the Royal Society B: Biological Sciences

http://publishing.royalsociety.org/philtransb

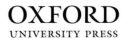

OXFORD
UNIVERSITY PRESS

OXFORD
UNIVERSITY PRESS

Great Clarendon Street, Oxford OX2 6DP

Oxford University Press is a department of the University of Oxford.
It furthers the University's objective of excellence in research, scholarship,
and education by publishing worldwide in

Oxford New York

Auckland Cape Town Dar es Salaam Hong Kong Karachi
Kuala Lumpur Madrid Melbourne Mexico City Nairobi
New Delhi Shanghai Taipei Toronto

With offices in

Argentina Austria Brazil Chile Czech Republic France Greece
Guatemala Hungary Italy Japan Poland Portugal Singapore
South Korea Switzerland Thailand Turkey Ukraine Vietnam

Oxford is a registered trade mark of Oxford University Press
in the UK and in certain other countries

Published in the United States
by Oxford University Press Inc., New York
© The Royal Society, 2010

A catalogue record for this title is available from the British Library
Data available

Library of Congress Cataloging in Publication Data
Data available

Typeset in Minion by Glyph International, Bangalore, India
Printed in Great Britain
on acid-free paper by
the MPG Books Group,
Bodmin and King's Lynn

ISBN 978–0–19–956215–2

10 9 8 7 6 5 4 3 2 1

Contents

Contributors

David Belin Behavioural and Clinical Neuroscience Institute, Department of Experimental Psychology, University of Cambridge, Cambridge, UK

Kent C. Berridge Department of Psychology (Biopsychology Program), East Hall, 530 Church Street, The University of Michigan, Ann Arbor, MI 48109, USA

Thomas J. R. Beveridge Department of Physiology and Pharmacology, Center for the Neurobiological Investigation of Drug Abuse, Wake Forest University School of Medicine, Medical Center Boulevard, Winston Salem, NC 27157-1083

Jennifer M. Bossert Behavioral Neuroscience Branch, Intramural Research Program, National Institute on Drug Abuse, NIH/DHHS, 251 Bayview Blvd, Baltimore, MD 21224

Toni-Kim Clarke MRC-SGDP-Centre, Institute of Psychiatry at King's College, 16 De Crespigny Park, London SE5 8AF

John C. Crabbe Department of Behavioral Neuroscience, Portland Alcohol Research Center, Oregon Health & Science University, VA Medical Center (R&D 12), 3710 Southwest US Veterans Hospital Road, Portland, OR 97239

Hans S. Crombag Behavioural and Clinical Neuroscience Group, Department of Psychology, School of Life Sciences, The University of Sussex, Brighton BN1 9RH

Paul W. Czoty Department of Physiology and Pharmacology, Wake Forest University School of Medicine, 546 NRC, Medical Center Boulevard, Winston-Salem, NC 27157-1083

Jeffrey W. Dalley Behavioural and Clinical Neuroscience Institute, Department of Experimental Psychology, and Department of Psychiatry, University of Cambridge, Cambridge, UK

Theodora Duka Department of Psychology, John Maynard Smith Building, University of Sussex, Falmer, Brighton BN1 9QG

Daina Economidou Behavioural and Clinical Neuroscience Institute, Department of Experimental Psychology, University of Cambridge, Cambridge, UK

Barry J. Everitt Behavioural and Clinical Neuroscience Institute, Department of Experimental Psychology, University of Cambridge, Downing street, Cambridge CB2 3EB UK

Joanna S. Fowler Medical Department, Brookhaven National Laboratory, Upton, NY 11973

Hugh Garavan Institute of Neuroscience, School of Psychology, Trinity College Dublin, Dublin 2, Ireland, and Department of Psychiatry and Behavioral Neuroscience, Medical College of Wisconsin, Milwaukee, WI 53226

Kathryn E. Gill Department of Physiology and Pharmacology, Wake Forest University School of Medicine, Medical Center Boulevard, Winston Salem, NC 27157-1083

Robert W. Gould Department of Physiology and Pharmacology, Wake Forest University School of Medicine, 546 NRC, Medical Center Boulevard, Winston-Salem, NC 27157-1083

Colleen A. Hanlon Department of Physiology and Pharmacology, Wake Forest University School of Medicine, Medical Center Boulevard, Winston Salem, NC 27157-1083

Robert Hester Institute of Neuroscience, School of Psychology, Trinity College Dublin, Dublin 2, Ireland, and Queensland Brain Institute and School of Psychology, University of Queensland, St. Lucia, QLD 4072, Australia

Jacqueline N. Kaufman Department of Psychiatry and Behavioral Neuroscience, Medical College of Wisconsin, Milwaukee, WI 53226, Department of Physical Medicine and Rehabilitation, University of Michigan, 325 East Eisenhower Suite 100, Ann Arbor, MI 48108

George F. Koob Committee on the Neurobiology of Addictive Disorders, The Scripps Research Institute, 10550 North Torrey Pines Road, SP30-2400, La Jolla, CA 92037

Eisuke Koya Behavioral Neuroscience Branch, Intramural Research Program, National Institute on Drug Abuse, NIH/DHHS, 251 Bayview Blvd, Baltimore, MD 21224

Athina Markou Department of Psychiatry, School of Medicine, University of California at San Diego, 9500 Gilman Drive, Mail Code 0603, La Jolla, CA 92093-0603, USA

Michel Le Moal Physiopathologie du Comportement, Institut National de la Santé et de la Recherche Médicale, Institut François Magendie, Université Victor Ségalen Bordeaux 2, 33076 Bordeaux, France

Michael A. Nader Department of Physiology and Pharmacology, Wake Forest University School of Medicine, 546 NRC, Medical Center Boulevard, Winston-Salem, NC 27157-1083

Eric J. Nestler Fishberg Department of Neuroscience, Mount Sinai School of Medicine, One Gustave L. Levy Place, Box 1065, New York, NY 10029

David J. Nutt Department of Neuropsychopharmacology and Molecular Imaging, Division of Neuroscience & Mental Health, Imperial College London, Burlington Danes Building, Hammersmith Campus, 160 Du Cane Road, London W12 0NN

Charles P. O'Brien Department of Psychiatry, University of Pennsylvania, 3900 Chestnut Street, Philadelphia, PA 19104–6178

Yann Pelloux Behavioural and Clinical Neuroscience Institute, Department of Experimental Psychology, University of Cambridge, Cambridge, UK

Linda J. Porrino Department of Physiology and Pharmacology, Center for the Neurobiological Investigation of Drug Abuse, Wake Forest University School of Medicine, Medical Center Boulevard, Winston Salem, NC 27157-1083

Marc N. Potenza Associate Professor, Departments of Psychiatry and Child Study Center, Yale University School of Medicine, Connecticut Mental Health Center, Room S-104, 34 Park Street, New Haven, CT 06519

Natallia V. Riddick Department of Physiology and Pharmacology, Wake Forest University School of Medicine, 546 NRC, Medical Center Boulevard, Winston Salem, NC 27157-1083

Trevor W. Robbins Department of Experimental Psychology, University of Cambridge, Downing Street, Cambridge CB2 3EB

Terry E. Robinson Biopsychology Program, Department of Psychology, University of Michigan, East Hall, 530 Church st., Ann Arbor, MI (USA) 48109

Gunter Schumann MRC-SGDP-Centre, Institute of Psychiatry at King's College, 16 De Crespigny Park, London SE5 8AF

Yavin Shaham Behavioral Neuroscience Branch, Intramural Research Program, National Institute on Drug Abuse, NIH/DHHS, 251 Bayview Blvd, Baltimore, MD 21224

David N. Stephens Department of Psychology, John Maynard Smith Building, University of Sussex, Falmer, Brighton BN1 9QG

Jane Stewart Center for Studies in Behavioral Neurobiology/Groupe de Recherche en Neurobiologie Comportementale, Department of Psychology, Concordia University, 7141 Sherbrooke Street West, Montreal, QC, Canada H4B 1R6

Frank Telang National Institute on Alcohol Abuse and Alcoholism, Bethesda, MD 20892

Nora D. Volkow National Institute on Drug Abuse, and National Institute on Alcohol Abuse and Alcoholism, Bethesda, MD 20892

Gene-Jack Wang Medical Department, Brookhaven National Laboratory, Upton, NY 11973

Chloe C. Y. Wong MRC-SGDP-Centre, Institute of Psychiatry at King's College, 16 De Crespigny Park, London SE5 8AF

Introduction: The neurobiology of drug addiction – new vistas

Trevor W. Robbins, Barry J. Everitt, and David J. Nutt

This Royal Society Discussion meeting, held on February 25 and 26 2008, reported first in the *Philosophical Transactions of the Royal Society, B, Biological Sciences*, (363, 3107–3286), and now captured by this volume, was intended to mark the enormous scientific progress that has been made in this field in the last decade or so, advances which can be measured from the time of a Frontiers Meeting of the Wellcome Trust (Altman et al. 1996). At that time, it was already clear that the nucleus accumbens in the ventral striatum of the basal forebrain was a key structure mediating some of the positive reinforcing ('rewarding') effects of several drugs of abuse, especially the psychomotor stimulant drugs, including cocaine and amphetamine. The innervation of the nucleus accumbens by the chemical neurotransmitter dopamine was also known to be a key mediator of some of these actions. However, although it was suspected that the nucleus accumbens was merely one node in a complex circuitry at the 'limbic-striatal interface', the full nature and functions of this circuitry was still unclear.

In parallel with these developments were new ideas emanating from the realization that certain forms of associative learning, including both Pavlovian and instrumental conditioning, depended upon elements of this system, for natural rewards such as food and sex, as well as for drugs of abuse. It was already clear that relapse derived in part from classical conditioning. Some theorists had begun to speculate that certain aspects of associative conditioning such as stimulus–response habit-learning were particularly relevant to understating drug abuse (e.g. White 1996), but the modern theory of habit-learning itself was still being developed in a way which was to prove crucial for understanding the functions of the striatum as a whole. Dopamine had previously been related to 'reward' functions (Wise 2004), but the shortcomings of this bold but simplistic notion were already becoming apparent, especially in relation to understanding how, for example, opiate drugs exerted their addictive actions. The concept of 'opponent motivational systems', originally developed as a notable psychological theory, was just beginning to be related to opponent neural systems, although the precise neural correlates of the 'negative' component were still not well understood. In addition to these basic issues of neural mediation, the question of why only certain individuals become addicted, even after exposure to drugs of abuse was only just being formulated and the consequences of drug addiction, including cognitive impairment and possibly lack of self-control, were also mainly a matter for speculation.

Many of these issues were addressed in the first part of the Discussion Meeting, '*Theories of drug addiction*'. Koob and LeMoal, following on from their 2005 synthesis, elaborate on the development of their neural opponent-motivational theory, which they relate closely to the concepts of homeostatsis and allostasis from stress research, and which appears especially relevant to the understanding of opiate abuse. Central to this theory is the concept that withdrawal leads to an aversive motivational state and that much drug-seeking behaviour is directed towards alleviating this state. Koob and LeMoal also subscribe to a staging of addiction that includes an initial 'impulsivity' phase followed by 'compulsivity', which forms the central theme of the paper by Everitt et al. These authors demonstrate how impulsive trait-like behaviour leads to compulsive-like cocaine dependence, paralleling a 'shift' in the locus of neural control from the ventral to the dorsal striatum, and embracing a possible behavioural transition in instrumental control to a dominance by Stimulus–Response habit-like representations. Robinson and Berridge counterpoint these two positions via their own 'incentive-salience' hypothesis with its focus on the sensitization by drugs of abuse of the mesolimbic dopamine system. Finally, Stewart reviews the considerable advances made in delineating the different and distinct neural systems underlying relapse, following exposure to stress, drug-related cues, or the drug itself.

Much of the advance in understanding of the neurobiology of drug abuse has come from the study of psychomotor stimulant and opiate drugs, but other forms of addiction have been recognized, notably in the case of nicotine, and now more controversially, in the form of the 'behavioural addictions' of gambling and compulsive eating. The questions now being asked are whether there are similar neural mechanisms underlying these extensions to the concept of addiction. Hence, in the section entitled '*Extending the concept of addiction*', Markou illustrates the utility of applying similar concepts and methods to the understanding of nicotine addiction, as have been used for the psychomotor stimulants. In particular, the advent of drugs with glutmatatergic or GABA-ergic actions is shown to have implications for the treatment of nicotine dependence. This is paralleled by Stephens and Duka's chapter on neural mechanisms underlying alcohol dependence, which shows how binge drinking in humans can be modelled in rodents to suggest important changes in glutamatergic-mediated excitability and reductions in neuronal plasticity (long-term potentiation) in limbic structures such as the amygdala and hippocampus. Potenza surveys the burgeoning information concerning compulsive gambling. Much of this concerns human behaviour and has emerged from the use of brain imaging techniques, which have revealed a remarkable commonality of neural systems mediating the reinforcing properties of drugs and money. He also considers the co-morbidity of gambling with substance dependence (e.g. especially alcoholism) and where similar issues of trait impulsivity are seen as contributing to individual vulnerability to gambling behaviour. Finally, the Director of the US National Institute on Drug Abuse, Nora Volkow, updates and extends her classic analysis (e.g. Volkow et al. 2003) of neuro-chemical changes present in substance abusers (using positron emission tomography, PET) to include obese individuals and animal models of obesity. These studies also raise the issue of the possibly causal role of baseline individual differences in striatal dopamine receptor binding that are also taken up in the contributions by Everitt et al. and by Nader et al. (see below). She also introduced an idea that has emerged from both the animal (e.g. Jentsch & Taylor 1999; Robbins & Everitt 1999) and the human literature (Rogers & Robbins 2002) that substance abuse can arise from an impairment of top–down inhibitory control, presumably arising from impairments in frontal lobe function.

The next group of papers, '*Vulnerability to drug abuse*', appropriately consider genetic and environmental factors contributing to the neurobiology of drug abuse, especially in the vanguard of the Human Genome Project. Crabbe focuses on the contribution of behavioural genetics, mainly in the mouse, to the understanding of alcoholism, where there is perhaps the best evidence of heritability. He also considers the likely importance of epigenetic factors. Wong and Schumann introduce strategies addressing the heterogeneity and polygenicity of substance use based on the identification of more homogenous subgroups of patients and the characterization of genes contributing to their phenotype via linkage and association studies. They also advocate functional genetic analysis based on endophenotyes and animal behavioural experimentation. By contrast, in work parallel to that of Volkow and colleagues, Nader et al. present the results of an exceptionally systematic series of PET studies of rhesus monkeys before and after their exposure to cocaine. The crucial findings were of reductions in striatal D2 dopamine receptor binding being found *before* drug exposure, implying that this change was not simply a consequence of drug abuse, but may be predisposing to it. Everitt et al. had earlier described the recent similar findings of Dalley et al. (2007) for the rat—where reductions in D2 dopamine receptor binding had been associated with enhanced impulsivity. Of course, the question arises about the origin of such predisposing changes, whether for example, they depend on specific genes or are the product of environmental factors. In the case of the non-human primates, Nader et al. stress the fact that the low DA binding is associated with the presumed stress that results from social neglect. Shaham and colleagues, in the paper by Crombag et al., return to the environmental factors through which individuals relapse to substance abuse, specifically according to contextual conditioning. This article thus complements the contribution by Stewart in defining the neural substrates of contextual reinstatement of drug-seeking behaviour.

The final section considers '*Causes and consequences of addiction*'. Nestler begins by reviewing the considerable advances over the last decade in understanding of the intracellular molecular changes associated with chronic exposure to drugs of abuse, in particular biochemical changes in proteins such as the transcription factor deltaFosB and its gene targets. He is approaching this question by use of DNA expression arrays coupled with the analysis of chromatin remodelling—changes in the posttranslational modifications of histones at drug-regulated gene promoters. His findings establish chromatin remodelling as an important regulatory mechanism underlying drug-induced behavioural plasticity, and promise to reveal fundamentally new insight into how ΔFosB contributes to addiction by regulating the expression of specific target genes in brain reward pathways. The paper by Porrino surveys the consequences of chronic drug exposure through self-administration in monkeys that provide further evidence for ramifying effects beyond the initial sites of drug action in the ventral striatum to the dorsal striatum and cortex, established by methods including autoradiography and the measurement of cerebral metabolism in the temporal and frontal lobes. These neuroanatomical changes are also accompanied by impairments in cognitive function such as visual recognition memory that are also demonstrated to occur in human drug abusers, using comparable neuropsychological tests. Garavan and colleagues also consider the sequelae of drug addiction in human substance abusers from the vantage of functional brain imaging using magnetic resonance (fMRI). They provide direct evidence that inhibitory control is impaired in cocaine abusers, associated with altered activity of the prefrontal cortex during performance of the stop-signal reaction time task. Moreover, they show surprisingly that intravenous cocaine actually *improves* performance in this task, not only in behavioural terms but also by normalizing brain activity in lateral and medial regions of the prefrontal cortex. These findings controversially suggest that one possible factor contributing to the susceptibility to stimulant addiction is a drive to self-medication. The last contribution by O'Brien focuses specifically on treatment of addiction and surveys the large number of strategies that are currently in vogue, particularly from a pharmaceutical viewpoint. New treatments have emerged over the past decade, many based on the advances derived from basic neurobiology, and there are obvious indications for opiate (e.g. buprenorphine), nicotine (e.g. patches), and alcohol (e.g. acamprosate and naltrexone) abuse, as well as more speculative candidate treatments such as vaccination. However, drug companies still needed encouragement to innovate in this area, and any treatment for cocaine dependence is still problematic.

The Discussion provoked by the Meeting was a measure of the contemporary interest in this field from the public, as well as the scientific community. Some of the current excitement has been engendered in the UK by a Technology Foresight Initiative in *Brain science, addiction and drugs*, published as *Drugs and the Future: Brain science, addiction, and society* (*2007*). This initiative has recently been the subject of a similarly named Academy of Medical Sciences publication, containing recommendations for UK government for future policy in the field of drug addiction and related fields, such as the treatment by drugs of mental illness, and cognitive enhancing drugs. The Discussion Meeting helped to highlight the vibrancy of this field in the UK and internationally and this volume is intended to mark this landmark. Many of the chapters published in the original *Philosophical Transactions* issue from had to be truncated for reasons of space. However, this collection consists of several revised and extended versions of the papers originally published in the *Philosophical Transactions*.

We would like to express our thanks to Nicola Richmond for her secretarial assistance with this volume, also to Chloe Sheppard and Claire Rawlinson of the Royal Society for facilitating the collation of the manuscripts, and to Martin Baum of Oxford University Press, for enabling the project.

References

Altman, J., Everitt, B. J., Glautier, S. et al. 1996 The biological, social and clinical bases of drug addiction: commentary and debate. *Psychopharmacology* **125**, 285–345.

Dalley, J. W., Fryer, T. D., Brichard, L. et al. 2007. Nucleus accumbens D2/3 receptors predict trait impulsivity and cocaine reinforcement. *Science* **315**, 1267–70.

Jentsch, J. D. & Taylor, J. R. 1999 Impulsivity resulting from frontostriatal dysfunction in drug abuse: Implications for the control of behavior by reward-related stimuli. *Psychopharmacology* **146**, 373–90.

Koob, G. F. & LeMoal, M. 2005 *The neurobiology of drug addiction*, Elsevier: Amsterdam.

Nutt, D., Robbins, T. W., Stimson, G. V., Ince, M. & Jackson, A. (eds.) 2007 *Drugs and the future: brain science, addiction and society*. Elsevier: Amsterdam.

Robbins, T. W. & Everitt, B. J. 1999 Drug addiction: bad habits add up. *Nature* **398**, 567–70.

Rogers, R. D. & Robbins, T. W. 2001 Investigating the neurocognitive deficits associated with chronic drug misuse. *Current Opinions in Neurobiology* **11**, 250–7.

Volkow, N. D., Fowler, J. S. & Wang, G. J. (2003) Positrom emission tomography and single-photon emission computed tomography in substance abuse research. *Seminars in Nuclear Medicine* **33**, 114–28.

White, N. M. 1996 Addictive drugs as reinforcers: multiple partial actions on memory systems. *Addiction* **91**, 921–49.

Wise, R. 2004 Dopamine, learning and motivation. *Nature Reviews Neuroscience* **5**, 483–94.

Part 1

Theories of Drug Addiction

2

Neurobiological mechanisms for opponent motivational processes in addiction

George F. Koob* and Michel Le Moal

The conceptualization of drug addiction as a compulsive disorder with excessive drug intake and loss of control over intake requires motivational mechanisms. Opponent process as a motivational theory for the negative reinforcement of drug dependence has long required a neurobiological explanation. Key neurochemical elements involved in reward and stress within basal forebrain structures involving the ventral striatum and extended amygdala are hypothesized to be dysregulated in addiction to convey the opponent motivational processes that drive dependence. Specific neurochemical elements in these structures include not only decreases in reward neurotransmission such as dopamine and opioid peptides in the ventral striatum, but also recruitment of brain stress systems such as corticotropin-releasing factor (CRF), noradrenaline, and dynorphin in the extended amygdala. Acute withdrawal from all major drugs of abuse produces increases in reward thresholds, anxiety-like responses, and extracellular levels of CRF in the central nucleus of the amygdala. CRF receptor antagonists block excessive drug intake produced by dependence. A brain stress response system is hypothesized to be activated by acute excessive drug intake, to be sensitized during repeated withdrawal, to persist into protracted abstinence, and to contribute to stress-induced relapse. The combination of loss of reward function and recruitment of brain stress systems provides a powerful neurochemical basis for the long hypothesized opponent motivational processes responsible for the negative reinforcement driving addiction.

Key Words: Addiction; opponent process; stress; extended amygdala; corticotropin-releasing factor.

2.1 Definitions and conceptual framework

Drug addiction, also known as substance dependence, is a chronically relapsing disorder characterized by (i) compulsion to seek and take the drug, (ii) loss of control in limiting intake, and (iii) emergence of a negative emotional state (e.g. dysphoria, anxiety, irritability) reflecting a motivational withdrawal syndrome when access to the drug is prevented (defined here as dependence; Koob & Le Moal 1997). *Addiction* is assumed to be identical to the syndrome of *substance dependence* (as currently defined by the *Diagnostic and statistical manual of mental disorders*, 4th edn., American Psychiatric Association 1994). Clinically, the occasional but limited use of a drug with the *potential* for abuse or dependence is distinct from escalated drug intake and the emergence of a chronic drug-dependent state.

Drug addiction has been conceptualized as a disorder that involves elements of both impulsivity and compulsivity (Koob & Le Moal 2008). The elements of impulsivity and compulsivity yield a composite addiction cycle comprising three stages—*preoccupation/anticipation*, *binge/intoxication*, and *withdrawal/negative affect* (Fig. 2.1)—in which impulsivity often dominates at the early stages and compulsivity dominates at the terminal stages. As an individual moves from impulsivity to compulsivity, a shift occurs from positive reinforcement

* gkoob@scripps.edu

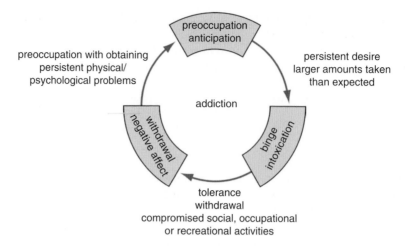

preoccupation
anticipation

preoccupation with obtaining
persistent physical/
psychological problems

persistent desire
larger amounts taken
than expected

addiction

withdrawal
negative affect

binge
intoxication

tolerance
withdrawal
compromised social, occupational
or recreational activities

Fig. 2.1 Diagram describing the addiction cycle—preoccupation/anticipation ('craving'), binge/intoxication and withdrawal/negative affect—with the different criteria for substance dependence incorporated from the *Diagnostic and statistical manual of mental disorders*, 4th edn. (Adapted from Koob 2008.)

driving the motivated behaviour to negative reinforcement driving the motivated behaviour (Koob 2004). These three stages are conceptualized as interacting with each other, becoming more intense and ultimately leading to the pathological state known as addiction (Koob & Le Moal 1997). Different drugs produce different patterns of addiction with an emphasis on different components of the addiction cycle (Koob et al. 2008). Common elements include binge/intoxication (dramatic with psychostimulants and ethanol but not present with nicotine), withdrawal/negative affect (dramatic with opioids and alcohol but common to all drugs of abuse), and preoccupation/anticipation (common to all drugs of abuse). The present review will focus on the role of the brain reward and stress systems in one key and common element of addiction: the withdrawal/negative affect stage of the addiction cycle.

2.2 Opponent process and addiction

2.2.1 Motivation and opponent process

Motivation is a state that can be defined as a 'tendency of the whole animal to produce organized activity' (Hebb 1972), and such motivational states are not constant but rather vary over time. The concept of motivation was linked inextricably with hedonic, affective, or emotional states in addiction in the context of temporal dynamics by Solomon's opponent process theory of motivation. Solomon & Corbit (1974) postulated that hedonic, affective, or emotional states, once initiated, are automatically modulated by the central nervous system with mechanisms that reduce the intensity of hedonic feelings. The opponent process theory of motivation is defined by two processes. The a-process consists of either positive or negative hedonic responses, occurs shortly after the presentation of a stimulus, correlates closely with the intensity, quality and duration of the reinforcer, and shows tolerance. By contrast, the b-process appears after the a-process has terminated and is sluggish in onset, slow to build up to an asymptote, slow to decay, and gets larger with repeated exposure. Thus, the affective dynamics of the opponent process generate new motives and new opportunities for reinforcing and energizing behaviour (Solomon 1980).

From a drug-taking perspective of brain motivational systems, the initial acute effect of a drug (the a-process or positive hedonic response) was hypothesized to be opposed or counteracted by the b-process as homeostatic changes in brain systems (Fig. 2.2). This affect control system was conceptualized as a single negative feedback or opponent loop that opposes the stimulus-aroused affective state and suppresses or reduces all departures from hedonic neutrality (Solomon & Corbit 1974; Siegel 1975; Poulos & Cappell 1991). Affective states, pleasant or aversive, were hypothesized to be automatically opposed by centrally mediated mechanisms that reduce the intensity of these affective states. In this opponent process theory, tolerance and dependence are inextricably linked (Solomon & Corbit 1974). In the context of drug dependence, Solomon argued that the first few self-administrations of an opiate drug produce a pattern of motivational changes similar to that of the a-process or euphoria, followed by a decline in intensity. After the effects of the drug wear off, an opposing, aversive negative emotional state emerges, i.e. the b-process.

More recently, opponent process theory has been expanded into the domains of the neurobiology of drug addiction from a neurocircuitry perspective. An allostatic model of the brain motivational systems has been proposed to explain the persistent changes in motivation that are associated with dependence in addiction (Koob & Le Moal 2001, 2008). In this formulation, addiction is conceptualized as a cycle of increasing dysregulation of brain reward/anti-reward mechanisms, which results in a negative emotional state contributing to the compulsive use of drugs. Counteradaptive processes such as the opponent b-process, which are part of the normal homeostatic limitation of reward function, fail to return to within the normal homeostatic range.

These counteradaptive processes are hypothesized to be mediated by two processes: within- and between-system neuroadaptations (Koob & Bloom 1988). In a within-system neuroadaptation, 'the primary cellular response element to the drug would itself adapt to neutralize the drug's effects; persistence of the opposing effects after the drug disappears

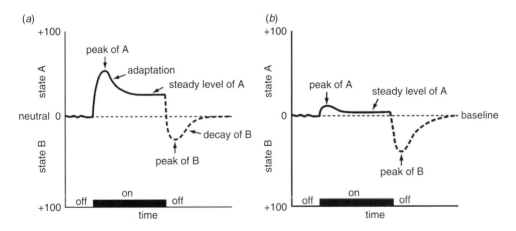

Fig. 2.2 Opponent process theory of affective dynamics relevant to addiction. (*a*) The standard pattern of affective dynamics produced by a relatively novel unconditioned stimulus (first few stimulations). (*b*) The standard pattern of affective dynamics produced by a familiar, frequently repeated unconditioned stimulus (after many stimulations). (Adapted from Solomon 1980.)

would produce the withdrawal response' (Koob & Bloom 1988, p. 720). Thus, a within-system neuroadaptation is a molecular or cellular change within a given reward circuit to accommodate the overactivity of hedonic processing associated with addiction resulting in a decrease in reward function.

In a between-system neuroadaptation, neurochemical systems other than those involved in the positive rewarding effects of drugs of abuse are recruited or dysregulated by chronic activation of the reward system (Koob & Bloom 1988). Thus, a between-system neuroadaptation is a circuitry change in which another different circuit (anti-reward circuit) is activated by the reward circuit and has opposing actions, again limiting the reward function. The purpose of this review is to explore the neuroadaptational changes that occur in the brain emotional systems to account for the neurocircuitry changes that produce opponent processes, which, we hypothesize, have a key role in the compulsivity of addiction.

2.2.2 Animal models of addiction relevant to opponent process

Animal models of addiction on specific drugs such as stimulants, opioids, alcohol, nicotine, and Δ^9-tetrahydrocannabinol can be defined by the models relevant to different stages of the addiction cycle. Animal models of reward and reinforcement (binge/intoxication stage) are extensive and well validated and include intravenous drug self-administration, conditioned place preference, and brain stimulation reward (Shippenberg & Koob 2002; Table 2.1). Animal models of the withdrawal/negative affect stage include measures of conditioned place aversion (rather than preference) to precipitated or spontaneous withdrawal from chronic administration of a drug, increases in reward thresholds using brain stimulation reward, and dependence-induced increased drug-taking and drug-seeking behaviours (Table 2.1). Such increased self-administration in dependent animals has now been observed with cocaine, methamphetamine, nicotine, heroin, and alcohol (Ahmed & Koob 1998; Ahmed et al. 2000; O'Dell et al. 2004; Kitamura et al. 2006; George et al. 2007; Fig. 2.3). This model will be a key element for evaluating the motivational significance of opponent process changes in the brain reward and stress systems in addiction outlined below. Animal models of the preoccupation/anticipation ('craving') stage involve reinstatement of drug seeking following extinction elicited by the drugs themselves, by cues linked to the drug and by exposure to stressors (Weiss et al. 2001; Shaham et al. 2003) and measures of protracted abstinence (Table 2.1). In stress-induced reinstatement, acute stressors can reinitiate drug-seeking behaviour in animals that have been extinguished. In rats with a history of drug dependence, protracted

Table 2.1 Stages of the addiction cycle.

Stage	Source of reinforcement	Animal models
Binge/intoxication	Positive reinforcement	Conditioned place preference, drug self-administration, decreased reward thresholds
Withdrawal/negative affect	Negative reinforcement	Conditioned place aversion, increased self-administration in dependence, increased reward thresholds
Preoccupation/anticipation	Conditioned positive and negative reinforcement	Drug-induced reinstatement, cue-induced reinstatement, stress-induced reinstatement, protracted abstinence

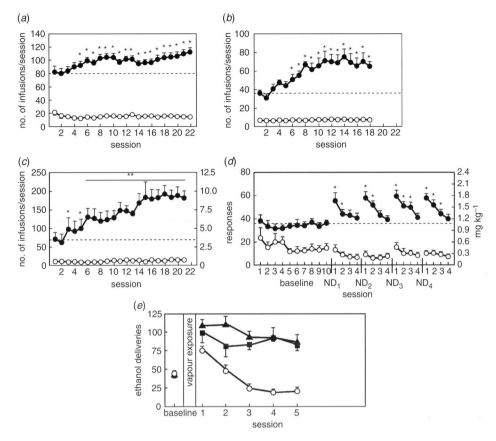

Fig. 2.3 Increases in drug intake associated with extended access and dependence. (*a*) Effect of drug availability on cocaine intake (mean ± s.e.m.). In long-access (LgA) rats ($n = 12$; filled circles) but not in short-access (ShA) rats ($n = 12$; open circles), mean total cocaine intake started to increase significantly from session 5 (*$p < 0.05$; sessions 5–22 compared with session 1) and continued to increase thereafter (*$p < 0.05$; session 5 compared with sessions 8–10, 12, 13, and 17–22). (Adapted from Ahmed & Koob 1998.) (*b*) Effect of drug availability on total intravenous heroin self-infusions (mean ± s.e.m.). During the escalation phase, rats had access to heroin (40 mg per infusion) for 1 hour (ShA rats, $n = 5$–6; open circles) or 11 hours per session (LgA rats, $n = 5$–6; filled circles). Regular 1-hour (ShA rats) or 11-hour (LgA rats) sessions of heroin self-administration were performed 6 days per week. The dotted line indicates the mean (±s.e.m.) number of heroin self-infusions of LgA rats during the first 11-hour session. *$p < 0.05$ compared with first session (paired *t*-test). (Adapted from Ahmed et al. 2000.) (*c*) Effect of extended access to intravenous methamphetamine self-administration as a function of daily sessions in rats trained to self-administer 0.05 mg kg^{-1} per infusion of intravenous methamphetamine during a 6-hour session. Short-access (open circles) group, 1-hour session ($n = 6$). Long-access (filled circles) group, 6-hour session ($n = 4$). All data were analysed using two-way ANOVA (dose × escalation session interaction within ShA or LgA group). *$p < 0.05$ and **$p < 0.01$ versus day 1. (Adapted from Kitamura et al. 2006.) (*d*) Total 23-hour active (filled circles) and inactive (open circles) responses after repeated cycles of 72 hours of nicotine deprivation (ND) followed by 4 days of self-administration (*$p < 0.05$ versus baseline). (Adapted from George et al. 2007.) (*e*) Ethanol deliveries (mean ± s.e.m.) in rats trained to respond for 10% ethanol and then either not exposed to ethanol vapour (control, $n = 5$; circles) or exposed to intermittent ethanol vapour (14 hours on/10 hours off) for two weeks and then tested either two hours ($n = 6$; squares) or eight hours ($n = 6$; triangles) after removal from ethanol vapour. No difference was observed between rats exposed to intermittent vapour and tested either two or eight hours after ethanol withdrawal. (Adapted from O'Dell et al. 2004.)

abstinence can be defined as a period after acute withdrawal has disappeared, usually two to eight weeks post-drug.

2.3 Within-system neuroadaptations in addiction

Electrical brain stimulation reward or intracranial self-stimulation has a long history as a measure of activity of the brain reward system and of the acute reinforcing effects of drugs of abuse. All drugs of abuse, when administered acutely, decrease brain stimulation reward thresholds (Kornetsky & Esposito 1979). Brain stimulation reward involves widespread neurocircuitry in the brain, but the most sensitive sites defined by the lowest thresholds involve the trajectory of the medial forebrain bundle connecting the ventral tegmental area (VTA) with the basal forebrain (Olds & Milner 1954). While much emphasis was focused initially on the role of the ascending monoamine systems in the medial forebrain bundle, other non-dopaminergic systems in the medial forebrain bundle clearly have a key role (Hernandez et al. 2006).

Measures of brain reward function during acute abstinence from all major drugs with dependence potential have revealed increases in brain reward thresholds measured by direct brain stimulation reward (Markou & Koob 1991; Schulteis et al. 1994, 1995; Epping-Jordan et al. 1998; Gardner & Vorel 1998; Paterson et al. 2000). These increases in reward thresholds may reflect decreases in the activity of reward neurotransmitter systems in the midbrain and forebrain implicated in the positive reinforcing effects of drugs.

The acute reinforcing effects of drugs of abuse are mediated by the activation of dopamine, serotonin, opioid peptides, and γ-aminobutyric acid (GABA) systems either by direct actions in the basal forebrain (notably the nucleus accumbens and central nucleus of the amygdala) or by indirect actions in the VTA (Koob & Le Moal 2001; Nestler 2005; Koob 2006). Much evidence supports the hypothesis that the mesolimbic dopamine system is dramatically activated by psychostimulant drugs during limited-access self-administration and to some extent by all drugs of abuse. Serotonin systems, particularly those involving serotonin 5-HT_{1B} receptor activation in the nucleus accumbens, also have been implicated in the acute reinforcing effects of psychostimulant drugs. Opioid peptides in the ventral striatum have been hypothesized to mediate the acute reinforcing effects of ethanol self-administration, largely based on the effects of opioid antagonists. μ-Opioid receptors in both the nucleus accumbens and the VTA mediate the reinforcing effects of opioid drugs. GABAergic systems are activated pre- and post-synaptically in the amygdala by ethanol at intoxicating doses, and GABA antagonists block ethanol self-administration (for reviews, see Nestler 2005; Koob 2006).

Within-system neuroadaptations to chronic drug exposure include decreases in function of the same neurotransmitter systems in the same neurocircuits implicated in the acute reinforcing effects of drugs of abuse. Decreases in activity of the mesolimbic dopamine system and decreases in serotonergic neurotransmission in the nucleus accumbens occur during drug withdrawal in animal studies (Weiss et al. 1992, 1996). Imaging studies in drug-addicted humans have consistently shown long-lasting decreases in the numbers of dopamine D_2 receptors in drug abusers compared with controls (Volkow et al. 2002). In addition, cocaine abusers have reduced dopamine release in response to a pharmacological challenge with a stimulant drug (Volkow et al. 1997; Martinez et al. 2007). Decreases in the number of dopamine D_2 receptors, coupled with the decrease in dopaminergic activity, in cocaine, nicotine and alcohol abusers, result in decreased sensitivity of reward circuits to stimulation by natural reinforcers (Volkow & Fowler 2000; Martin-Solch et al. 2001). These findings suggest an overall reduction in the sensitivity of the dopamine component of reward circuitry to natural reinforcers and other drugs in drug-addicted individuals.

Substantial evidence for increased sensitivity of receptor transduction mechanisms in the nucleus accumbens, including activation of adenylate cyclase, protein kinase A, cyclic adenosine monophosphate response-element binding protein (CREB), and ΔFosB, has been observed during administration of drugs of abuse (Self et al. 1995; Nye & Nestler 1996; Shaw-Lutchman et al. 2002; Nestler 2004; see Nestler 2008), and the ΔFosB response is hypothesized to represent a neuroadaptive change that extends long into protracted abstinence (Nestler & Malenka 2004).

Alcohol dependence has long been associated with changes in GABAergic neurotransmission. Chronic ethanol decreases $GABA_A$ receptor function (Morrow et al. 1988) and increases in GABA release in interneurons in the central nucleus of the amygdala (Roberto et al. 2004). The observation that very low doses of the $GABA_A$ agonist muscimol, when injected into the central nucleus of the amygdala, block the increased ethanol intake associated with acute withdrawal suggests that the changes in GABAergic function in the central nucleus of the amygdala may have some motivational significance in ethanol dependence (Roberts et al. 1996).

Thus, decreases in reward neurotransmission have been hypothesized to reflect a within-system neuroadaptation and contribute significantly to the negative motivational state associated with acute drug abstinence. Decreased reward system function also may persist in the form of long-term biochemical changes that contribute to the clinical syndrome of protracted abstinence and vulnerability to relapse. For example, while the activation of CREB and c-*fos* triggered by the activation of dopamine systems is relatively short lived, more stable changes in other transcription factors such as ΔFosB may persist for weeks (Nestler et al. 2001).

2.4 Between-system neuroadaptations in addiction

The neuroanatomical entity termed the extended amygdala (Heimer & Alheid 1991) may represent a common anatomical substrate integrating brain arousal-stress systems with hedonic processing systems to produce the between-system opponent process elaborated above. The extended amygdala is composed of the central nucleus of the amygdala, the bed nucleus of the stria terminalis, and a transition zone in the medial (shell) subregion of the nucleus accumbens. Each of these regions has cytoarchitectural and circuitry similarities (Heimer & Alheid 1991). The extended amygdala receives numerous afferents from limbic structures such as the basolateral amygdala and hippocampus and sends efferents to the medial part of the ventral pallidum and a large projection to the lateral hypothalamus, thus further defining the specific brain areas that interface classical limbic (emotional) structures with the extrapyramidal motor system (Alheid et al. 1995). The extended amygdala has long been hypothesized to have a key role not only in fear conditioning (Le Doux 2000) but also in the emotional component of pain processing (Neugebauer et al. 2004).

Brain neurochemical systems involved in arousal-stress modulation also may be engaged within the neurocircuitry of the brain stress systems in an attempt to overcome the chronic presence of the perturbing drug and to restore normal function despite the presence of drug. Both the hypothalamic–pituitary–adrenal axis and the brain stress system mediated by corticotropin-releasing factor (CRF) are dysregulated by the chronic administration of all major drugs with dependence or abuse potential, with a common response of elevated adrenocorticotropic hormone, corticosterone, and amygdala CRF during acute withdrawal (Rivier et al. 1984; Koob et al. 1994; Merlo-Pich et al. 1995; Delfs et al. 2000; Rasmussen et al. 2000; Olive et al. 2002). Acute withdrawal from all drugs of abuse produces an anxiety-like state that can be reversed by CRF antagonists, and CRF antagonists also block the increased intake of drug associated with dependence (Table 2.2).

A particularly dramatic example of the motivational effects of CRF in dependence can be observed in animal models of increased ethanol self-administration in dependent animals (Rimondini et al. 2002; O'Dell et al. 2004). During ethanol withdrawal, extra-hypothalamic CRF systems become hyperactive, with an increase in extracellular CRF within the central nucleus of the amygdala and bed nucleus of the stria terminalis of dependent rats (Merlo-Pich et al. 1995; Olive et al. 2002; Funk et al. 2006; Table 2.2). The dysregulation of brain CRF systems is hypothesized to underlie both the enhanced anxiety-like behaviours and the enhanced ethanol self-administration associated with ethanol withdrawal. Supporting this hypothesis, the subtype non-selective CRF receptor antagonists α-helical CRF_{9-41} and D-Phe CRF_{12-41} (intracerebroventricular administration) reduce both ethanol withdrawal-induced anxiety-like behaviour and ethanol self-administration in dependent animals (Baldwin et al. 1991; Valdez et al. 2004). When administered directly into the central nucleus of the amygdala, CRF receptor antagonists also attenuate anxiety-like behaviour (Rassnick et al. 1993) and ethanol self-administration in ethanol-dependent rats (Funk et al. 2007; Fig. 2.4). These data suggest an important role for CRF, primarily within the central nucleus of the amygdala, in mediating the increased self-administration associated with dependence.

Systemic injections of small-molecule CRF_1 antagonists also block both the anxiety-like responses and the increased ethanol intake associated with acute withdrawal (Knapp et al. 2004; Overstreet et al. 2004; Funk et al. 2007; Gehlert et al. 2007). Similar interactions with CRF have been observed with the dependence associated with extended access to intravenous self-administration of cocaine (Specio et al. 2008), nicotine (George et al. 2007), and heroin (Greenwell et al., 2009a).

Although less well developed, functional noradrenaline (NA) antagonists that block the anxiogenic-like and aversive effects of opiate withdrawal also block excessive drug intake associated with ethanol dependence (Walker et al. 2008), cocaine (Wee et al. 2008), and opioids (Greenwell et al., 2009b). A focal point for many of these effects also is the extended amygdala but at the level of the bed nucleus of the stria terminalis.

The dynamic nature of the brain stress system response to challenge is illustrated by the pronounced interaction of central nervous system-CRF systems and central nervous

Table 2.2 Role of CRF in dependence.

Drug	CRF antagonist effects on withdrawal-induced anxiety-like responses	Withdrawal-induced changes in extracellular CRF in CeA	CRF antagonist effects on dependence-induced increases in self-administration
Cocaine	↓	↑	↓
Opioids	↓[a]	↑	↓
Ethanol	↓	↑	↓
Nicotine	↓	↑	↓
Δ^9-Tetrahydrocannabinol	↓	↑	nt

nt, not tested; CeA, central nucleus of the amygdale.

[a]Aversive effects with place conditioning.

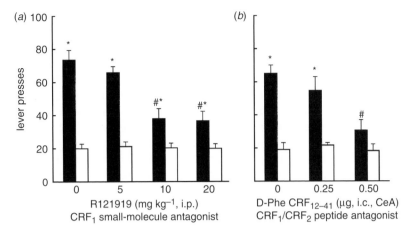

Fig. 2.4 (*a*) Effects of CRF$_1$ receptor small-molecule antagonist R121919 on ethanol self-administration in dependent (filled bars) and non-dependent (opened bars) rats. Ethanol dependence was induced by intermittent exposure to ethanol vapours for four weeks. Animals were subsequently tested for ethanol and water self-administration following 2 hours of acute withdrawal. Withdrawn, ethanol-dependent animals displayed a significant increase in ethanol lever pressing compared with non-dependent animals. R121919 significantly decreased ethanol self-administration in withdrawn, dependent but not non-dependent animals. Neither ethanol vapour exposure nor R121919 altered water responding. *$p < 0.001$ compared with same drug dose in non-dependent animals. #$p < 0.0001$ compared with vehicle treatment in dependent animals. (Adapted from Funk et al. 2007.) (*b*) Effects of CRF$_1$/CRF$_2$ peptide antagonist D-Phe CRF$_{12-41}$ administered directly into the central nucleus of the amygdala on ethanol and water self-administration in ethanol-dependent (filled bars) and non-dependent (open bars) rats. Ethanol dependence was induced by intermittent exposure to ethanol vapours for four weeks. Animals were subsequently tested for ethanol and water self-administration after 2 hours of acute withdrawal. Withdrawn, ethanol-dependent animals displayed a significant increase in ethanol lever pressing compared with non-dependent animals. D-Phe CRF$_{12-41}$ significantly decreased ethanol self-administration in withdrawn, dependent but not non-dependent animals when administered directly into the central nucleus of the amygdala. Neither ethanol vapour exposure nor D-Phe CRF$_{12-41}$ altered water responding. *$p < 0.0001$ compared with same drug dose in non-dependent animals. #$p < 0.0001$ compared with vehicle treatment in dependent animals. Error bars indicate s.e.m. (Adapted from Funk et al. 2006.)

system-NA systems. Conceptualized as a feed-forward system at multiple levels (e.g. in the pons and basal forebrain), CRF activates NA and NA in turn activates CRF (Koob 1999). Such feed-forward systems were further hypothesized to have powerful functional significance for mobilizing an organism's response to environmental challenge, but such a mechanism may be particularly vulnerable to pathology (Koob 1999).

Much evidence shows that dynorphin is increased in the nucleus accumbens in response to dopaminergic activation and, in turn, that overactivity of the dynorphin systems can decrease dopaminergic function. κ-Opioid agonists are aversive (Pfeiffer et al. 1986; Land et al. 2008), and withdrawal from cocaine, opioids, and ethanol is associated with increased dynorphin in the nucleus accumbens and/or amygdala (Rattan et al. 1992; Spangler et al. 1993; Lindholm et al. 2000). A κ-antagonist blocks the excessive drinking associated with ethanol withdrawal and dependence (Walker & Koob 2008). Evidence demonstrates that κ-receptor activation can activate CRF systems (Valdez et al. 2007; Taylor et al. 1996), but recently some have argued that the effects of dynorphin in producing negative emotional states are mediated via the activation of CRF systems (Land et al. 2008).

Significant evidence also suggests that the activation of neuropeptide Y (NPY) in the central nucleus of the amygdala can block the motivational aspects of dependence associated with chronic ethanol administration. NPY administered intracerebroventricularly blocks the anxiogenic-like effects of withdrawal from ethanol (Woldbye et al. 2002) and blocks the increased drug intake associated with ethanol dependence (Thorsell et al. 2005a,b). Injection of NPY directly into the central nucleus of the amygdala (Gilpin et al. 2008) and viral vector-enhanced expression of NPY in the central nucleus of the amygdala also block the increased drug intake associated with ethanol dependence (Thorsell et al. 2007).

Thus, acute withdrawal from drugs increases CRF in the central nucleus of the amygdala that has motivational significance for the anxiety-like effects of acute withdrawal and the increased drug intake associated with dependence (Fig. 2.5). Acute withdrawal also may increase the release of NA in the bed nucleus of the stria terminalis and dynorphin in the nucleus accumbens, both of which possibly contributing to the negative emotional state associated with dependence (Fig. 2.5). Decreased activity of NPY in the central nucleus of the amygdala also may contribute to the anxiety-like state associated with ethanol dependence. The activation of brain stress systems (CRF, NA, dynorphin) combined with the inactivation of brain anti-stress systems (NPY) in the extended amygdala may elicit the powerful emotional dysregulation associated with addiction. Such dysregulation of emotional processing may be a significant contribution to the between-system opponent processes that help

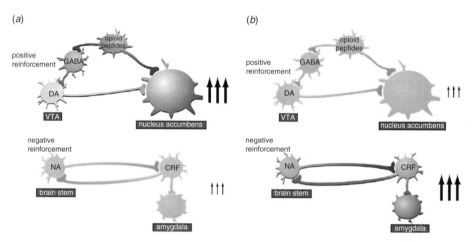

Fig. 2.5 Neurocircuitry associated with the acute positive reinforcing effects of drugs of abuse and the negative reinforcement of dependence and how it changes in the transition from (a) non-dependent drug taking to (b) dependent drug taking. Key elements of the reward circuit are DA and opioid peptide neurons that intersect at both the VTA and the nucleus accumbens and are activated during initial use and the early binge/intoxication stage. Key elements of the stress circuit are CRF and noradrenergic neurons that converge on GABA interneurons in the central nucleus of the amygdala that are activated during the development of dependence. CRF, corticotropin-releasing factor; DA, dopamine; GABA, γ-aminobutyric acid; NA, noradrenaline; VTA, ventral tegmental area. (Adapted from Koob & Le Moal 2008.)

maintain dependence and also set the stage for more prolonged state changes in emotionality such as protracted abstinence.

The neuroadaptations outlined above also may contribute to the critical problem in drug addiction, that of chronic relapse, where individuals with addiction return to compulsive drug taking long after acute withdrawal. The preoccupation/anticipation (craving) stage of the addiction cycle has long been hypothesized to be a key element of relapse in humans and defines addiction as a chronic relapsing disorder. Craving can be defined as the memory of the rewarding effects of a drug superimposed upon a negative emotional state.

From a within-system framework, changes in the dopaminergic system that persist well past acute withdrawal are hypothesized to contribute to craving and include psychomotor sensitization and increases in incentive salience (Robinson & Berridge 1993), decreases in dopamine D_2 receptors (Volkow et al. 2002) and persistent changes in signal transduction factors that may contribute to both chronic dysphoria (CREB activation) and sensitization of craving (ΔFosB; Nestler 2005). Evidence that subordinate primates socially isolated during development showed increased vulnerability to intravenously self-administer cocaine and had significantly reduced dopamine D_2 receptors provides compelling evidence that dopaminergic tone can regulate hedonic set point outside of acute withdrawal from drugs of abuse (Morgan et al. 2002).

From the perspective of between-system neuroadaptations, the brain stress systems outlined above are hypothesized to contribute directly to the preoccupation/anticipation (craving) stage via protracted abstinence. Protracted abstinence can be defined as the persistence of a negative emotional state long past acute withdrawal. This state in humans is characterized by low-level dysphoria, sleep disturbances, and increased sensitivity to stress and pain. In animals, protracted abstinence is characterized by increased sensitivity to a stressor and increased drug seeking long after acute withdrawal, both of which having been observed in alcohol studies (Valdez & Koob 2004, Sommer et al. 2008). Using CRF as an example in protracted abstinence, CRF is hypothesized to contribute to a residual negative emotional state that provides a basis for drug seeking (Valdez et al. 2002; Valdez & Koob 2004).

2.5 Opponent process, reward set point, and allostasis

The development of the aversive emotional state that drives the negative reinforcement of addiction has been defined as the 'dark side' of addiction (Koob & Le Moal 2005, 2008) and is hypothesized to be the b-process of the hedonic dynamic known as opponent process when the a-process is euphoria. The negative emotional state that comprises the withdrawal/negative affect stage defined above consists of key motivational elements, such as chronic irritability, emotional pain, malaise, dysphoria, alexithymia, and loss of motivation for natural rewards, and is characterized in animals by increases in reward thresholds during withdrawal from all major drugs of abuse. Two processes are hypothesized to form the neurobiological basis for the b-process: loss of function in the reward systems (within-system neuroadaptation) and recruitment of the brain stress or anti-reward systems (between-system neuroadaptation; Koob & Bloom 1988; Koob & Le Moal 1997). Anti-reward is a construct based on the hypothesis that brain systems are in place to limit reward (Koob & Le Moal 2008). As dependence and withdrawal develop, brain stress systems such as CRF, NA, and dynorphin are recruited (Fig. 2.5), producing aversive or stress-like states

(Aston-Jones et al. 1999; Nestler 2001; Koob 2003). At the same time, within the motivational circuits of the ventral striatum-extended amygdala, reward function decreases. The combination of decreases in reward neurotransmitter function and recruitment of anti-reward systems provides a powerful source of negative reinforcement that contributes to compulsive drug-seeking behaviour and addiction (Fig. 2.5).

The overall conceptual theme argued here is that drug addiction represents a break with homeostatic brain regulatory mechanisms that regulate the emotional state of the animal. However, the view that drug addiction represents a simple break with homeostasis is not sufficient to explain a number of key elements of addiction. Drug addiction, similar to other chronic physiological disorders such as high blood pressure that worsens over time, is subject to significant environmental influences and leaves a residual neuroadaptive trace that allows rapid 're-addiction' even months and years after detoxification and abstinence. These characteristics of drug addiction imply more than simply a homeostatic dysregulation of hedonic function and executive function, but rather a dynamic break with homeostasis of these systems, which have been termed allostasis.

Allostasis, originally conceptualized to explain persistent morbidity of arousal and autonomic function, is defined as 'stability through change' and a continuous readjustment of all parameters towards a new set point (Sterling & Eyer 1988). As such, an *allostatic state* can be defined as a state of chronic deviation of the regulatory system from its normal (homeostatic) operating level. Thus, the very physiological mechanism that allows rapid responses to environmental challenge becomes the engine of pathology if adequate time or resources are not available to shut off the response.

Two components are hypothesized to reflect adjustment to challenges to the brain produced by drugs of abuse to engage an allostatic-like state: (i) underactivation of brain reward transmitters and circuits and (ii) recruitment of the brain anti-reward or brain stress systems (Fig. 2.5). Repeated challenges, such as the case with drugs of abuse, lead to attempts of the brain via molecular, cellular, and neurocircuitry changes to maintain stability but at a cost. For the drug addiction framework elaborated here, the residual deviation from normal brain reward threshold regulation is termed the allostatic state. This state represents a combination of chronic elevation of reward set point fueled from the opponent process, motivational perspective by decreased function of reward circuits and recruitment of anti-reward systems, both of which contribute to the compulsivity of drug seeking and drug taking. How these systems are modulated by other known brain emotional systems localized to the extended amygdala (e.g. vasopressin, orexin, nociceptin), where the extended amygdala projects to convey emotional valence, and how individuals differ at the molecular-genetic level of analysis to convey loading on these circuits remain challenges for future research.

Achnowledgements

The author would like to thank Mike Arends for his outstanding assistance with the preparation of the manuscript. Research was supported by the National Institutes of Health grants AA06420 and AA08459 from the National Institute on Alcohol Abuse and Alcoholism, DA10072, DA04043, DA023597, and DA04398 from the National Institute on Drug Abuse, and DK26741 from the National Institute of Diabetes and Digestive and Kidney Diseases. Research was also supported by the Pearson Center for Alcoholism and Addiction Research. This is publication no. 19396 from The Scripps Research Institute.

References

Ahmed, S. H. & Koob, G. F. 1998 Transition from moderate to excessive drug intake: change in hedonic set point. *Science* **282**, 298–300. (doi:10.1126/science.282.5387.298)

Ahmed, S. H., Walker, J. R. & Koob, G. F. 2000 Persistent increase in the motivation to take heroin in rats with a history of drug escalation. *Neuropsychopharmacology* **22**, 413–21. (doi:10.1016/S0893-133X(99)00133-5)

Alheid, G. F., De Olmos, J. S. & Beltramino, C. A. 1995 Amygdala and extended amygdala. In *The rat nervous system* (ed. G. Paxinos), pp. 495–578. San Diego, CA: Academic Press.

American Psychiatric Association 1994 *Diagnostic and statistical manual of mental disorders*, 4th edn. Washington, DC: American Psychiatric Press.

Aston-Jones, G., Delfs, J. M., Druhan, J. & Zhu, Y. 1999 The bed nucleus of the stria terminalis: a target site for noradrenergic actions in opiate withdrawal. In *Advancing from the ventral striatum to the extended amygdala: implications for neuropsychiatry and drug abuse*, vol. 877 (ed. J. F. McGinty). Annals of the New York Academy of Sciences, pp. 486–98. New York, NY: New York Academy of Sciences.

Baldwin, H. A., Rassnick, S., Rivier, J., Koob, G. F. & Britton, K. T. 1991 CRF antagonist reverses the "anxiogenic" response to ethanol withdrawal in the rat. *Psychopharmacology* **103**, 227–32. (doi:10.1007/BF02 244208)

Delfs, J. M., Zhu, Y., Druhan, J. P. & Aston-Jones, G. 2000 Noradrenaline in the ventral forebrain is critical for opiate withdrawal-induced aversion. *Nature* **403**, 430–4. (doi:10.1038/35000212)

Epping-Jordan, M. P., Watkins, S. S., Koob, G. F. & Markou, A. 1998 Dramatic decreases in brain reward function during nicotine withdrawal. *Nature* **393**, 76–9. (doi:10. 1038/30001)

Funk, C. K., O'Dell, L. E., Crawford, E. F. & Koob, G. F. 2006 Corticotropin-releasing factor within the central nucleus of the amygdala mediates enhanced ethanol self-administration in withdrawn, ethanol-dependent rats. *J. Neurosci.* **26**, 11 324–11 332. (doi:10.1523/JNEUR-OSCI.3096-06.2006)

Funk, C. K., Zorrilla, E. P., Lee, M. J., Rice, K. C. & Koob, G. F. 2007 Corticotropin-releasing factor 1 antagonists selectively reduce ethanol self-administration in ethanol-dependent rats. *Biol. Psychiatry* **61**, 78–86. (doi:10.1016/ j.biopsych.2006.03.063)

Gardner, E. L. & Vorel, S. R. 1998 Cannabinoid transmission and reward-related events. *Neurobiol. Dis.* **5**, 502–33. (doi:10.1006/nbdi.1998.0219)

Gehlert, D. R., Cippitelli, A., Thorsell, A. et al. 2007 3-(4-Chloro-2-morpholin-4-y1)-8-(1-ethylpropyl)-2,6-dimethyl-imidazo [1,2-b]pyridazine: a novel brain-penetrant, orally available corticotropin-releasing factor receptor 1 antagonist with efficacy in animal models of alcoholism. *J. Neurosci.* **27**, 2718–26.

George, O., Ghozland, S., Azar, M. R. et al. 2007 CRF-CRF1 system activation mediates withdrawal-induced increases in nicotine self-administration in nicotine-dependent rats. *Proc. Natl Acad. Sci. USA* **104**, 17198–203. (doi:10. 1073/pnas.0707585104)

Gilpin, N. W., Richardson, H. N., Lumeng, L. & Koob, G. F. 2008 Dependence-induced alcohol drinking by P rats selectively bred for high alcohol preference and outbred Wistar rats. *Alcoho. Clin. Exp. Res.* **32**, 1688–96 (doi:10.1111/j.1530-0277.2008.00678.x)

Greenwell, T. N., Funk, C. K., Cottone, P. et al. 2009 a Corticotropin-releasing factor-1 receptor antagonists decrease heroin self-administration in long-, but not short-access rats. *Addict. Biol.* **14**, 130–143.

Greenwell, T. N., Walker, B. M., Cottone, P., Zorrilla, E. P. & Koob, G. F. 2009b The α_1 adrenergic receptor antagonist prazosin reduces heroin self-administration in rats with extended access to heroin administration. *Pharmacol. Biochem. Behav.* **91**, 295–302.

Hebb, D. O. 1972 *Textbook of psychology*, 3rd edn. Philadelphia, PA: W. B. Saunders.

Heimer, L. & Alheid, G. 1991 Piecing together the puzzle of basal forebrain anatomy. In *The basal forebrain: anatomy to function*, vol. 295 (eds T. C. Napier, P. W Kalivas & I. Hanin). Advances in experimental medicine and biology, pp. 1–42. New York, NY: Plenum Press.

Hernandez, G., Hamdani, S., Rajabi, H. et al. 2006 Prolonged rewarding stimulation of the rat medial forebrain bundle: neurochemical and behavioral consequences. *Behav. Neurosci.* **120**, 888–904. (doi:10.1037/ 0735-7044.120.4.888)

Kitamura, O., Wee, S., Specio, S. E., Koob, G. F. & Pulvirenti, L. 2006 Escalation of methamphet-amine self-administration in rats: a dose-effect function. *Psychopharmacology* **186**, 48–53. (doi:10.1007/s00213-006-0353-z)

Knapp, D. J., Overstreet, D. H., Moy, S. S. & Breese, G. R. 2004 SB242084, flumazenil, and CRA1000 block ethanol withdrawal-induced anxiety in rats. *Alcohol* **32**, 101–11. (doi:10.1016/j.alcohol.2003.08.007)

Koob, G. F. 1999 Corticotropin-releasing factor, nor-epinephrine and stress. *Biol. Psychiatry* **46**, 1167–80. (doi:10.1016/S0006-3223(99)00164-X)

Koob, G. F. 2003 Neuroadaptive mechanisms of addiction: studies on the extended amygdala. *Eur. Neuropsychopharmacology* **13**, 442–52. (doi:10.1016/j.euro neuro.2003.08.005)

Koob, G. F. 2004 Allostatic view of motivation: implications for psychopathology. In *Motivational factors in the etiology of drug abuse*, vol. 50 (eds R. A. Bevins & M. T. Bardo). Nebraska sympo-sium on motivation, pp. 1–18. Lincoln, NE: University of Nebraska Press.

Koob, G. F. 2006 The neurobiology of addiction: a neuroadaptational view relevant for diagnosis. *Addiction* **101**(Suppl. 1), 23–30.

Koob, G. F. 2008 Neurobiology of addiction. In *Textbook of substance abuse treatment* (eds M. Galanter & H. D. Kleber), pp. 3–16, 4th edn. American Psychiatric Press.

Koob, G. F. & Bloom, F. E. 1988 Cellular and molecular mechanisms of drug dependence. *Science* **242**, 715–23. (doi:10.1126/science.2903550)

Koob, G. F. & Le Moal, M. 1997 Drug abuse: hedonic homeostatic dysregulation. *Science* **278**, 52–8. (doi:10. 1126/science.278.5335.52)

Koob, G. F. & Le Moal, M. 2001 Drug addiction, dysregulation of reward, and allostasis. *Neuropsychopharmacology* **24**, 97–129. (doi:10.1016/S0893-133X(00)00195-0)

Koob, G. F. & Le Moal, M. 2005 Plasticity of reward neurocircuitry and the 'dark side' of drug addic-tion. *Nat. Neurosci.* **8**, 1442–4. (doi:10.1038/nn1 105-1442)

Koob, G. F. & Le Moal, M. 2008 Addiction and the brain antireward system. *Annu. Rev. Psychol.* **59**, 29–53. (doi:10. 1146/annurev.psych.59.103006.093548)

Koob, G. F., Heinrichs, S. C., Menzaghi, F., Pich, E. M. & Britton, K. T. 1994 Corticotropin releasing factor, stress and behavior. *Semin. Neurosci.* **6**, 221–9. (doi:10.1006/ smns.1994.1029)

Koob, G. F., Kandel, D. & Volkow, N. D. 2008 Pathophy-siology of addiction In *Psychiatry* (eds A. Tasman J. Kay, J. A. Lieberman M. B. First & M. Maj), pp. 354–78, 3rd edn. Philadelphia, PA: W. B. Saunders.

Kornetsky, C. & Esposito, R. U. 1979 Euphorigenic drugs: effects on the reward pathways of the brain. *Fed. Proc.* **38**, 2473–6.

Land, B. B., Bruchas, M. R., Lemos, J. C., Xu, M., Melief, E. J. & Chavkin, C. 2008 The dysphoric component of stress is encoded by activation of the dynorphin k-opioid system. *f. Neurosci.* **28**, 407–14. (doi:10.1523/JNEURO SCI.4458-07.2008)

Le Doux, J. E. 2000 Emotion circuits in the brain. *Annu. Rev. Neurosci.* **23**, 155–84. (doi:10.1146/annurev.neuro. 23.1.155)

Lindholm, S., Ploj, K., Franck, J. & Nylander, I. 2000 Repeated ethanol administration induces short- and long-term changes in enkephalin and dynorphin tissue concentrations in rat brain. *Alcohol* **22**, 165–71. (doi:10.1016/ S0741-8329(00)00118-X)

Markou, A. & Koob, G. F. 1991 Post-cocaine anhedonia: an animal model of cocaine withdrawal. *Neuropsychopharma-cology* **4**, 17–26.

Martinez, D., Narendran, R., Foltin, R. W. et al. 2007 Amphetamine-induced dopamine release: markedly blunted in cocaine dependence and predictive of the choice to self-administer cocaine. *Am. f. Psychiatry* **164**, 622–9. (doi:10.1176/appi.ajp. 164.4.622)

Martin-Solch, C., Magyar, S., Kunig, G., Missimer, J., Schultz, W. & Leenders, K. L. 2001 Changes in brain activation associated with reward processing in smokers and non-smokers: a positron emis-sion tomography study. *Exp. Brain Res.* **139**, 278–86. (doi:10.1007/s002210100751)

Merlo-Pich, E., Lorang, M., Yeganeh, M. et al. 1995 Increase of extracellular corticotropin-releasing factor-like immunoreactivity levels in the amygdala of awake rats during restraint stress and ethanol withdrawal as measured by microdialysis. *J. Neurosci.* **15**, 5439–47.

Morgan, D., Grant, K. A., Gage, H. D. et al. 2002 Social dominance in monkeys: dopamine D_2 recep-tors and cocaine self-administration. *Nat. Neurosci.* **5**, 169–74. (doi:10.1038/nn798)

Morrow, A. L., Suzdak, P. D., Karanian, J. W. & Paul, S. M. 1988 Chronic ethanol administration alters γ-aminobutyric acid, pentobarbital and ethanol-mediated ^{36}Cl⁻ uptake in cerebral cortical synaptoneurosomes. *J. Pharmacol. Exp. Ther.* **246**, 158–64.

Nestler, E. J. 2001 Molecular basis of long-term plasticity underlying addiction. *Nat. Rev. Neurosci.* **2**, 119–28. (doi: 10.1038/35053570)

Nestler, E. J. 2004 Historical review: molecular and cellular mechanisms of opiate and cocaine addiction. *Trends Pharmacol. Sci.* **25**, 210–18. (doi:10.1016/j.tips.2004. 02.005)

Nestler, E. J. 2005 Is there a common molecular pathway for addiction? *Nat. Neurosci.* **8**, 1445–9. (doi: 10.1038/ nn1578)

Nestler, E. J. 2008 Transcriptional mechanisms of addiction: role of ΔFosB. *Phil. Trans. R. Soc. B* **363**, 3245–55. (doi:10.1098/rstb.2008.0067)

Nestler, E. J. & Malenka, R. C. 2004 The addicted brain. *Sci. Am.* **290**, 78–85.

Nestler, E. J., Barrot, M. & Self, D. W. 2001 ΔFosB: a sustained molecular switch for addiction. *Proc. NatlAcad. Sci. USA* **98**, 11042–6. (doi:10.1073/pnas.191352698)

Neugebauer, V., Li, W., Bird, G. C. & Han, J. S. 2004 The amygdala and persistent pain. *Neuroscientist* **10**, 221–34. (doi: 10.1177/1073858403261077)

Nye, H. E. & Nestler, E. J. 1996 Induction of chronic Fos-related antigens in rat brain by chronic morphine administration. *Mol. Pharmacol.* **49**, 636–45.

O'Dell, L. E., Roberts, A. J., Smith, R. T. & Koob, G. F. 2004 Enhanced alcohol self-administration after intermittent versus continuous alcohol vapor exposure. *Alcohol. Clin. Exp. Res.* **28**, 1676–82. (doi: 10.1097/01.ALC.000014 5781.11923.4E)

Olds, J. &.Milner, P. 1954 Positive reinforcement produced by electrical stimulation of septal area and other regions of rat brain. *J. Comp. Physiol. Psychol.* **47**, 419–27. (doi:10. 1037/h0058775)

Olive, M. F., Koenig, H. N., Nannini, M. A. & Hodge, C. W. 2002 Elevated extracellular CRF levels in the bed nucleus of the stria terminalis during ethanol withdrawal and reduction by subsequent ethanol intake. *Pharmacol. Biochem. Behav.* **72**, 213–20. (doi:10.1016/S0091-3057(01)00748-1)

Overstreet, D. H., Knapp, D. J. & Breese, G. R. 2004 Modulation of multiple ethanol withdrawal-induced anxiety-like behavior by CRF and CRF$_1$ receptors. *Pharmacol. Biochem. Behav.* **77**, 405–13. (doi:10.1016/ j.pbb.2003.11.010)

Paterson, N. E., Myers, C. & Markou, A. 2000 Effects of repeated withdrawal from continuous amphetamine administration on brain reward function in rats. *Psychopharma-cology* **152**, 440–6. (doi:10.1007/s002130000559)

Pfeiffer, A., Brantl, V., Herz, A. & Emrich, H. M. 1986 Psychotomimesis mediated by κ opiate receptors. *Science* **233**, 774–6. (doi:10.1126/science.3016896)

Poulos, C. X. & Cappell, H. 1991 Homeostatic theory of drug tolerance: a general model of physio-logical adaptation. *Psychol. Rev.* **98**, 390–408. (doi:10.1037/0033-295X.98.3.390)

Rasmussen, D. D., Boldt, B. M., Bryant, C. A., Mitton, D. R., Larsen, S. A. & Wilkinson, C. W 2000 Chronic daily ethanol and withdrawal: 1. Long-term changes in the hypothalamo-pituitary-adrenal axis. *Alcohol. Clin. Exp. Res.* **24**, 1836–49. (doi:10.1111/j.1530-0277.2000.tb01988.x)

Rassnick, S., Heinrichs, S. C., Britton, K. T. & Koob, G. F. 1993 Microinjection of a corticotropin-releasing factor antagonist into the central nucleus of the amygdala reverses anxiogenic-like effects of ethanol withdrawal. *Brain Res.* **605**, 25–32. (doi:10.1016/0006-8993(93)91352-S)

Rattan, A. K., Koo, K. L., Tejwani, G. A. & Bhargava, H. N. 1992 The effect of morphine tolerance dependence and abstinence on immunoreactive dynorphin (1–13) levels in discrete brain regions, spinal cord, pituitary gland and peripheral tissues of the rat. *Brain Res.* **584**, 207–12. (doi:10.1016/0006-8993(92)90896-H)

Rimondini, R., Arlinde, C., Sommer, W. & Heilig, M. 2002 Long-lasting increase in voluntary ethanol consumption and transcriptional regulation in the rat brain after intermittent exposure to alcohol. *FASEB J.* **16**, 27–35. (doi:10.1096/fj.01-0593com)

Rivier, C., Bruhn, T. & Vale, W. 1984 Effect of ethanol on the hypothalamic-pituitary-adrenal axis in the rat: role of corticotropin-releasing factor (CRF). *J. Pharmacol. Exp. Ther.* **229**, 127–31.

Roberto, M., Madamba, S. G., Stouffer, D. G., Parsons, L. H. & Siggins, G. R. 2004 Increased GABA release in the central amygdala of ethanol-dependent rats. *J. Neurosci.* **24**, 10159–66. (doi: 10.1523/ JNEUR-OSCI.3004-04.2004)

Roberts, A. J., Cole, M. & Koob, G. F. 1996 Intra-amygdala muscimol decreases operant ethanol self-administration in dependent rats. *Alcohol. Clin. Exp. Res.* **20**, 1289–98. (doi: 10.1111/j. 1530-0277.1996.tb01125.x)

Robinson, T. E. & Berridge, K. C. 1993 The neural basis of drug craving: an incentive-sensitization theory of addiction. *Brain Res. Rev.* **18**, 247–91. (doi:10.1016/0165-0173(93)90013-P)

Schulteis, G., Markou, A., Gold, L. H., Stinus, L. & Koob, G. F. 1994 Relative sensitivity to naloxone of multiple indices of opiate withdrawal: a quantitative dose-response analysis. *J. Pharmacol. Exp. Ther.* **271**, 1391–8.

Schulteis, G., Markou, A., Cole, M. & Koob, G. 1995 Decreased brain reward produced by ethanol withdrawal. *Proc. Natl Acad. Sci. USA* **92**, 5880–4. (doi:10.1073/ pnas.92.13.5880)

Self, D. W., McClenahan, A. W., Beitner-Johnson, D., Terwilliger, R. Z. & Nestler, E. J. 1995 Biochemical adaptations in the mesolimbic dopamine system in response to heroin self-administration. *Synapse* **21**, 312–18. (doi:10. 1002/syn.890210405)

Shaham, Y., Shalev, U., Lu, L., De Wit, H. & Stewart, J. 2003 The reinstatement model of drug relapse: history, methodology and major findings. *Psychopharmacology* **168**, 3–20. (doi:10.1007/ s00213-002-1224-x)

Shaw-Lutchman, T. Z., Barrot, M., Wallace, T. et al. J. 2002 Regional and cellular mapping of cAMP response element-mediated transcription during naltrexone-precipitated morphine withdrawal. *J. Neurosci.* **22**, 3663–72.

Shippenberg, T. S. & Koob, G. F. 2002 Recent advances in animal models of drug addiction and alcoholism. In *Neuropsychopharmacology: the fifth generation of progress* (eds K. L. Davis, D. Charney, J. T. Coyle & C. Nemeroff), pp. 1381–97. Philadelphia, PA: Lippincott Williams and Wilkins.

Siegel, S. 1975 Evidence from rats that morphine tolerance is a learned response. *J. Comp. Physiol. Psychol.* **89**, 498–506. (doi:10.1037/h0077058)

Solomon, R. L. 1980 The opponent-process theory of acquired motivation: the costs of pleasure and the benefits of pain. *Am. Psychol.* **35**, 691–712. (doi:10.1037/0003-066X.35.8.691)

Solomon, R. L. & Corbit, J. D. 1974 An opponent-process theory of motivation: 1. Temporal dynamics of affect. *Psychol. Rev.* **81**, 119–45. (doi:10.1037/h0036128)

Sommer, W. H., Rimondini, R., Hansson, A. C. et al. 2008 Upregulation of voluntry alcohol intake, behavioral sensitivity to stress, and amygdala crhrl expression following a history of dependence. *Biol. Psychiatry* **63**, 139–45.

Song, Z. H. & Takemori, A. E. 1992 Stimulation by corticotropin-releasing factor of the release of immuno-reactive dynorphin A from mouse spinal cords *in vitro*. *Eur. J. Pharmacol.* **222**, 27–32. (doi:10.1016/0014-2999(92) 90458-G)

Spangler, R., Unterwald, E. M. & Kreek, M. J. 1993 "Binge" cocaine administration induces a sustained increase of prodynorphin mRNA in rat caudate-putamen. *Mol. Brain Res.* **19**, 323–327. (doi:10.1016/0169-328X(93)90133-A)

Specio, S. E., Wee, S., O'Dell, L. E., Boutrel, B., Zorrilla, E. P. & Koob, G. F. 2008 CRF$_1$ receptor antagonists attenuate escalated cocaine self-administration in rats. *Psychopharmacology* **196**, 473–82. (doi:10.1007/s00213-007-0983-9)

Sterling, P. & Eyer, J. 1988 Allostasis: a new paradigm to explain arousal pathology. In *Handbook of life stress, cognition and health* (eds S. Fisher & J. Reason), pp. 629–49. Chichester, UK: Wiley.

Taylor, C. C., Wu, D., Soong, Y., Yee, J. S. & Szeto, H. H. 1996 κ-Opioid agonist, U50, 488H, stimulates ovine fetal pituitary-adrenal function via hypothalamic arginine-vasopressin and corticotropin-releasing factor. *J. Pharmacol. Exp. Ther.* **277**, 877–84.

Thorsell, A., Slawecki, C. J. & Ehlers, C. L. 2005a Effects of neuropeptide Y and corticotropin-releasing factor on ethanol intake in Wistar rats: interaction with chronic ethanol exposure. *Behav. Brain Res.* **161**, 133–40. (doi:10.1016/j.bbr.2005.01.016)

Thorsell, A., Slawecki, C. J. & Ehlers, C. L. 2005b Effects of neuropeptide Yon appetitive and consummatory behaviors associated with alcohol drinking in wistar rats with a history of ethanol exposure. *Alcohol. Clin. Exp. Res.* **29**, 584–90. (doi:10.1097/01.ALC.0000160084.13148.02)

Thorsell, A., Rapunte-Canonigo, V., O'Dell, L. et al. 2007 Viral vector-induced amygdala NPY overexpression reverses increased alcohol intake caused by repeated deprivations in Wistar rats. *Brain* **130**, 1330–7. (doi:10.1093/brain/ awm033)

Valdez, G. R. & Koob, G. F. 2004 Allostasis and dysregulation of corticotropin-releasing factor and neuropeptide Y systems: implications for the development of alcoholism. *Pharmacol. Biochem. Behav.* **79**, 671–89. (doi:10.1016/j.pbb.2004.09.020)

Valdez, G. R., Platt, D. M., Rowlett, J. K. Ruedi-Bettschen, D. & Spealman, R. D. 2007 κ Agonist-induced reinstatement of cocaine seeking in squirrel monkeys: a role for opioid and stress-related mechanisms. *J Pharmacol. Exp. Ther.* **323**, 525–33.

Valdez, G. R., Roberts, A. J., Chan, K. et al. 2002 Increased ethanol self-administration and anxiety-like behavior during acute withdrawal and protracted abstinence: regulation by corticotropin-releasing factor. *Alcohol. Clin. Exp. Res.* **26**, 1494–501.

Valdez, G. R., Sabino, V. & Koob, G. F. 2004 Increased anxiety-like behavior and ethanol self-administration in dependent rats: reversal via corticotropin-releasing factor-2 receptor activation. *Alcohol. Clin. Exp. Res.* **28**, 865–72.

Volkow, N. D. & Fowler, J. S. 2000 Addiction, a disease of compulsion and drive: involvement of the orbitofrontal cortex. *Cereb. Cortex* **10**, 318–25. (doi:10.1093/cercor/10. 3.318)

Volkow, N. D., Wang, G. J., Fowler, J. S. et al. 1997 Decreased striatal dopaminergic responsiveness in detoxified cocaine-dependent subjects. *Nature* **386**, 830–3. (doi:10.1038/386830a0)

Volkow, N. D., Fowler, J. S. & Wang, G. J. 2002 Role of dopamine in drug reinforcement and addiction in humans: results from imaging studies. *Behav. Pharmacol.* **13**, 355–66.

Walker, B. M. & Koob, G. F. 2008 Pharmacological evidence for a motivational role of κ-opioid systems in ethanol dependence. *Neuropsychopharmacology* **33**, 643–52. (doi:10.1038/sj.npp.1301438)

Walker, B. M., Rasmussen, D. D., Raskind, M. A. & Koob, G. F. 2008 a1-Noradrenergic receptor antagonism blocks dependence-induced increases in responding for ethanol. *Alcohol* **42**, 91–7. (doi:10.1016/j.alcohol.2007.12.002)

Wee, S., Mandyam, C. D., Lekic, D. M. & Koob, G. F. 2008 α_1-Noradrenergic system role in increased motivation for cocaine intake in rats with prolonged access. *Eur. Neuropsychopharmacol.* **18**, 303–11. (doi:10.1016/ j.euroneuro.2007.08.003)

Weiss, F., Markou, A., Lorang, M. T. & Koob, G. F. 1992 Basal extracellular dopamine levels in the nucleus accumbens are decreased during cocaine withdrawal after unlimited-access self-administration. *Brain Res.* **593**, 314–18. (doi:10.1016/0006-8993(92)91327-B)

Weiss, F., Parsons, L. H., Schulteis, G. et al. 1996 Ethanol self-administration restores withdrawal-associated deficiencies in accumbal dopamine and 5-hydroxytryptamine release in dependent rats. *J. Neurosci.* **16**, 3474–3485.

Weiss, F. et al. 2001 Compulsive drug-seeking behavior and relapse: neuroadaptation, stress, and conditioning factors. In *The biological basis of cocaine addiction*, vol. 937 (ed. V. Quinones-Jenab). Annals of the New York Academy of Sciences, pp. 1–26. New York, NY: New York Academy of Sciences.

Woldbye, D. P., Ulrichsen, J., Haugbol, S. & Bolwig, T. G. 2002 Ethanol withdrawal in rats is attenuated by intracerebroventricular administration of neuropeptide Y. *Alcohol. Alcohol.* **37**, 318–321.

Neural mechanisms underlying the vulnerability to develop compulsive drug-seeking habits and addiction

Barry J. Everitt,* David Belin, Daina Economidou, Yann Pelloux, Jeffrey W. Dalley, and Trevor W. Robbins

3.1 Introduction

The central hypothesis guiding our research during the past decade or more has been that drug addiction can be understood in terms of the operation of the brain's learning and memory systems (Everitt et al. 2001, 2008; Everitt & Robbins 2005; Robbins & Everitt 1999). In particular, that chronically self-administered drugs may in some way pathologically subvert these memory systems and so lead to the establishment of compulsive drug-seeking habits (Everitt & Robbins 2005). Initially, our approach to the understanding of drug addiction built upon the clinical insight embodied within the DSM-IV (DSM-IV 1994) criteria for 'substance abuse' and 'substance dependence' (although it is perhaps to be regretted that this widely used diagnostic manual did not adopt the word 'addiction' to describe the state in which individuals compulsively seek and take drugs, often in the face of profoundly negative consequences). Therefore, we began experimentally to decompose and augment the DSM-IV diagnostic framework in terms of specified learning and cognitive processes deriving from animal learning theory and which increasingly have been attributed to the operation of specific neural, especially limbic cortical-striatal, systems (Everitt et al. 2001).

The early focus of much experimental drug addiction research was to understand the reinforcing, or 'rewarding', effects of abused drugs; this has led to enormous advances in defining the primary molecular targets of addictive drugs as well as, more recently, the adaptations in these targets that develop with chronic drug self-administration (Koob & Le Moal 2005; Nestler 2004). However, it has been appreciated for some time that the molecular and neurochemical correlates of acute and chronic drug administration must be interpreted in behavioural and cognitive terms if the psychological processes and neurobiological mechanisms determining human drug addiction are to be specified. Therefore, we and others have increasingly come to view drug addiction as the endpoint of a series of transitions from initial drug use—when a drug is voluntarily taken because it has reinforcing, often hedonic, effects—through loss of control over this behavior, such that it becomes habitual and ultimately compulsive. We have recently reviewed the evidence that these transitions depend upon interactions between Pavlovian and instrumental learning processes (Everitt & Robbins 2005). Furthermore, we have hypothesized that the 'switch' from voluntary drug use to habitual and progressively compulsive drug use represents a transition at the neural level

* bje10@cam.ac.uk

from prefrontal cortical to striatal control over drug-seeking and drug-taking behaviour, as well as a progression from ventral to more dorsal domains of the striatum, mediated at least in part by its stratified dopaminergic innervation (Everitt & Robbins 2005; Everitt et al. 2008).

We summarize here recent evidence in support of the hypothesis that drug-seeking habits are associated with a shift from ventral to dorsal striatal control over behaviour. We also address the major issue of vulnerability to drug addiction—that some individuals are more likely than others to take drugs, lose control over, and escalate their drug intake, ultimately seeking drugs compulsively. Experimental models of addiction, rather than drug self-administration, must reflect such individual differences and also incorporate extended periods of drug taking in order to understand the underlying neural mechanisms of addiction (Koob & Le Moal 2005).

3.2 From voluntary to habitual drug seeking: the shift from ventral to dorsal striatum

With drugs such as cocaine, there is wide, though not universal, agreement that the dopaminergic innervation of the nucleus accumbens shell (AcbS), and even more ventral regions of the striatum, such as the olfactory tubercle, underlies its primary reinforcing effects in simple drug self-administration procedures where each response on a lever results in an intravenous or intracerebral drug infusion (Di Chiara et al. 2004; Ikemoto et al. 2005; Wise 2004). We term this 'drug taking' to distinguish it from 'drug-seeking' behaviour that must often be maintained over long periods of time and is profoundly influenced by environmental stimuli associated with self-administered drugs through Pavlovian conditioning (Everitt et al. 2001). In humans, such stimuli can induce subjective states such as craving, as well as drug seeking and relapse after abstinence (Childress et al. 1999; Garavan et al. 2000; Grant et al. 1996). We have therefore developed a general model of drug seeking, a second-order schedule of cocaine reinforcement, in which this behaviour is sensitive not only to the contingency between instrumental responses and drug administration, but also to the presence of drug-associated stimuli (conditioned stimuli, CSs), which have a powerful effect on performance by acting as conditioned reinforcers (Everitt & Robbins 2000). We have established that the acquisition of this cocaine-seeking behaviour depends upon the integrity of the nucleus accumbens core (AcbC) and its afferents from the basolateral amygdala (BLA). Thus, selective lesions of the BLA prevented the acquisition of cocaine seeking under a second-order schedule (Whitelaw et al. 1996), as expected given its fundamental role in conditioned reinforcement (Cador et al. 1989; Cardinal et al. 2002; Robbins et al. 1989). Similarly, selective lesions of the AcbC also greatly impaired the acquisition of cocaine seeking (Ito et al. 2004). Simple drug taking, on the other hand, was unimpaired in these animals, which both acquired and maintained cocaine self-administration following lesions of either the BLA or AcbC (Ito et al. 2004). As we have reviewed elsewhere, the AcbC region of the ventral striatum is also a key locus not only for conditioned reinforcement, but also for other Pavlovian influences on appetitive behaviour, including approach, as measured in autoshaping procedures, and also Pavlovian-instrumental transfer, the process by which Pavlovian CSs energize ongoing instrumental behaviour, an example of conditioned motivation, each of which also depends upon processing in sub-regions of the amygdala (Cardinal et al. 2002, 2004).

These observations indicate that the BLA and AcbC may function together as nodes within a limbic cortical-ventral striatopallidal system that underlies the acquisition of drug seeking. This notion is further supported by the observation that disconnecting these structures by unilateral pharmacological blockade of dopamine and AMPA receptors in the BLA and AcbC, respectively, on opposite sides of the brain also greatly diminished cocaine seeking (Di Ciano & Everitt 2004). Thus, the acquisition and early performance of cocaine seeking that is maintained over protracted periods of time by the contingent presentation of drug-associated conditioned reinforcers depends upon the integrity of the AcbC and its afferent input from the BLA. It is likely that at this stage, drug seeking is under the control of instrumental response–outcome contingencies in which animals respond in a voluntary and goal-directed way for intravenous cocaine infusions. Indeed, we have clear evidence that this is so from studies using a 'seeking-taking' chained schedule in which animals perform a drug-seeking response in the initial link of the chain, which then gives access to a drug-taking response in the second link, performance of which delivers cocaine (Olmstead et al. 2000). After limited experience with the drug, cocaine seeking was shown to be a goal-directed action in that its performance was sensitive to devaluation of the drug-taking link (Olmstead et al. 2001). This devaluation effect demonstrates that cocaine seeking at early stages of acquisition and performance is mediated by knowledge of the contingency between the seeking response and its outcome.

This response–outcome process can be contrasted with a second, stimulus–response (S–R) instrumental process in which seeking behaviour is a response habit triggered and main-tained by drug-associated stimuli (Everitt et al. 2001). Tiffany (1990), O'Brien and McClellan (1996), and ourselves (Everitt et al. 2001; Everitt & Robbins 2005; Robbins & Everitt 1999) have all advanced the hypothesis that drug addiction encompasses changes in the associative structure underlying drug seeking such that it becomes 'automatic' or habitual. We have additionally hypothesized the progressive engagement of dorsal striatal mechanisms under-lying this transition (Everitt & Robbins 2005), based upon evidence that the dorsal striatum mediates S–R habit learning—evidence that has been considerably strengthened through studies of instrumental responding for food and its resistance to reinforcer devaluation, a canonical test of the development of S–R habits (Yin et al. 2004, 2006). What then is the evidence that the dorsal striatum mediates the performance of well-established drug-seeking habits that depend initially upon ventral striatal, or ventromedial dorsal striatal, mechanisms during acquisition? Correlative evidence came from *in vivo* microdialysis measurement of extracellular dopamine in rats that had attained stable responding under a second-order schedule of cocaine seeking over a two-month period. While self-administered cocaine increased dopamine release in the AcbS, AcbC, and dorsal striatum, extracellular dopamine was only increased in the AcbC in response to unexpected (i.e. non-response-contingent) presentations of a cocaine-associated stimulus. However, during a prolonged period of cocaine seeking maintained by contingent presentations of the same cocaine-associated CS, dopamine release was increased only in the dorsal striatum, not in the AcbC or AcbS (Ito et al. 2000, 2002). Furthermore, dopamine release in the dorsal striatum was subsequently shown to be causally important for the *maintenance* of drug seeking by the observation that dopamine receptor blockade at this site dose-dependently reduced cocaine seeking, whereas the same infusions into the AcbC were without effect (Vanderschuren et al. 2005). This apparent shift from ventral to dorsal striatal control over drug seeking provides support for the hypothesis that it is under S–R, or 'habit', control because of accumulated evidence implicating the dorsal striatum in habit learning (Yin et al. 2004, 2006). Moreover, the fact that the second-order schedule we have principally used overall is of a fixed-interval type encourages this view, since interval schedules, as compared to ratio schedules, are known to result in the more rapid development of S–R habits through the weaker relationship between response and outcome that obtains (Dickinson 1985; Dickinson & Balleine 1994). In addition, studies with orally self-administered cocaine and alcohol have shown the more rapid development of habitual drug seeking compared with the seeking of a natural sweet reward, as evidenced by the failure of reinforcer devaluation through ingestive malaise to reduce the seeking of the drug reward, whilst at the same time-point greatly reducing responding for sucrose (Dickinson et al. 2002; Miles et al. 2003).

These observations supporting the increasing importance of the dorsal striatum in well-established, or habitual, drug seeking raise the issue of how, in neural terms, such a shift in the locus of control from ventral to dorsal striatum might occur. The observations of Haber et al. (2000) in primates and, more recently, Ikemoto (2007) in rats provide a possible neuro-anatomical basis for this shift. Their data show that ventral tiers of the striatal complex regulate the dopaminergic innervation of more dorsal tiers through so-called 'spiralling' connections with the midbrain (Fig. 3.1A). Thus, the AcbS projects to dopamine neurons in

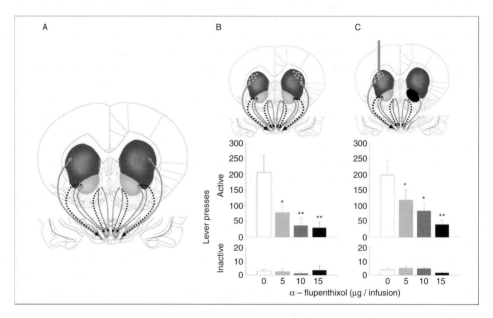

Fig. 3.1 (See also Plate 1) Within striatum, serial processing underlies the establishment of cocaine seeking habits. **A** Schematic representation of the intrastriatal dopamine-dependent spiralling circuitry functionally connecting the ventral with the dorsal striatum in the rat (modified from Belin & Everitt 2008). The spiralling loop organization is depicted as the alternation of pink and black arrows from the ventral to the more dorsal parts of the circuit, i.e. from the Acb Shell (yellow) to the AcbC (light blue) via the ventral tegmental area (pink) and from the AcbC via the substantia nigra to the dorsal striatum (dark blue). **B** Cocaine-seeking is dose-dependently impaired by bilateral infusions of the DA receptor antagonist α-flupenthixol (depicted as green dots in the diagram) into the DL striatum. α-flupenthixol infusions into the DL striatum dose-dependently decreased responding on the active lever under a second-order schedule of cocaine reinforcement, but had no effect on responding on the inactive lever (Belin & Everitt, 2008). **C** Disconnecting the AcbC from the dopaminergic innervation of the dorsal striatum impairs habitual cocaine-seeking. In unilateral AcbC-lesioned rats, the AcbC relay of the loop is lost on one side of the brain. However, on the non-lesioned side, the spiralling circuitry is intact and functional. When α-flupenthixol (green dots in the diagram) is infused in the DL striatum contralateral to the lesion it blocks the DAergic innervation from the midbrain, impairing the output structure of the spiralling circuitry on the non-lesioned side of the brain. Therefore, this asymmetric manipulation disconnects the core of the nucleus accumbens from the DL striatum and greatly diminishes cocaine seeking (Belin & Everitt 2008).

the ventral tegmental area that innervate not only the shell, but also the more dorsally situated AcbC. Neurons in the AcbC innervate dopamine neurons projecting both to the AcbC and the immediately dorsal regions of the dorsomedial caudate-putamen and so on, in a serially cascading pattern ultimately to encompass more lateral parts of the dorsal striatum—the site at which dopamine release is increased during habitual drug seeking and where dopamine receptor antagonist infusions impair this behaviour.

To test the hypothesis that the serial cascade of striato-nigro-striatal connectivity under-lies this progressively greater control over well-established cocaine-seeking behaviour by the DL striatum, we have used a novel intrastriatal 'disconnection' procedure in which the AcbC was selectively lesioned on one side of the brain and combined with dopamine receptor blockade in the contralateral DL striatum, thereby functionally disconnecting serial inter-actions between these ventral and dorsal striatal domains bilaterally (Belin et al. 2008). This disconnection greatly and selectively decreased cocaine seeking in rats trained to respond for cocaine under a second-order schedule of reinforcement tested some weeks after stable responding had been attained (Fig. 3.1B,C). Two important, additional observations under-line the specificity of the effects of this ventral-dorsal striatal disconnection: (1) the same animals were trained to perform a novel chain-pulling response for sucrose under continuous reinforcement and underwent the disconnection manipulation, or bilateral dorsal striatal dopamine receptor antagonist infusions (in non-lesioned rats), immediately after acquisi-tion when the behaviour was under response–outcome control (Adams & Dickinson 1981); neither manipulation had any effect (Belin et al. 2008). (2) In separate groups of animals, either bilateral dorsal striatal dopamine receptor blockade or AcbC-dorsal striatal discon-nection was performed at a much earlier stage of acquisition of the cocaine seeking, second-order schedule when responding was under ratio, rather than interval, control and when response–outcome mechanisms dominated performance. Again, neither manipulation had any effect on cocaine seeking (Belin & Everitt 2008; unpublished observations).

Taken together, the above results clearly indicate devolution of control over drug seeking from ventral to dorsal striatum and also strongly suggest that this shift is progressive. Other data also support the notion of this shift. For example, using autoradiographic methods, Porrino and colleagues showed the progressive development of neuroadaptations in dopamine D2 receptors and other neurochemical or metabolic markers in the dorsal striatum follow-ing chronic, but not acute, cocaine self-administration by monkeys (Letchworth et al. 2001, 1999; Porrino et al. 2004). At earlier stages of training, these adaptations were largely restricted to the more ventral, nucleus accumbens region. The dorsolateral striatum has also been shown to be involved in 'relapse' to a cocaine-seeking habit, since neural inhibition induced by GABA receptor agonist infusion into this area, but not into the AcbS or AcbC, prevented the reinstatement of cocaine seeking after protracted withdrawal (Fuchs et al. 2006; See et al. 2007). Moreover, the presentation of drug cues to human cocaine addicts not only induces drug craving that is correlated with activation of the amygdala and limbic prefrontal cortical areas (Childress et al. 1999; Garavan et al. 2000; Grant et al. 1996; Volkow et al. 2002), but also results in marked activation of the dorsal striatum (Garavan et al. 2000; Volkow et al. 2006). These observations, therefore, strongly indicate a link between limbic cortical mechanisms and engagement of the dorsal striatum in long-term drug abusers exposed to drug cues, whereas the results of our ventral/dorsal striatal disconnection experi-ments reveal that this recruitment is mediated by antecedent activity in the AcbC and its regulation of dorsal striatal dopaminergic projections originating in the midbrain.

It seems likely that the ventral to dorsal striatum shift is not specific to drug seeking, but would apply equally to the control over instrumental responding for natural reinforcers under appropriate conditions. Indeed, lesions or inactivation of the AcbC, dorsomedial or dorsolateral striatum, in rats responding for ingestive reinforcers do not globally impair instrumental behaviour, but instead have major effects that depend upon the response–outcome or S–R associative structure underlying the behaviour. Lesions or NMDA receptor blockade of the AcbC (Corbit et al. 2001; Kelley et al. 1997) or DM striatum (Yin et al. 2004, 2005) impair instrumental behaviour under response–outcome control, but actually enhance the development of S–R habits in which responding persists after reinforcer devaluation (Yin et al. 2004). In contrast, dorsolateral striatal lesions, inactivation, or dopamine denervation return previously habitual responding to response–outcome control, reinstating sensitivity to reinforcer devaluation (Faure et al. 2005; Yin et al. 2004) or action–outcome contingency degradation (Yin et al. 2006). These observations emphasize that response–outcome and S–R learning mechanisms are probably engaged not serially, but in parallel, with dorsolateral striatum-dependent S–R mechanisms eventually dominating the control over behaviour.

However, it is possible that the shift from ventral to dorsal striatal control occurs more rapidly in animals seeking drugs because of the direct, pharmacological effects of these agents on the plasticity mechanisms involved, particularly in the case of psychomotor stimulants, which so powerfully increase dopamine transmission. Thus, an amphetamine sensitization treatment regimen leads to the more rapid instantiation of habit learning in animals responding for food (Nelson & Killcross 2006). Moreover, animals that had escalated their cocaine intake showed, when subsequently challenged with cocaine, a marked enhancement ('sensitization') of stereotyped behavioural responses that have long been known to depend upon the dorsal, rather than the ventral, striatal dopaminergic innervation (Ferrario et al. 2005). Finally, Schoenbaum and colleagues have demonstrated a shift in the balance of associative encoding from ventral to dorsal striatum correlated with concomitant enhancement of cue-evoked neuronal firing in the dorsal striatum (Takahashi et al. 2007). The latter finding resonates with the observation of drug-associated CS-induced activation of the dorsal striatum in human cocaine abusers (Garavan et al. 2000; Volkow et al. 2006). Therefore, the unique properties of drugs as reinforcers, especially stimulant drugs, might accelerate, or more effectively *consolidate*, the development of drug seeking as a S–R habit (Everitt et al. 2001).

However, it should also be appreciated that whilst all animals responding for drugs or natural reinforcers will engage the dorsal striatal habit mechanism under appropriate reinforcement contingencies, not all individuals that take addictive drugs will become addicted. That is, not all individuals self-administering drugs will escalate their intake and go on to develop compulsive drug seeking that persists in the face of negative or aversive outcomes, the key characteristics of addiction, or 'substance dependence', in DSM-IV. Thus, some individuals are vulnerable in terms of these characteristics, a proportion that is often estimated to be about 20% or less of those initially exposed to addictive drugs (Anthony et al. 1994). We have recently shown that impulsivity is a behavioural characteristic that both predicts the escalation of cocaine intake and the progression to compulsive drug seeking as well as an increased propensity to relapse after abstinence.

3.3 Impulsivity, ventral striatal dopamine receptors, and vulnerability to addiction

Studies of human addicts have implicated individual differences in impulsivity, or other traits, such as 'sensation-seeking', in the vulnerability to drug use and abuse (Chakroun et al. 2004; Verdejo-Garcia & Perez-Garcia 2007), although it has never been clear whether the impulsivity observed in drug addicts pre-dates the onset of addiction, or is a consequence of protracted periods of drug taking (Dom et al. 2006; Zilberman et al. 2007). We have investigated this issue experimentally by defining in rats an operational measure of the human trait of impulsivity as premature responses in a 5-choice serial reaction-time task (5-CSRTT), a test of visual attentional function (Dalley et al. 2007). A proportion (<10%) of the outbred, Lister-hooded strain of rats in our study were impulsive on this task in that they showed high levels of anticipatory responses made before the presentation of a food-predictive, brief light stimulus—especially under conditions when the stimulus presentation was delayed after trial onset (Dalley et al. 2007). This impulsivity we term 'waiting impulsivity', as it is related to impulsivity measured as an inability to tolerate delays of reinforcement (Robinson et al. 2009), but appears different from the response impulsivity measured in STOP signal reaction time tasks (Eagle et al. 2008).

When given access to intravenous cocaine in a self-administration setting, the impulsive subjects showed a marked escalation of their cocaine intake compared to non-impulsive controls. They did not acquire cocaine self-administration at a faster rate, but responded at a much higher rate for their cocaine infusions than did non-impulsive subjects (Dalley et al. 2007). This is in marked contrast to subjects showing high locomotor responses to novelty (a 'sensation-seeking' phenotype), which self-administer cocaine at low doses that do not sustain self-administration in subjects showing low locomotor responses to novelty (Piazza et al. 1989, 2000). Thus, high impulsivity predicts the tendency to escalate cocaine intake and is reminiscent of one of the diagnostic characteristics of substance dependence in DSM-IV, which describes as a core symptom the taking of drugs in larger quantities than intended.

Highly impulsive animals were investigated neurobiologically using positron emission tomography to measure dopamine D2/3 receptor binding in the striatum using the selective, high-affinity dopamine D2/3 receptor antagonist [18F]fallypride (Mukherjee et al. 1999). Impulsive animals showed markedly reduced fallypride binding within the ventral, but not the dorsal, striatum (Fig. 3.2). Moreover, the reduced dopamine D2/3 receptor availability in the ventral striatum was correlated with impulsivity on the 5CSRTT (Dalley et al. 2007). Thus, low dopamine D2/3 receptors in the ventral striatum, encompassing the nucleus

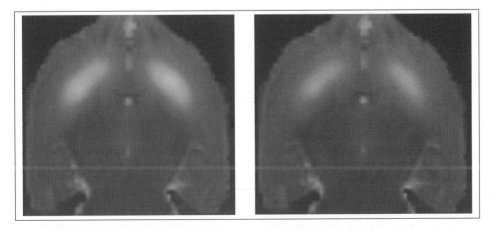

Fig. 3.2 (See also Plate 8) Reduced [18F]fallypride binding in the ventral striatum of highly impulsive (right panel) compared to non-impulsive (left panel) rats (Dalley et al., 2007).

accumbens core and shell regions, is not only correlated with the impulsive tendency, but is also associated with a marked propensity to escalate cocaine intake when rats are given the opportunity to self-administer the drug during long access sessions. This observation, taken together with the role of the Acb shell in the reinforcing and stimulant effects of cocaine, as well as involvement of the AcbC in the acquisition of drug-seeking behaviour (Ito et al. 2004) and the ability to tolerate delays to reinforcement (Cardinal et al. 2001), indicates the importance of the ventral striatum in the neural mechanisms underlying the propensity to seek and work for extended periods of time in order to self-administer cocaine. Nader et al. (2008), in studies of socially housed monkeys, have also demonstrated the significant relationship between D2 dopamine receptors in the striatum and cocaine self-admininstration (Czoty et al. 2004; Nader et al. 2006).

An additional observation in the study by Dalley et al. (2007) was that impulsive rats having self-administered cocaine showed reduced levels of impulsivity—perhaps related to the reduction in impulsive behaviour following treatment with the stimulant methylphenidate in subjects with attention-deficit hyperactivity disorder. Moreover, during a subsequent period in which animals had no access to cocaine self-administration ('enforced abstinence'), impulsivity returned to near pre-cocaine self-administration levels (Fig. 3.3). Since impulsivity predicts the escalation of drug intake, we investigated whether the return of impulsivity during abstinence might also be associated with a greater propensity to relapse, as suggested by de Wit and Richards (de Wit et al. 2004). In these experiments (Economidou et al. 2009), rats were trained in a cocaine-seeking-taking task. Once responding had stabilized, a punishment contingency was introduced, whereby on a random basis, 50% of the seeking responses were followed by presentation of the cocaine taking link in the chain, but 50% were followed by mild footshock (Pelloux et al. 2007). This schedule of unpredictable cocaine taking and aversive footshock outcomes results in the suppression of drug-seeking responses, especially after a limited, or non-escalated, history of cocaine self-administration and can therefore be viewed as the development of 'abstinence', in that animals voluntarily withhold their drug-seeking responses when the punishment contingency is present. After having attained abstinence in this way and some two weeks after their last cocaine infusion, groups of impulsive

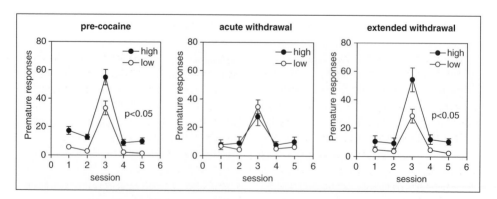

Fig. 3.3 The return of impulsive behaviour in highly impulsive rats following withdrawal and abstinence from cocaine self-administration. The data shown are premature responses in a 5-choice serial reaction-time task. Highly impulsive rats respond prematurely before any cocaine experience (left panel) and their impulsivity is *reduced* following sessions of cocaine self-administration (middle panel), but premature responding returns to pre-cocaine levels following an extended period of withdrawal (Dalley et al., unpublished observations).

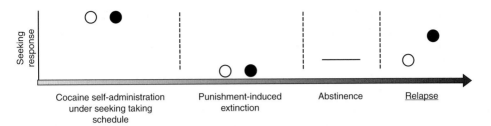

Fig. 3.4 Impulsive rats show an increased propensity to relapse after abstinence. Impulsive and non-impulsive rats were trained to seek and take cocaine under a chained schedule (left panel). Subsequently, 50% of the seeking responses were followed unpredictably by punishment and 50% by access to the taking lever; this results in the suppression of drug seeking (2nd panel). Following a further period of abstinence, when no cocaine is available (3rd panel), rats are returned to the self-admininistration setting in which seeking responses result in presentation of a cocaine-associated conditioned reinforcer, but no drug. Impulsive rats show much higher numbers of seeking responses than low impuslive rats (4th panel) and hence show a greater propensity to 'relapse'.

and non-impulsive rats were re-introduced to the test boxes and again allowed to respond on the seeking lever, which always resulted in access to the taking lever, responses upon which resulted in the presentation of the cocaine-associated CS, but no drug. Thus, in many respects, this relapse or reinstatement test is similar to that used in related procedures in which withdrawal of drug access, rather than extinction of the instrumental drug-taking response, is used to achieve abstinence prior to assessing the propensity to relapse (Fuchs et al. 2006; Lu et al. 2005). While both groups of animals reinstated their drug-seeking responses, i.e. 'relapsed', responding by impulsive rats was markedly and significantly greater than that of non-impulsive subjects (Fig. 3.4). Thus, impulsivity not only confers an increased predisposition to escalate cocaine self-administration, but also an increased propensity to relapse to a drug-seeking habit after abstinence. The neurobiological mechanisms underlying this persisting vulnerability to seek and take drugs after abstinence is an important area for future research.

3.4 From impulsivity to compulsive drug seeking in addiction

Demonstrating that impulsivity is a factor underlying the propensity to escalate drug intake and to relapse after abstinence leaves open the important issue of whether impulsivity is also a vulnerability marker for drug addiction and the compulsive drug seeking this entails. There are relatively few accepted models of compulsive drug seeking, or indeed compulsive behaviour in general in animals. Perseverative responding in reversal learning tasks may provide one interesting example because this form of compulsion is persistently enhanced following even relatively brief periods of cocaine treatment (Calu et al. 2007; Jentsch et al., 2002). In theoretical terms, we have suggested (Everitt & Robbins 2005) that compulsive drug seeking can be characterized as a maladaptive S–R habit in which the ultimate goal of the behavior has been devalued, perhaps through tolerance to the rewarding effects of the drug, so that the behaviour is not directly under the control of the goal. Instead, responding is increasingly controlled by a succession of drug-associated discriminative stimuli, which also function as conditioned reinforcers when presented as a consequence of instrumental responses, as in the second-order, drug-seeking schedule described above. Central to drug addiction, then, is the persisting quality of these habits, which we have suggested (Everitt & Robbins 2005) may correspond to the subjective state of 'must do!'—the persistent reinitiation of habitual acts—not least to distinguish it from the subjective state of excessive 'wanting' embodied in the incentive salience sensitization view of addiction (Robinson et al. 1993, 2000).

In attempting to model drug addiction in animals, we have tried to capture the *compulsive* quality of drug seeking by measuring its persistence despite negative or aversive outcomes, thereby also capturing a key aspect of addiction, or 'substance dependence', in DSM-IV. In developing such behavioural procedures, we have shown that compulsive drug seeking only emerges following an extended, or chronic, history of cocaine taking (Deroche-Gamonet et al. 2004; Pelloux et al. 2007; Vanderschuren et al. 2004). In the study by Deroche-Gamonet et al. (2004), three addiction-like behavioural criteria were measured in rats, namely, (i) increased motivation to take the drug, (ii) inability to refrain from drug seeking, and (iii) maintained drug use despite aversive consequences. After about 40 days of cocaine self-administration, but not at earlier times, some 17% of subjects developed these addiction-like criteria, showing increased breakpoints under a progressive ratio of cocaine reinforcement, persistent responding during signalled periods of drug unavailability, and, perhaps most importantly, persisting in the instrumental nosepoke response for cocaine even when it was punished by mild footshock. In the study by Pelloux et al. (2007), rats were trained on the seeking-taking chained schedule with intermittent punishment of the seeking response (i.e. on 50% of the seeking bouts, randomly occurring) to achieve suppression of drug seeking, or abstinence as described above. In this study too, all rats suppressed their cocaine seeking after a limited history of cocaine self-administration, after an extended period some 17–20% of subjects were completely resistant to punishment, continuing to seek and take drugs despite the ongoing, daily experience of the negative outcome. The proportion of rats compulsively seeking drugs, then, was similar both to that in the study by Deroche-Gamonet et al. (2004) and to the addiction-vulnerable sub-group of human subjects, often estimated to be less than 20% of the population that initially use drugs (Anthony et al. 1994). Thus, independently conducted experiments from our laboratory and that in Bordeaux have successfully modelled in animals compulsive drug seeking and other characteristics of addiction in humans and also have shown that this behaviour does not develop in all rats, but only in a vulnerable sub-group and only after a chronic drug-taking history.

However, the origins of this propensity to seek cocaine compulsively have not been established. We hypothesized that impulsivity, which we have shown to be associated with low dopamine D2/3 receptor availability in the ventral striatum and to predict the escalation of cocaine intake (Dalley et al. 2007), might also confer the vulnerability to develop compulsive drug seeking and addiction following extended access to cocaine. Rats were screened both for impulsivity in the 5CSSRT and also for the sensation-seeking phenotype of high locomotor responsiveness to novelty (HR rats), which has earlier been suggested to be an addiction vulnerability phenotype (Piazza et al. 1989). The resultant groups were then studied in the acquisition of cocaine self-administration, and for the emergence of the three addiction-like behavioural criteria (Deroche-Gamonet et al. 2004), but especially persistent responding for the drug in the face of punishment. As expected, and as reported previously (Piazza et al. 1989, 2000), the HR rats more readily acquired cocaine self-administration and showed an upward shift in the cocaine dose-response curve as compared both to rats with low responses to novelty and also high impulsivity. We also confirmed our earlier finding that impulsivity is not associated with more rapid acquisition of cocaine self-administration, but instead to the more rapid escalation of cocaine intake (Dalley et al. 2007). However, and in marked contrast, it was high impulsivity, but not high reactivity to novelty, that predicted the 'switch' (Leshner 1997) from controlled to compulsive cocaine taking (Belin et al. 2008; Fig. 3.5).

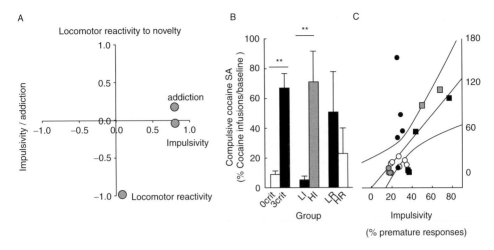

Fig. 3.5 Impulsivity predicts the shift to compulsive cocaine self-administration. **A** Impulsivity and addiction-like behaviour, but not high locomotor responses to novelty, co-associate. Factor analysis on 23 rats grouped according to their impulsivity or locomotor reactivity to novelty after 40 days of cocaine self-administration revealed that addiction-like behaviour (as measured by the sum of the normalized distributions of each of three addiction-like behaviours (see text and Deroche-Gamonet et al. 2004) and impulsivity (Dalley et al. 2007) are clustered along the same dimension that is orthogonal to novelty-seeking. **B–C** Impulsivity predicts the transition to compulsive cocaine self-administration. **B** When compared for their persistence of cocaine-taking responses despite punishment by mild electric footshock, rats showing 3 addiction-like criteria show greater scores than animals that were selected for their resistance to addiction, or 0 criteria rats. Similarly, highly impulsive rats showed a much greater resistance to punishment than low impulsive rats and displayed a level of compulsive responding that was similar to 3 criteria rats. However, rats showing high locomotor responses to novelty ('sensation-seeking') did not show greater resistance to punishment than rats with low locomotor reactivity to novelty. These two groups being highly heterogeneous but still sensitive to aversive consequences of drug-taking responses. C: Spearman correlation analysis revealed that impulsivity was highly predictive of the subsequent development of compulsive cocaine self-administration. It is noteworthy that highly impulsive rats (squares) are clustered in the top-right corner of the correlation, and overlap with 3 criteria rats (black-filled circles).

Highly impulsive rats displayed higher addiction scores and, especially, much greater resistance to punishment than rats with high or low responses to novelty or low impulsivity. In fact, highly impulsive rats did not differ from rats showing the three addiction-like behavioural criteria in any of their addiction-like behaviours after the extended period of cocaine self-administration. The pattern of results of this experiment clearly suggest that the relationship between high impulsivity and drug addiction is independent of the initial propensity to acquire cocaine self-administration. Therefore it seems, perhaps counter-intuitively, that the sensitivity to the reinforcing properties of cocaine on initial exposure to the drug, and the vulnerability to develop compulsive cocaine intake (addiction), depend upon distinct and seemingly orthogonal behavioural characteristics, each of which might have a genetic or environmental basis. The results of this study also provide experimental evidence that high levels of impulsivity can antedate the onset of compulsive drug use, thereby emphasizing the importance of pre-existing impulsivity observed in individuals addicted to drugs (Dom et al. 2006; Jentsch & Taylor 1999).

Now that we have established models of compulsive drug seeking and addiction, it is possible to investigate not only predisposing factors, such as impulsivity, but also the underlying neurobiological mechanisms. There are several current views about the origins of compulsion within the brain, which are often seen to be, but in reality are not, mutually exclusive. The neuroadaptations occurring during behavioural sensitization to stimulant drugs have been argued to underlie an extreme incentive motivational state of drug 'wanting' (Robinson et al. 1993; Robinson & Berridge 2000). According to this view, addicts experience this state in particular when exposed to drug-associated cues, which leads to over-activation of the sensitized dopaminergic innervation of the nucleus accumbens, in which plasticity-associated structural changes in dendritic spines have also been observed (Ferrario et al. 2005). This hypothesis is discussed in detail by Robinson & Berridge (2008). One interpretation of compulsive drug seeking, then, is that it is a behavioural manifestation of this potentiated motivational state, although its impact on the motivation to seek drugs has been demonstrated in rather few studies measuring increased breakpoints in progressive ratio schedules of reinforcement (for a review, see Vezina 2004). However, as noted above, a sensitization treatment regimen with amphetamine also leads to the more rapid instantiation of S–R habits (Nelson & Killcross 2006) and it is not easy to differentiate at the behavioural level between an increased tendency to repeat drug-seeking responses elicited and maintained by drug-associated stimuli—the must do! of *compulsive* habits discussed above—from an increased desire for a drug, which might also seem counter-intuitive, given the development of tolerance to its rewarding or reinforcing effects. Of course, both mechanisms may co-occur.

Perhaps, more directly related to the notion of drug seeking as a compulsive habit, however, is the observation of progressive reductions in dopamine D2 receptors in the dorsal striatum in abstinent addicts (Volkow et al. 2001; Volkow et al. 2004) and following chronic, but not acute, cocaine self-administration in monkeys (Moore et al. 1998; Nader et al. 2002). The consequences of this change in striatal dopamine transmission for the plasticity underlying instrumental learning and performance are unclear, but a putative sequential mechanism within the striatum and involving its dopaminergic innervation might be considered. Thus, the early vulnerability to escalate cocaine intake seen in impulsive rats is predicted by low dopamine D2/3 receptor levels in the *ventral*, but not the dorsal, striatum (Dalley et al. 2007). However, this escalated intake may lead to more rapid neuroadaptations, including down-regulated D2 dopamine receptors, in the *dorsal* striatum mediated by aberrant engagement of the spiralling striato–nigro–striatal circuitry. This would lead to more rapid consolidation of drug-seeking habits that are difficult to relinquish, despite negative outcomes and are more readily re-instantiated after abstinence following exposure to response-eliciting drug-associated stimuli.

An alternative account may be provided by the impact of negative reinforcement, as has been suggested to underlie obsessive-compulsive disorder, whereby drug-seeking habits are maintained by the motivation to alleviate or avoid (self-medicate) the negative emotional state and dysregulation resulting from tolerance to, and withdrawal from, drugs taken in increasing amounts over time (Koob et al. 2001). These counter-adaptations are prevalent in the central and extended amygdala and their motivational impact on drug self-administration is described in detail by Koob & Le Moal (2008). These mechanisms are not of course mutually exclusive. Addiction to drugs may reflect a combination of increased incentive motivation mediated by the up-regulation of ventral striatal dopamine transmission, by 'hyper-consolidated' habit learning mediated by aberrantly engaged dorsal striatum, dopamine-dependent mechanisms, and the drive engendered by negative emotional states in extra-striatal networks.

However, we and others have hypothesized an additional neurobiological mechanism, perhaps, arising in part as the direct or indirect consequence of toxic drug effects. This mechanism may be implicated in the balance of behavioural control processes from the prefrontal cortex to the striatum, thereby promoting *compulsive* habitual behaviour. There are abundant data suggesting prefrontal cortical, especially orbitofrontal (OFC), dysfunction in addicts, which are also increasingly supported by experimental studies in animals (Everitt et al. 2007; Olausson et al. 2007; Schoenbaum et al., 2006) and humans (see Garavan et al. 2008). Thus, in cocaine and methamphetamine abusers, reduced activity of the OFC (which correlates with reduced dopamine D2 receptors in the striatum) (Volkow et al. 2001) and also reduced grey matter volume in this region (Matochik et al. 2003) have been reported. There are also growing numbers of reports of impaired behavioural and cognitive functions, including poor behavioural adjustment (Bechara 2005; Fillmore et al. 2003) and impaired probabilistic reversal learning in cocaine abusers (Ersche et al., in press), possibly due to reduced inhibitory control. Deficits have been reported in decision-making cognition on computerized versions of a gambling task, when stimulant abusers chose the most favourable option less frequently than control subjects and chose significantly against the odds in risky conditions, suggesting difficulties in estimating outcome probabilities (Ersche et al. 2005; Rogers et al. 1999). Similar changes in behaviour are seen in individuals with OFC damage (Rogers et al. 1999) and this has encouraged the view that chronic drug taking may actually be a causal factor in inducing these prefrontal cortex-dependent deficits. But suboptimal prefrontal cortical, including OFC and anterior cingulate cortex, function (Hester & Garavan 2004; Kaufman et al. 2003; Volkow & Fowler 2000) may also represent a pre-existing vulnerability trait that results in poor decisions and/or a lack of sensitivity to the consequences of such decisions, and hence drug abuse leading to addiction. Prefrontal cortical dysfunction in addicts might also be a limiting factor in attempts by addicted individuals to abstain, or in their responsiveness to cognitive–behavioural therapeutic interventions when seeking treatment. However, it is difficult to establish cause and effect by studying already drug-addicted individuals alone (Everitt et al. 2007).

Experimental studies primarily involving psychostimulant treatment of rats and monkeys even after brief periods of exposure have supported the view that disrupted OFC function may indeed be a consequence of toxic drug effects during an addict's history of drug abuse (Jentsch & Taylor 1999; Schoenbaum et al. 2006). Short-term, usually experimenter-, and not self, administered cocaine or amphetamine have been reported to enhance the development of impulsivity (Jentsch & Taylor 1999; Roesch et al. 2007). Impaired reversal learning following cocaine treatment has been reported in monkeys (Jentsch et al. 2002) and in rats (Schoenbaum et al. 2004). A particularly important study by Schoenbaum and colleagues showed that rats having self-administered and then been withdrawn from cocaine exhibited both increased extinction responding 1 and 30 days into withdrawal, and also a marked deficit in reversal learning some 2 months into withdrawal (Calu et al. 2007). Schoenbaum and colleagues not only emphasized the similarity between OFC lesions and these apparently long-lasting effects of relatively short-term treatment with cocaine, but also showed that the deficit in reversal learning is reflected in a change in the properties of OFC neurons, which do not develop appropriate responses to cues predicting outcomes (Stalnaker et al. 2006).

It is clearly impressive that even brief periods of drug exposure, whether experimenter- or self-administered, can result in enduring changes in behaviour indicative of OFC dysfunction. However, in the great majority of imaging and neuropsychological investigations of addicts, there has been an exceptionally long history of drug abuse and often poly-drug abuse. These drug-addicted individuals must represent, therefore, a relatively small proportion of the much larger number of individuals in a population who have abused drugs over vary-ing periods, but who have not made the transition to an addicted state as characterized by compulsive drug seeking. Thus, it would seem unlikely that the experimental groups of rats receiving the fairly modest exposure to stimulant drugs in the experiments described above would in any sense fulfill the criteria for addiction, yet the changes in behaviour indicative of OFC dysfunction are seen in the entire population of treated experimental animals. It will be important, therefore, to investigate neurobiologically those models that capture chronic drug self-administration (Dalley et al. 2005, 2007; Pelloux et al. 2007; Belin et al. 2008) and the compulsive drug seeking that develops in vulnerable sub-populations of rats. In this way, we may seek to understand the neurobiological mechanisms underlying the interaction between pre-disposing traits and chronic drug exposure in the development of drug addiction.

3.5 Conclusions

We have discussed evidence that drug addiction can be viewed as the endpoint of a series of transitions from initial voluntary drug use through loss of control over this behavior, such that it becomes habitual and ultimately compulsive. We have described evidence that the switch from controlled to compulsive drug seeking represents a transition at the neural level from prefrontal cortical to striatal control over drug-seeking and drug-taking behavior as well as a progression from ventral to more dorsal domains of the striatum, mediated by its serially interconnecting dopaminergic circuitry. These neural transitions depend upon the neuroplasticity in both cortical and striatal structures that is induced by chronic self-administration of drugs, including long-lasting changes that are the consequence of toxic drug effects. However, caution must be exercised when considering the degree to which the underlying hypotheses and experimental data reviewed here can be generalized to addiction to other drugs. Much of the theorizing and evidence comes from studies of stimulant drugs such as cocaine. There is a major need for studies of other drugs, especially opiates and alcohol, at both the psychological and neurobiological level before the gaps in our under-standing are filled.

Acknowledgements

This research was supported by grants from the Medical Research Council and Wellcome Trust and was conducted within the Behavioural and Clinical Neuroscience Institute in the University of Cambridge.

References

Adams, C.D. and Dickinson, A. 1981 Instrumental responding following reinforcer devaluation. *Quarterly Journal of Experimental Psychology Section B-Comparative and Physiological Psychology*, **33**, 109–121.

Anthony, J.C., Warner, L.A. and Kessler, R.C. 1994 Comparative epidemiology of dependence on tobacco, alcohol, controlled substances, and inhalants. *Experimental and Clinical Psychopharmacology*, **2**, 244.

Bechara, A. 2005 Decision making, impulse control and loss of willpower to resist drugs: a neurocog-nitive perspective. *Nature Neuroscience*, **8**, 1458–63.

Belin, D. and Everitt, B.J. 2008 Cocaine seeking habits depend upon doparnine-dependent serial connectivity linking the ventral with the dorsal striatum. *Neuron*, **57**, 432–441.

Belin, D, Mar, A.C., Dalley, J.W., Robbins, T.W. and Everitt, B.J. 2008 Impulsivity predicts the switch to compulsive cocaine seeking. *Science* **320**, 1352–5.

Cador, M., Robbins, T.W. and Everitt, B.J. 1989 Involvement of the amygdala in stimulus–reward associations: interaction with the ventral striatum. *Neuroscience*, **30**, 77–86.

Calu, D.J., Stalnaker, T.A., Franz, T.F., Singh, T., Shaham, Y. and Schoenbaum, G. 2007 Withdrawal from cocaine self-administration produces long-lasting deficits in orbitofrontal-dependent revearsal learning in rats. *Learning and Memory*, **14**, 325–8.

Cardinal, R.N. and Everitt, B.J. 2004 Neural and psychological mechanisms underlying appetitive learning: links to drug addiction. *Current Opinions in Neurobiology*, **14**, 156–62.

Cardinal, R.N., Parkinson, J.A., Hall, J. and Everitt, B.J. 2002 Emotion and motivation: the role of the amygdala, ventral striatum, and prefrontal cortex. *Neuroscience and Biobehavioral Reviews*, **26**, 321–52.

Cardinal, R.N., Pennicott, D.R., Sugathapala, C.L., Robbins, T.W. and Everitt, B.J. 2001 Impulsive choice induced in rats by lesions of the nucleus accumbens core. *Science*, **292**, 2499–501.

Chakroun, N., Doron, J. and Swendsen, J. 2004 Substance use, affective problems and personality traits: test of two association models. *Encephale-Revue De Psychiatrie Clinique Biologique Et Therapeutique*, **30**, 564–9.

Childress, A.R., Mozley, P.D., McElgin, W., Fitzgerald, J., Reivich, M. and O'Brien, C.P. 1999 Limbic activation during cue-induced cocaine craving. *American Journal of Psychiatry*, **156**, 11–18.

Corbit, L.H., Muir, J.L. and Balleine, B.W. 2001 The role of the nucleus accumbens in instrumental conditioning: evidence of a functional dissociation between accumbens core and shell. *Journal of Neuroscience*, **21**, 3251–60.

Czoty, P.W., Morgan, D., Shannon, E.E., Gage, H.D. and Nader, M.A. 2004 Characterization of dopamine D-1 and D-2 receptor function in socially housed cynomolgus monkeys self-administering cocaine. *Psychopharmacology*, **174**, 381–8.

Dalley, J.W., Fryer, T.D., Brichard, L. et al. 2007 Nucleus accumbens D2/3 receptors predict trait impulsivity and cocaine reinforcement. *Science*, **315**, 1267–70.

Dalley, J.W., Laane, K., Pena, Y., Theobald, D.E.H., Everitt, B.J. and Robbins, T.W. 2005 Attentional and motivational deficits in rats withdrawn from intravenous self-administration of cocaine or heroin. *Psychopharmacology*, **182**, 579–87.

Dalley, J.W., Laane, K., Theobald, D.E.H. et al. 2007 Enduring deficits in sustained visual attention during withdrawal of intravenous methylenedioxymethamphetamine self-administration in rats: results from a comparative study with d-amphetamine and methamphetamine. *Neuropsychopharmacology*, **32**, 1195–206.

Dalley, J.W., Theobald, D.E.H., Berry, D. et al. 2005 Cognitive sequelae of intravenous amphetamine self-administration in rats: Evidence for selective effects on attentional performance. *Neuropsychopharmacology*, **30**, 525–37.

de Wit, H. and Richards, J.B. (2004) In Bevins, R. A. and Bardo, M. T. (eds.), *Motivational Factors in the Etiology of Drug Abuse*. University of Nebraska Press, Lincoln, Nebraska, Vol. 50, pp. 19–56.

Deroche-Gamonet, V., Belin, D. and Piazza, P.V. 2004 Evidence for addiction-like behavior in the rat. *Science*, **305**, 1014–17.

Di Chiara, G., Bassareo, V., Fenu, S. et al. 2004 Dopamine and drug addiction: the nucleus accumbens shell connection. *Neuropharmacology*, **47**, 227–41.

Di Ciano, P. and Everitt, B.J. 2004 Direct interactions between the basolateral amygdala and nucleus accumbens core underlie cocaine-seeking behavior by rats. *Journal of Neuroscience*, **24**, 7167–73.

Dickinson, A. 1985 Actions and habits: the development of behavioural autonomy. *Philosophical Transactions of the Royal Society of London B*, **308**, 67–78.

Dickinson, A. and Balleine, B. 1994 Motivational control of goal-directed action. *Animal Learning & Behavior*, **22**, 1–18.

Dickinson, A., Wood, N. and Smith, J.W. 2002 Alcohol seeking by rats: Action or habit? *Quarterly Journal of Experimental Psychology Section B- Comparative and Physiological Psychology*, **55**, 331–48.

Dom, G., D'Haene, P., Hulstijn, W. and Sabbe, B. 2006 Impulsivity in abstinent early- and late-onset alcoholics: differences in self-report measures and a discounting task. *Addiction*, **101**, 50–9.

DSM-IV. (1994) *Diagnostic and Statistical Manual of Mental Disorders*. American Psychiatric Association, Washington.

Eagle, D.M., Baunez, C., Hutcheson, D.M., Lehmann, O., Shah, A.P. and Robbins, T.W. 2008 Stop-signal reaction-time task performance: role of prefrontal cortex and subthalamic nucleus. *Cerebral Cortex*, **18**, 178–88.

Economidou, D., Pelloux, Y., Robbins, T.W., Dalley, J.W. and Everitt, B.J. 2009 High impulsivity predicts relapse to cocaine seeking following punishment-induced abstinence. *Biological Psychiatry*, **65**, 851–6.

Ersche, K.D., Fletcher, P.C., Lewis, S.J.G. et al. 2005 Abnormal frontal activations related to decision-making in current and former amphetamine and opiate dependent individuals *Psychopharmacology*, **180**, 612–23.

Ersche, K.D., Roiser, J.P., Robbins, T.W. and Sahakian, B.J. In press. Chronic cocaine, but not chronic amphetamine consumption impairs probabilistic reversal learning and produces perseverative responding. *Psychopharmacology*.

Everitt, B.J., Dickinson, A. and Robbins, T.W. 2001 The neuropsychological basis of addictive behaviour. *Brain Research Reviews*, **36**, 129–38.

Everitt, B.J., Hutcheson, D.M., Ersche, K.D. et al. (eds.), *Linking Affect to Action*: *Critical Contributions of the Orbitofrontal Cortex*. Blackwell, Boston, Vol. 1121, pp. 576–97.

Everitt, B.J. and Robbins, T.W. 2000 Second-order schedules of drug reinforcement in rats and monkeys: measurement of reinforcing efficacy and drug-seeking behaviour. *Psychopharmacology*, **153**, 17–30.

Everitt, B.J. and Robbins, T.W. 2005 Neural systems of reinforcement for drug addiction: from actions to habits to compulsion. *Nature Neuroscience*, **8**, 1481–9.

Everitt, B.J., Belin, D., Economidou, D., Pelloux, Y., Dalley, J.W. and Robbins, T.W. 2008 Neural mechanisms underlying the vulnerability to develop compulsive drug seeking habits and addiction. *Philosophical Transactions of the Royal Society of London, B: Biological Science*, **363**, 3125–35 (doi:10.1098/rstb.2008.0089).

Faure, A., Haberland, U., Conde, F. and El Massioui, N. 2005 Lesion to the nigrostriatal dopamine system disrupts stimulus–response habit formation. *Journal of Neuroscience*, **25**, 2771–80.

Ferrario, C.R., Gorny, G., Crombag, H.S., Li, Y.L., Kolb, B. and Robinson, T.E. 2005 Neural and behavioral plasticity associated with the transition from controlled to escalated cocaine use. *Biological Psychiatry*, **58**, 751–9.

Fillmore, M.T., Rush, C.R. and Marczinski, C.A. 2003 Effects of D-amphetamine on behavioral control in stimulant abusers: the role of prepotent response tendencies. *Drug and Alcohol Dependence*, **71**, 143–52.

Fuchs, R.A., Branham, R.K. and See, R.E. 2006 Different neural substrates mediate cocaine seeking after abstinence versus extinction training: A critical role for the dorsolateral caudate-putamen. *Journal of Neuroscience*, **26**, 3584–8.

Garavan, H., Pankiewicz, J., Bloom, A. et al. 2000 Cue-induced cocaine craving: neuroanatomical specificity for drug users and drug stimuli. *American Journal of Psychiatry*, **157**, 1789–98.

Garavan, H., Kaufman, J.N. and Hester, R. 2008 Acute effects of cocaine on the neurobiology of cognitive control. *Philosophical Transactions of the Royal Society of London, B: Biological Science*, **363**, 3267–76

Grant, S., London, E.D., Newlin, D.B. et al. 1996 Activation of memory circuits during cue-elicited cocaine craving. *Proceedings of the National Academy of Sciences of the United States of America*, **93**, 12040–5.

Haber, S.N., Fudge, J.L. and McFarland, N.R. 2000 Striatonigral pathways in primates form an ascending spiral from the shell to the dorsolateral striatum. *Journal of Neuroscience*, **20**, 2369–82.

Hester, R. and Garavan, H. 2004 Executive dysfunction in cocaine addiction: evidence for discordant frontal, cingulate, and cerebellar activity. *Journal of Neuroscience*, **24**, 11017–22.

Ikemoto, S. 2007 Dopamine reward circuitry: Two projection systems from the ventral midbrain to the nucleus accumbens-olfactory tubercle complex. *Brain Research Reviews*, **56**, 27–78.

Ikemoto, S., Qin, M. and Liu, Z.H. 2005 The functional divide for primary reinforcement of D-amphetamine lies between the medial and lateral ventral striatum: Is the division of the accumbens core, shell, and olfactory tubercle valid? *Journal of Neuroscience*, **25**, 5061–5.

Ito, R., Dalley, J.W., Howes, S.R., Robbins, T.W. and Everitt, B.J. 2000 Dissociation in conditioned dopamine release in the nucleus accumbens core and shell in response to cocaine cues and during cocaine-seeking behavior in rats. *Journal of Neuroscience*, **20**, 7489–95.

Ito, R., Dalley, J.W., Robbins, T.W. and Everitt, B.J. 2002 Dopamine release in the dorsal striatum during cocaine-seeking behavior under the control of a drug-associated cue. *Journal of Neuroscience*, **22**, 6247–53.

Ito, R., Robbins, T.W. and Everitt, B.J. 2004 Differential control over cocaine-seeking behavior by nucleus accumbens core and shell. *Nature Neuroscience*, **7**, 389–97.

Jentsch, J.D., Olausson, P., De la Garza, R. and Taylor, J.R. 2002 Impairments of reversal learning and response perseveration after repeated, intermittent cocaine administrations to monkeys. *Neuropsychopharmacology*, **26**, 183–90.

Jentsch, J.D. and Taylor, J.R. 1999 Impulsivity resulting from frontostriatal dysfunction in drug abuse: implications for the control of behavior by reward-related stimuli. *Psychopharmacology*, **146**, 373–90.

Kaufman, J.N., Ross, T.J., Stein, E.A. and Garavan, H. 2003 Cingulate hypoactivity in cocaine users during a GO-NOGO task as revealed by event-related functional magnetic resonance imaging. *Journal of Neuroscience*, **23**, 7839–43.

Kelley, A.E., SmithRoe, S.L. and Holahan, M.R. 1997 Response-reinforcement learning is dependent on N-methyl-n-aspartate receptor activation in the nucleus accumbens core. *Proceedings of the National Academy of Sciences of the United States of America*, **94**, 12174–9.

Koob, G.F. and Le Moal, M. 2001 Drug addiction, dysregulation of reward, and allostasis. *Neuropsychopharmacology*, **24**, 97–129.

Koob, G.F. and Le Moal, M. (2005) *Neurobiology of Addiction*. Academic Press, San Diego.

Koob, G.F. and Le Moal, M 2008 Neurobiological mechanisms for opponent motivational processes in addiction. *Philosophical Transactions of the Royal Society of London, B: Biological Science*, **363**, 3113–23

Leshner, A.I. 1997 Addiction is a brain disease, and it matters. *Science*, **278**, 45–7.

Letchworth, S.R., Nader, M.A., Smith, H.R., Friedman, D.P. and Porrino, L.J. 2001 Progression of changes in dopamine transporter binding site density as a result of cocaine self-administration in rhesus monkeys. *Journal of Neuroscience*, **21**, 2799–807.

Letchworth, S.R., Sexton, T., Childers, S.R. et al. 1999 Regulation of rat dopamine transpoter mRNA and protein by chronic cocaine administration. *Journal of Neurochemistry*, **73**, 1982–9.

Lu, L., Hope, B.T., Dempsey, J., Liu, S.Y., Bossert, J.M. and Shaham, Y. 2005 Central amygdala ERK signaling pathway is critical to incubation of cocaine craving. *Nature Neuroscience*, **8**, 212–19.

Matochik, J.A., London, E.D., Eldreth, D.A., Cadet, J.L. and Bolla, K.I. 2003 Frontal cortical tissue composition in abstinent cocaine abusers: a magnetic resonance imaging study. *Neuroimage*, **19**, 1095-102.

Miles, F.J., Everitt, B.J. and Dickinson, A. 2003 Oral cocaine seeking by rats: action or habit? *Behavioural Neuroscience*, **117**, 927–38.

Moore, R.J., Vinsant, S.L., Nader, M.A., Porrino, L.J. and Friedman, D.P. 1998 Effect of cocaine self-administration on dopamine D-2 receptors in rhesus monkeys. *Synapse*, **30**, 88–96.

Mukherjee, J., Yang, Z.Y., Brown, T. et al. 1999 Preliminary assessment of extrastriatal dopamine D-2 receptor binding in the rodent and nonhuman primate brains using the high affinity radioligand, 18F-fallypride. *Nuclear Medicine and Biology*, **26**, 519–27.

Nader, M.A., Daunais, J.B., Moore, T. et al. 2002 Effects of cocaine self-administration on striatal dopamine systems in rhesus monkeys: Initial and chronic exposure. *Neuropsychopharmacology*, **27**, 35–46.

Nader, M.A., Morgan, D., Gage, H.D. et al. 2006 PET imaging of dopamine D2 receptors during chronic cocaine self-administration in monkeys. *Nature Neuroscience*, **9**, 1050–6.

Nader, M.A., Czoty, P.W., Gould, R.W. and Riddick, N.V. 2008 Positron emission tomography imaging studies of dopamine receptors in primate models of addiction. *Philosophical Transactions of the Royal Society of London, B: Biological Science*, **363**, 3223–32

Nelson, A. and Killcross, S. 2006 Amphetamine exposure enhances habit formation. *Journal of Neuroscience*, **26**, 3805–12.

Nestler, E.J. 2004 Molecular mechanisms of drug addiction. *Neuropharmacology*, **47**, 24–32.

O'Brien, C.P. and McLellan, A.T. 1996 Myths about the treatment of addiction. *Lancet*, **347**, 237–40.

Olausson, P., Jentsch, J.D., Krueger, D.D., Tronson, N.C., Nairn, A.C. and Taylor, J.R. 2007 Orbitofrontal cortex and cognitive-motivational impairments in psychostimulant addiction. *Linking Affect to Action: Critical Contributions of the Orbitofrontal Cortex*, **1121**, 610–38.

Olmstead, M.C., Lafond, M.V., Everitt, B.J. and Dickinson, A. 2001 Cocaine seeking by rats is a goal-directed action. *Behavioral Neuroscience*, **115**, 394–402.

Olmstead, M.C., Parkinson, J.A., Miles, F.J., Everitt, B.J. and Dickinson, A. 2000 Cocaine-seeking by rats: regulation, reinforcement and activation. *Psychopharmacology*, **152**, 123–31.

Pelloux, Y., Everitt, B.J. and Dickinson, A. 2007 Compulsive drug seeking by rats under punishment: effects of drug taking history. *Psychopharmacology*, **194**, 127–37.

Piazza, P.V., Deminière, J.M., Le Moal, M. and Simon, H. 1989 Factors that predict individual vulnerability to amphetamine self-administration. *Science*, **245**, 1511–13.

Piazza, P.V., Deroche-Gamonent, V., Rouge-Pont, F. and Le Moal, M. 2000 Vertical shifts in self-administration dose-response functions predict a drug-vulnerable phenotype predisposed to addiction. *Journal of Neuroscience*, **20**, 4226–32.

Porrino, L.J., Daunais, J.B., Smith, H.R. and Nader, M.A. 2004 The expanding effects of cocaine: studies in a nonhuman primate model of cocaine self-administration. *Neuroscience and Biobehavioral Reviews*, **27**, 813–20.

Robbins, T.W., Cador, M., Taylor, J.R. and Everitt, B.J. 1989 Limbic-striatal interactions in reward-related processes. *Neuroscience and Biobehavioral Reviews*, **13**, 155–62.

Robbins, T.W. and Everitt, B.J. 1999 Drug addiction: bad habits add up. *Nature*, **398**, 567–70.

Robinson, E.S.J., Eagle, D.M., Economidou, D. et al. 2009 Behavioural characterisation of high impulsivity on the five-choice serial reaction time task: specific deficits in 'waiting' versus 'stopping'. *Behavioural Brain Research*, **196**, 310–16.

Robinson, T.E. and Berridge, K.C. 1993 The neural basis of drug craving: an incentive-sensitization theory of addiction. *Brain Research Reviews*, **18**, 247–91.

Robinson, T.E. and Berridge, K.C. 2000 The psychology and neurobiology of addiction: an incentive-sensitization view. *Addiction*, **95**, S91–117.

Robinson, T.E. and Berridge, K.C. 2008 The incentive sensitization theory of addiction: some current issues. *Philosophical Transactions of the Royal Society of London, B: Biological Science*, **363**, 3137–46.

Roesch, M.R., Takahashi, Y., Gugsa, N., Bissonette, G.B. and Schoenbaum, G. 2007 Previous cocaine exposure makes rats hypersensitive to both delay and reward magnitude. *Journal of Neuroscience*, **27**, 245–50.

Rogers, R.D., Everitt, B.J., Baldacchino, A. et al. 1999 Dissociable deficits in the decision-making cognition of chronic amphetamine abusers, opiate abusers, patients with focal damage to prefrontal cortex, and tryptophan-depleted normal volunteers: Evidence for monoaminergic mechanisms. *Neuropsychopharmacology*, **20**, 322–39.

Schoenbaum, G., Roesch, M.R. and Stalnaker, T.A. 2006 Orbitofrontal cortex, decision-making and drug addiction. *Trends in Neurosciences*, **29**, 116–24.

Schoenbaum, G., Saddoris, M.P., Ramus, S.J., Shaham, Y. and Setlow, B. 2004 Cocaine-experienced rats exhibit learning deficits in a task sensitive to orbitofrontal cortex lesions. *European Journal of Neuroscience*, **19**, 1997–2002.

See, R.E., Elliott, J.C. and Feltenstein, M.W. 2007 The role of dorsal vs. ventral striatal pathways in cocaine-seeking behavior following prolonged abstinence in rats. *Psychopharmacology*, **195**, 321–31.

Stalnaker, T.A., Roesch, M.R., Franz, T.M., Burke, K.A. and Schoenbaum, G. 2006 Abnormal associative encoding in orbitofrontal neurons in cocaine-experienced rats during decision-making. *European Journal of Neuroscience*, **24**, 2643–53.

Takahashi, Y., Roesch, M.R., Stanlaker, T.A. and Schoenbaum, G. 2007 Cocaine shifts the balance of cue-evoked firing from ventral to dorsal striatum. *http://frontiersin.org/neuroscience/abstract/10.3389/neuro.07/011.2007*.

Tiffany, S.T. 1990 A cognitive model of drug urges and drug-use behavior: role of automatic and non-automatic processes. *Psychological Reviews*, **97**, 146–68.

Vanderschuren, L., Di Ciano, P. and Everitt, B.J. 2005 Involvement of the dorsal striatum in cue-controlled cocaine seeking. *Journal of Neuroscience*, **25**, 8665–70.

Vanderschuren, L.J. and Everitt, B.J. 2004 Drug seeking becomes compulsive after prolonged cocaine self-administration. *Science*, **305**, 1017–19.

Verdejo-Garcia, A. and Perez-Garcia, M. 2007 Ecological assessment of executive functions in substance dependent individuals. *Drug and Alcohol Dependence*, **90**, 48–55.

Vezina, P. 2004 Sensitization of midbrain dopamine neuron reactivity and the self-administration of psychomotor stimulant drugs. *Neuroscience and Biobehavioral Reviews*, **27**, 827–39.

Volkow, N.D., Chang, L., Wang, G.J. et al. 2001 Low level of brain dopamine D-2 receptors in methamphetamine abusers: association with metabolism in the orbitofrontal cortex. *American Journal of Psychiatry*, **158**, 2015–21.

Volkow, N.D. and Fowler, J.S. 2000 Addiction, a disease of compulsion and drive: involvement of the orbitofrontal cortex. *Cerebral Cortex*, **10**, 318–25.

Volkow, N.D., Fowler, J.S. and Wang, G.J. 2004 The addicted human brain viewed in the light of imaging studies: brain circuits and treatment strategies. *Neuropharmacology*, **47**, 3–13.

Volkow, N.D., Fowler, J.S., Wang, G.J. and Goldstein, R.Z. 2002 Role of dopamine, the frontal cortex and memory circuits in drug addiction: Insight from imaging studies. *Neurobiology of Learning and Memory*, **78**, 610–24.

Volkow, N.D., Wang, G.J., Telang, F. et al. 2006 Cocaine cues and dopamine in dorsal striatum: mechanism of craving in cocaine addiction. *Journal of Neuroscience*, **26**, 6583–8.

Whitelaw, R.B., Markou, A., Robbins, T.W. and Everitt, B.J. 1996 Excitotoxic lesions of the basolateral amygdala impair the acquisition of cocaine-seeking behaviour under a second-order schedule of reinforcement. *Psychopharmacology*, **127**, 213–24.

Wise, R.A. 2004 Dopamine, learning and motivation. *Nature Reviews Neuroscience*, **5**, 483–94.

Yin, H.H., Knowlton, B.J. and Balleine, B.W. 2004 Lesions of dorsolateral striatum preserve outcome expectancy but disrupt habit formation in instrumental learning. *European Journal of Neuroscience*, **19**, 181–9.

Yin, H.H., Knowlton, B.J. and Balleine, B.W. 2006 Inactivation of dorsolateral striatum enhances sensitivity to changes in the action-outcome contingency in instrumental conditioning. *Behavioural Brain Research*, **166**, 189–96.

Yin, H.H., Ostlund, S.B., Knowlton, B.J. and Balleine, B.W. 2005 The role of the dorsomedial striatum in instrumental conditioning. *European Journal of Neuroscience*, **22**, 513–23.

Zilberman, M.L., Tavares, H., Hodgins, D.C. and El-Guebaly, N. 2007 The impact of gender, depression, and personality on craving. *Journal of Addictive Diseases*, **26**, 79–84.

4

The incentive-sensitization theory of addiction: Some current issues

Terry E. Robinson* and Kent C. Berridge

We present a brief overview of the incentive-sensitization theory of addiction. This posits that one major cause of addiction is drug-induced changes in brain mesocorticolimbic systems that attribute incentive salience to reward-associated stimuli and changes that render this neural circuitry hypersensitive ('sensitised'). When rendered hypersensitive, these systems cause pathological incentive motivation ('wanting') for drugs. We address some of the following current questions: What is the role of learning in incentive sensitization and addiction? Does incentive-sensitization occur in human addicts? Is the development of addiction-like behaviour in animals associated with sensitization? What is the best way to model addiction symptoms using animal models? And finally, what are the roles of affective pleasure or withdrawal in addiction?

Key Words: Sensitization; dopamine; habits; cocaine; amphetamine; motivation.

4.1 Introduction

At some time in their life, most people try a potentially addictive drug (e.g. alcohol). However, few become addicts. Addiction implies a pathological and compulsive pattern of drug-seeking and drug-taking behaviour, which occupies an inordinate amount of an individual's time and thoughts and persists despite adverse consequences (Hasin et al. 2006). Addicts also find it difficult to reduce or terminate drug use, even when they desire to do so. Finally, addicts are highly vulnerable to relapse even after long abstinence and well after symptoms of withdrawal have disappeared. Thus, this is a key question in addiction research: what is responsible for the transition to addiction in those few susceptible individuals?

Over the last 20 years or so, there has been increasing recognition that drugs change the brain of addicts in complex and persistent ways, so persistent that they far outlast other changes associated with tolerance and withdrawal. It is important to identify brain changes that contribute to the transition from casual or recreational drug use to addiction, and the features that make particular individuals especially susceptible to the transition (Hyman et al. 2006; Kalivas & O'Brien 2008; Nestler 2001; Robinson & Berridge 1993). Persistent drug-induced changes in the brain alter a number of psychological processes, resulting in various symptoms of addiction. We suggested in the incentive-sensitization theory of addiction, originally published in 1993, that the most important of these psychological changes is a *'sensitization' or hypersensitivity to the incentive motivational effects of drugs and drug-associated stimuli* (Robinson & Berridge 1993). *Incentive-sensitization* produces a bias of attentional processing towards drug-associated stimuli and pathological motivation for drugs (compulsive 'wanting'). When combined with impaired executive control over behaviour, incentive-sensitization culminates in the core symptoms of addiction (Robinson & Berridge

* ter@umich.edu

1993, 2000, 2003). The concept of incentive-sensitization has drawn considerable interest in the past 15 years; therefore, we thought it worthwhile to update our perspective. We present here a brief and idiosyncratic overview of this view of addiction and raise some current issues.

4.2 What is incentive-sensitization theory and what is the role of learning?

The central thesis of the incentive-sensitization theory of addiction (Robinson & Berridge 1993) is that repeated exposure to potentially addictive drugs can, in susceptible individuals and under particular circumstances, persistently change brain cells and circuits that normally regulate the attribution of incentive salience to stimuli, a psychological process involved in motivated behaviour. The nature of these 'neuroadaptations' is to render these brain circuits hypersensitive ('sensitized') in a way that results in pathological levels of incentive salience being attributed to drugs and drug-associated cues. Persistence of incentive-sensitization makes pathological incentive motivation ('wanting') for drugs last for years, even after the discontinuation of drug use. Sensitized incentive salience can be manifested in behaviour via either implicit or explicit processes (as unconscious 'wanting' or as conscious craving), depending on circumstances. Finally, the *focus* on drugs, in particular in addicts, is produced by an interaction between incentive salience mechanisms with associative learning mechanisms that normally direct motivation to specific and appropriate targets. Learning specifies the object of desire, but it is important to note that learning *per se* is not enough for pathological motivation to take drugs. Thus, we argue that pathological motivation arises from sensitization of brain circuits that mediate Pavlovian-conditioned incentive motivational processes (i.e. incentive-sensitization). However, it is important to emphasize that associative learning processes can *modulate* the expression of neural sensitization in behaviour at particular places or times (and not others), as well as guide the direction of incentive attributions. This is why behavioural sensitization is often expressed only in contexts in which drugs have been previously experienced (Anagnostaras & Robinson 1996; Robinson et al. 1998; Stewart & Vezina 1991) and may reflect the operation of an 'occasion-setting' type of mechanism (Anagnostaras et al. 2002). Learning might be viewed as layered onto basic sensitization processes in a top–down fashion, similar to how learning regulates the expression of such non-associative motivation process as stress and pain. The contextual control over the expression of sensitization provides an additional mechanism that accounts for why addicts 'want' drugs most particularly when they are in drug-associated contexts.

Finally, by spreading beyond the associative focus of 'wanting' on drug targets, incentive-sensitization can also sometimes spillover in animals or humans to other targets such as food, sex, gambling, etc. (Fiorino & Phillips 1999a, b; Mitchell & Stewart 1990; Nocjar & Panksepp 2002; Taylor & Horger 1999). For example, treatment with dopaminergic medications in some patient populations can lead to a 'dopamine dysregulation syndrome' (DDS) that is manifested not only by compulsive drug use, but also sometimes by 'pathological gambling, hypersexuality, food bingeing . . . and punding, a form of complex behavioural stereotypy' (Evans et al. 2006, p. 852).

4.2.1 Incentive-sensitization: more than just learning

It has become popular to refer to addiction as a 'learning disorder' (Hyman 2005), but we think this phrase may be too narrow to fit reality. Learning is only one part of the process and probably not the one that contributes most to the pathological pursuit of drugs.

The most influential type of 'learning hypothesis' suggests that drugs promote the learning of strong 'automatized' stimulus–response (S–R) *habits*, and it is then supposed that by their nature S–R habits confer compulsivity to behaviour (Berke & Hyman 2000; Everitt et al. 2001; Hyman et al. 2006; Tiffany 1990). However, it is difficult to imagine how any influence of drugs on *learning* processes alone could confer compulsivity on behaviour, unless an additional motivational component was also involved, and S–R habits by definition are not modulated by motivational factors (Robinson & Berridge 2003). Do automatic S–R habits really become compulsive merely by virtue of being extremely well learned? We have doubts. Strong S–R habits do not necessarily lead to compulsive behaviour: tying your shoe, brushing your teeth, etc., are not performed compulsively by most people, even after being performed more than 10,000 times. Additional motivational processes seem needed to explain why an addict waking up in the morning with no drug spends the day engaging in a complex and sometimes new series of behaviours—scamming, stealing, negotiating—all seemingly motivated to procure drug. Addicts do what they have to do and go where they have to go to get drugs, even if actions and routes that never have been performed before are required. Such focused yet flexible behaviour in addiction shows pathological motivation for drugs that cannot be explained by evoking S–R habits. Indeed, a strict S–R habit theory would require the addict, upon waking up in the morning with no drug available, to engage 'automatically' in exactly the same old sequence of habitual actions they used previously to get drugs, whether the actions were currently effective or not. Yet addicts in the real world are not S–R automatons; they are, if nothing else, quite resourceful.

On the other hand, everyone must agree that S–R habits probably contribute to the 'automatized' behaviours and rituals involved in *consuming* drugs once obtained (Tiffany 1990), and it has been shown that treatment with drugs facilitates the development of S–R habits in animals (Miles et al. 2003; Nelson & Killcross 2006), perhaps via recruitment of the dorsal striatum (Everitt et al. 2001; Porrino et al. 2007). We also note that habits may be especially prominent in standard animal self-administration experiments, where only a single response is available to be performed (e.g. press a lever) thousands of times in a very impoverished environment to earn injections of drugs. Thus, we think the studies on how drugs promote the learning of S–R habits will provide important information about the regulation of *drug consumption behaviour* in addicts, but this is not the core problem in addiction.

4.2.2 *Relation of incentive-sensitization to cognitive dysfunction*

The incentive-sensitization theory focuses on sensitization-induced changes in incentive motivational processes and related changes in brain, but we have acknowledged that other brain changes contribute importantly to addiction too, including damage or dysfunction in cortical mechanisms that underlie cognitive choice and decision-making (Robinson & Berridge 2000, 2003). Many studies have documented that changes in 'executive functions', involving how alternative outcomes are evaluated and decisions and choices made, occur in addicts and in animals given drugs (Bechara et al. 2002; Jentsch & Taylor 1999; Rogers & Robbins 2001; Schoenbaum & Shaham 2008). We agree that impairment of executive control plays an important role in making bad choices about drugs, especially when combined with the pathological incentive motivation for drugs induced by incentive-sensitization.

4.3 What is sensitization?

It is easy to get the impression from the literature that behavioural sensitization might be equivalent to 'sensitization of locomotor activity', but locomotion is only one of many different psychomotor effects of drugs that undergo sensitization, most of which are dissociable (Robinson & Becker 1986). It is important to remember that in this context, the word 'sensitization' simply refers to an increase in a drug effect caused by repeated drug administration. What is critical for the incentive sensitization theory is not 'locomotor sensitization', or even 'psychomotor sensitization', but *'incentive-sensitization'*. Insofar as psychomotor activation is thought to reflect the engagement of brain incentive systems, including mesotelencephalic dopamine systems (Wise & Bozarth 1987), psychomotor sensitization may be often used as evidence (albeit indirect evidence) for hypersensitivity in relevant motivation circuitry. However, it is the hypersensitivity in this motivation circuitry—not the locomotion circuitry—that contributes most to addictive 'wanting' for drugs.

4.3.1 Direct evidence for incentive-sensitization

What evidence is there for this main postulate of incentive-sensitization theory—that repeated drug use sensitizes neural substrates responsible for the attribution of incentive salience to reward-related stimuli? First, prior exposure to a number of drugs of abuse enhances the incentive effects of drugs measured using a variety of behavioural paradigms. Thus, sensitization facilitates the later acquisition of drug self-administration behaviour, conditioned preferences for locations paired with drug, and the motivation to work for drug, as indicated by 'breakpoint' on a progressive ratio schedule (Lett 1989; Vezina 2004; Ward et al. 2006).

More specific evidence for incentive-sensitization comes from studies designed to more directly assess drug-induced changes in the incentive salience attributed to reward-related stimuli, to exclude alternative explanations for increases in reward-directed behaviour based on habit learning, etc. Stimuli acquire incentive properties by being associatively paired with a reward, and 'conditioned stimuli' that have been imbued with incentive salience have three fundamental characteristics (Berridge 2001; Cardinal et al. 2002). (1) They can elicit approach towards them (become 'wanted'), acting as 'motivational magnets' (measurable by Pavlovian conditioned approach behaviour or 'sign-tracking'). (2) They can energize ongoing actions by eliciting cue-triggered 'wanting' for their associated unconditioned rewards (measurable by Pavlovian-instrumental transfer). (3) They can act as reinforcers in their own right, reinforcing the acquisition of a new instrumental response (measurable by conditioned reinforcement). Thus, the most direct evidence for incentive-sensitization comes from studies showing that past drug treatment, which produces psychomotor sensitization, also facilitates all three features of incentive stimuli: Pavlovian-conditioned approach behaviour (Harmer & Phillips 1998), Pavlovian-instrumental transfer (Wyvell & Berridge 2001), and conditioned reinforcement (Di Ciano 2008; Taylor & Horger 1999).

It should be acknowledged, however, that in most studies on incentive-sensitization pairing with natural rewards (usually food or water), not a drug reward, was used to confer CSs with incentive motivational properties. It is difficult to address the question of whether prior sensitization directly facilitates the incentive properties of *drug*-associated stimuli in animal experiments because the pairing of a stimulus with drug administration may itself produce sensitization. In fact, it has only been reported very recently that a cue paired with drug administration in a Pavlovian manner (i.e. independent of any action) can come to elicit approach towards itself (Uslaner et al. 2006). It is important, therefore, to note that in a recent study, Di Ciano (2008) found that cocaine sensitization did facilitate the conditioned reinforcing effects of a cocaine-associated stimulus, consistent with incentive-sensitization. Of course, the fact that patients with 'dopamine dysregulation syndrome' pathologically 'want' drugs is also consistent with the concept of incentive-sensitization (Evans et al. 2006). Nevertheless, this is an area that deserves much more investigation.

Another way of approaching whether incentive-sensitization occurs is to ask the question from the brain's point of view. That is, does sensitization increase neural activations in brain systems that code the incentive value of a reward stimulus? Several studies indicate that it does (Boileau et al. 2006; Evans et al. 2006; Tindell et al. 2005). For example, amphetamine sensitization in rats increases specific firing patterns of neurons in mesolimbic structures that code the incentive salience of a reward CS (Tindell et al. 2005). In humans, repeated amphetamine treatment is reported to sensitize amphetamine-stimulated dopamine 'release' in the ventral striatum, even a year after the last drug treatment (Boileau et al. 2006), and a 'sensitization' of dopamine 'release' has also been reported in patients with 'dopamine dysregulation syndrome' (Evans et al. 2006). In conclusion, even if we are unsure at this point about exactly which of the many changes in brain produced by drugs underlie the psychological change of incentive-sensitization, we suggest that the evidence provided above indicating that repeated drug exposure alters the relevant behaviours, psychological processes, and brain structures themselves in the predicted directions is *prima facie* evidence for the thesis.

4.4 Does sensitization occur in humans?

One criticism we heard frequently about incentive-sensitization theory in its first decade was that there was no evidence that humans showed behavioural or neural sensitization. However, in the last few years, several studies have now demonstrated both behavioural and neural sensitization in people (we refer readers to a thoughtful review of the subject by Marco Leyton, 2007). Of course, even earlier it was recognized that humans showed sensitization to the paranoia-related psychotomimetic and stereotypy-inducing ('punding') effects of psychostimulant drugs, though the relevance of this to incentive salience was not widely recognized. It is interesting, therefore, that a 'sensitized' incentive salience type mechanism has been proposed to contribute to the symptoms of schizophrenia and stimulant psychoses (Kapur et al. 2005).

Briefly, regarding evidence in humans for incentive sensitization, the repeated intermittent administration of amphetamine in humans can produce persistent behavioural sensitization (e.g. eye-blink responses, vigor, and energy ratings), especially at high doses (Boileau et al. 2006; Strakowski & Sax 1998; Strakowski et al. 1996). Also, in drug addicts, attention is biased to visual drug-associated cues at an immediate and implicit level, as measured by eye-tracking, as though drug cues were more attractive and attention-grabbing in a way consistent with incentive-sensitization (see Wiers & Stacy 2006). Neural evidence of sensitization has also been described recently in humans, as mentioned above. Repeated intermittent administration of amphetamine causes sensitization of dopamine 'release' in humans, even when a drug challenge is given a year later (Boileau et al. 2006), and drug cues also elicit a vigorous dopamine response in the same reward-related brain structures (Boileau et al. 2007; also see Childress et al. 2008). Intriguingly, a similar sensitized dopamine response to L-Dopa occurs in Parkinson's patients with so-called 'dopamine dysregulation syndrome' (Evans et al. 2006).

In these patients, L-Dopa induces unusually high levels of dopamine release in the ventral striatum, as though sensitized. Behaviourally, patients with DDS compulsively take dopaminergic drugs at excessive levels and show other compulsive activities, including gambling and 'punding' (a complex form of behavioural stereotypy). Perhaps most interesting, increased dopamine release is associated with increased ratings of drug 'wanting' but not drug 'liking' in patients who take excessive amounts of their drug (Evans et al. 2006). All of these effects are consistent with incentive-sensitization and are difficult to explain by other views of addiction.

However, it must be acknowledged that the current literature contains conflicting results about brain dopamine changes in addicts. For example, it has been reported that detoxified cocaine addicts actually show a decrease in evoked dopamine 'release', rather than the sensitized increase described above (Martinez et al. 2007; Volkow et al. 1997). However, these reports need to be interpreted with caution, because many variables interact in complex ways to determine if sensitization is expressed at any particular place or time. In particular, as discussed by Leyton (2007), the role of context is crucial in gating the expression of sensitization in general, and thus of sensitized increases in dopamine release. Animal studies have shown that the expression of sensitization is powerfully modulated by the context in which drugs are administered (Robinson et al. 1998), and humans are likely to be even more sensitive to psychological contexts (Leyton 2007). For example, sensitization and enhanced dopamine release typically are *not* manifested if animals are tested in a context where drugs have never before been experienced (Anagnostaras & Robinson 1996; Duvauchelle et al. 2000; Fontana et al. 1993). Therefore, based on the animal literature, human drug addicts should not be expected to display behavioural sensitization or sensitized dopamine release if the environment in which they are given a drug 'challenge' (e.g. a scanner) is dramatically different from contexts where drugs were taken before. It is noteworthy that in the best demonstration so far of sensitized dopamine 'release' in humans, investigators took care to keep contexts similar by giving sensitizing drug treatments in the same context later used for testing (the scanner; Boileau et al. 2006). Thus, in future studies context needs to be considered before assuming that what is seen in the laboratory setting reflects what happens when addicts take drugs in their usual setting. Lastly, it is also important not to test for sensitization too soon after the discontinuation of drug use, but rather to wait until tolerance has subsided, both because tolerance can mask the expression of sensitization (Dalia et al. 1998) and because sensitization is expressed best after a period of 'incubation' (Robinson & Becker 1986).

Another finding in humans that seems inconsistent with sensitization is that cocaine addicts are reported to have low levels of striatal dopamine D2 receptors even after long abstinence (Martinez et al. 2004; Volkow et al. 1990). This suggests a hypo-dopaminergic state rather than a 'sensitized' state (Volkow et al. 2004). However, again, there are grounds for caution. First, psychostimulant treatments in rats, including cocaine self-administration, cause behavioural supersensitivity to direct-acting D2 agonists—as though D2 receptors were increased or more sensitive (De Vries et al. 2002; Edwards et al. 2007; Ujike et al. 1990). The reason for this discrepancy is not clear, but one potential resolution is raised by considering that dopamine D2 receptors can exist in one of two interconvertible affinity states: a high-affinity state ($D2^{High}$) and a low-affinity state ($D2^{Low}$), and dopamine exerts its functional effects by action on only $D2^{High}$ receptors (Seeman et al. 2005). Many treatments that produce D2 supersensitivity also cause increases in striatal $D2^{High}$ receptors in rats, but do not change or even decrease total D2 binding (Seeman et al. 2005). Most important for the discussion here, cocaine self-administration experience (Briand et al. 2008b) and sensitization to amphetamine (Seeman et al. 2007; 2002) have also been reported to produce a persistent increase in the number of striatal D2^{High} receptors, with no change in total D2 binding (and therefore presumably a proportionate decrease in D2^{Low} receptors). Ligands used thus far for *in vivo* studies of dopamine D2 receptors in humans do not discriminate between the low- and high-affinity states of the D2 receptor; therefore, it could miss changes that are specific to D2^{High} receptors and give a misleading impression about dopamine function (Seeman et al. 2005). Thus, it will be important to conduct studies with ligands that can specifically quantify D2^{High} receptors in humans before concluding that addicts have increased or reduced D2 receptor signalling.

4.5 Do procedures that produce 'addiction-like' behaviour in animals also produce sensitization?

Most animal studies of addictive drugs have used procedures and methods that do not necessarily mimic human addiction. For example, evidence now indicates that limited access to self-administered drugs is not as effective in producing symptoms of addiction in animals as giving more extended access—either by extending the number of days animals are allowed to self-administer drugs (Deroche-Gamonet et al. 2004; Heyne & Wolffgramm 1998; Wolffgramm & Heyne 1995) or by extending to several hours the amount of time drugs are available each day (Ahmed & Koob 1998). In one study, it took several months of IV cocaine self-administration before some rats began to develop addiction-like symptoms (Deroche-Gamonet et al. 2004), including continued drug-seeking in the face of punishment or when drugs were known to be unavailable, increased motivation to obtain drugs, and a greater propensity to 'relapse' after enforced abstinence. Similarly, Ahmed and Koob (1998) reported that rats allowed to self-administer IV cocaine for 6 h/day (extended access), but not 1 h/day (limited access), developed 'addiction-like' behaviours. These included an escalation of intake (Ahmed & Koob 1998; Ferrario et al. 2005; Mantsch et al. 2004), increased motivation to take drug (Paterson & Markou 2003), continued drug-seeking in the face of adverse consequences (Pelloux et al. 2007; Vanderschuren & Everitt 2004), and a greater propensity for reinstatement (Ahmed & Koob 1998; Ferrario et al. 2005; Knackstedt & Kalivas 2007). Some of these effects have also been described after extended access to heroin (Ahmed et al. 2000).

4.5.1 Cognitive deficits after extended access

Extended access to cocaine also produces symptoms of prefrontal cortex dysfunction in animals, apparently similar to those reported in human addicts (Jentsch & Taylor 1999; Rogers et al. 1999). For example, Briand et al. (2008a) recently found a persistent decrease in dopamine D2 (not D1) receptor mRNA and protein in the medial prefrontal cortex in rats given extended, but not limited, access to cocaine (0.4 mg/kg/injection), accompanied by persistent deficits on a sustained-attention task that were indicative of decreased cognitive flexibility. George et al. (2008) have reported that extended, but not limited, access to cocaine (0.5 mg/kg/injection) produced deficits on a working memory task that requires the frontal cortex, which was associated with cellular alterations in that brain region. Finally, using higher doses (0.75 mg/kg/injection), Calu et al. (2007) found that rats allowed to self-administer cocaine for 3 h/day showed persistent deficits in reversal learning.

In summary, there is now considerable evidence that extending access to drugs facilitates the development of 'addiction-like' symptoms and cognitive deficits in animals. This is presumably because extended access facilitates greater drug intake than limited access and produces greater corresponding changes in brain responsible for addiction-like behaviour (Ahmed et al. 2005; Briand et al. 2008a; Ferrario et al. 2005; Mantsch et al. 2004).

4.5.2 Does extended access to self-administered cocaine produce sensitization?

The incentive sensitization theory posits that sensitization-related changes in brain are important for the transition from casual to compulsive drug use. Therefore, given that extended access procedures provide the best models for this transition, we would predict that extended access should also produce robust behavioural sensitization and related changes in brain. We have some evidence to suggest this is indeed the case. Ferrario et al. (2005) allowed rats extended access to cocaine (6 h/day for about 3 weeks) and then tested for sensitization later, one month after the last exposure to drug. Rats that had extended access to cocaine showed more robust psychomotor sensitization than rats given limited access (1 h/day) and greater changes in their brains: a much larger increase in the density of dendritic spines on medium spiny neurons in the core of the nucleus accumbens. Such increases in spine density specifically in the accumbens core (but not shell) have been previously associated with the development of psychomotor sensitization (Li et al. 2004).

Conversely, if sensitization-related changes in the brain help cause addiction, it might be predicted that prior sensitizing treatments with drug would facilitate the subsequent development of addiction-like behaviours when rats were given extended access to drugs. This seems to be the case. We have found that an amphetamine treatment regimen that produced psychomotor sensitization accelerated the subsequent escalation of cocaine intake, when animals were later allowed to self-administer cocaine (Ferrario & Robinson 2007). Of course, as mentioned above, repeated treatment with a number of drugs increases subsequent motivation for drug (Nordquist et al. 2007; Vezina 2004) and even facilitates the development of S–R habits, which are a symptom of addiction (Nelson & Killcross 2006; Nordquist et al. 2007). These studies suggest that the neural changes underlying sensitization may be sufficient to promote subsequent 'addiction-like' behaviours.

However, it is worth noting that there is some confusion in the literature about whether extended access to self-administered cocaine produces psychomotor sensitization. A few reports claim that extended access to cocaine produces psychomotor sensitization, but no greater sensitization than limited access (Ahmed & Cador 2006; Knackstedt & Kalivas 2007), and there is even one report that extended access results in a 'loss' of sensitization (Ben-Shahar et al. 2004). However, these latter studies may have measured the wrong behaviours: behavioural sensitization was over-narrowly defined as increases in locomotor activity alone. The studies failed to measure other behaviours that reflect even more intense psychomotor sensitization (e.g. the emergence of qualitative changes in behaviour, including motor stereotypies, which at high levels may compete with locomotion). Consistent with these studies, we also found no differential effect of limited vs. extended access when locomotor activity was the only measure used (Ferrario et al. 2005). However, at the same time, we found that extended access to cocaine actually produced much more robust psychomotor sensitization than limited access when drug-induced stereotyped head movements were also measured. As pointed out long ago by Segal (1975, p. 248), one of the pioneers in research on behavioural sensitization, 'Characterization of the various components of the behavioural response is required because drug effects on behaviour may be competitively related'. Locomotor measures alone are often not sensitive to the transition from behaviour dominated by forward locomotion to that involving motor stereotypy, as occurs with robust sensitization (Post & Rose 1976; Segal 1975), and thus, the sole use of locomotor behaviour as an index of psychomotor sensitization can lead to erroneous conclusions.

Over-interpretation of negative results in cases like this can plague the field because negative results are next to impossible to interpret without additional information. Only in the case of a positive result can a single measure like locomotion alone be decisive. Flagel and Robinson (2007) reiterated this point recently, showing that at a given dose, there might be no group difference in cocaine-induced locomotor activity (e.g. distance travelled or crossovers), but large group differences in both the pattern of locomotion (velocity of each bout of locomotion) and in other behaviours (e.g. the frequency and number of head movements; see Crombag et al. 1999; Flagel & Robinson 2007 for an extensive discussion of this issue). Future studies of sensitization after extended access would benefit from keeping in mind that sensitization can manifest in several different ways and measure more than one.

4.6 Does experimenter-administered drug produces changes in the brain relevant to addiction?

Another controversy concerns whether it is possible to produce changes in brain and behaviour in animals relevant to human addiction when drugs are given by an experimenter, rather than self-administered by the animal. In thinking about this, it may be more important to consider the similarity of *symptom outcomes* to human addiction than the *mode of administration*. Of course, the most appropriate models or procedures are those that produce behavioural, psychological, or neurobiological outcomes most similar to those in human addiction. Therefore, the question is which procedures can do this in animals.

We suggest that both experimenter-administered drug and self-administered drug can produce relevant outcomes—*as long as they produce neural sensitization*. Indeed, one can make a case for an even more radical proposition: if experimenter-administered drug produces robust sensitization, this may more effectively model addiction than self-administration procedures that fail to produce robust sensitization (such as limited access procedures). For example, limited access self-administration may fail to produce either robust sensitization or symptoms of addiction, as discussed above. Conversely, sensitizing treatments with experimenter-administered drugs are sufficient to produce increased motivation for drug reward (Vezina 2004), incentive-sensitization of cue 'wanting' (Di Ciano 2008; Robinson & Berridge 2000), cognitive impairment (Schoenbaum & Shaham 2008), and stronger S–R habits (Miles et al. 2003; Nelson & Killcross 2006), all of which may contribute to the transition to addiction. In addition, experimenter-administered drug that induces sensitization also changes the brain in ways related to the propensity to 'relapse', such as enhancing glutamate release in the core of the accumbens (Pierce et al. 1996). Sensitization induced by experimenter-administered drugs even shows a kind of 'incubation effect' (growing over a period of drug-free abstinence; Paulson & Robinson 1995) that seems to facilitate the propensity to relapse (Grimm et al. 2001) and can accelerate the escalation of drug intake (Ferrario & Robinson 2007). It is possible, therefore, that under conditions that result in robust sensitization, experimenter-administered drugs may be not only effective in producing behavioural, psychological, or neurobiological outcomes relevant to addiction, but also even more effective than self-administration procedures that fail to produce robust sensitization.

There are many reasons why this may be the case, but one could be that some self-administration procedures are not especially effective in producing robust sensitization-related changes in brain. Many interacting factors influence whether exposure to a drug produces sensitization-related changes in the brain, including dose, number of exposures, pattern of exposure (intermittency), rate of drug administration, the context in which the drug is experienced, individual predispositions, etc. Take just intermittency. Injections given close together in time are relatively ineffective in producing sensitization (Post 1980; Robinson & Becker 1986). This may be why limited access self-administration procedures produce only relatively modest sensitization: this would produce a sustained increase in plasma levels of cocaine throughout a test session, which is not optimal for producing sensitization. Of course, 6 h of extended access each day also would result in sustained plasma levels of drug, but in this situation the escalation of intake, and the large amount of drug eventually consumed, may overwhelm other factors that would otherwise limit sensitization. Experimenter-administration may circumvent those limiting factors by combining relatively high doses with intermittent treatment (Robinson & Becker 1986). In fact, this may better capture the situation early in the development of addiction when drugs use may be erratic and intermittent.

4.7 What is the role of affective processes in addiction—'wanting' vs. 'liking'?

Many potentially addictive drugs initially produce feelings of pleasure (euphoria), encouraging users to take drugs again. However, with the transition to addiction there appears to be a decrease in the role of drug pleasure. How can it be that drugs come to be 'wanted' more and more even if they become 'liked' less? According to incentive sensitization theory, the reason for this paradox is that the repeated drug use sensitizes only the neural systems that mediate the motivational process of incentive salience ('wanting'), but not neural systems that mediate the pleasurable effects of drugs ('liking'). Thus, the degree to which drugs are 'wanted' increases disproportionately to the degree to which they are 'liked' and this dissociation between 'wanting' and 'liking' progressively increases with the development of addiction. The dissociation between 'wanting' and 'liking' solves the puzzle that otherwise has led some neuroscientists to conclude that, 'one prominent prediction of an incentive sensitization view would be that with repeated use, addicts would take less drug' (Koob & Le Moal 2006, p. 445). Of course, that is the opposite of what we predict: if sensitization makes addicts 'want' more drugs, then they should take more drugs – not less.

In a related but opposite way, the separation of 'wanting' from 'liking' also frees the control of addiction from being driven solely by the negative affective dysphoria that often follows cessation of drug use, at least for a few days or weeks. Withdrawal states may well contribute to drug-taking while they last (Koob & Le Moal 2006). However, addiction typically persists long after withdrawal states dissipate. Sensitization-related changes in the brain, which can persist long after withdrawal ends, provide a mechanism to explain why addicts continue to 'want' drugs and are liable to relapse even after long periods of abstinence and even in the absence of a negative affective state.

4.8 Conclusion

In conclusion, addiction involves drug-induced changes in many different brain circuits, leading to complex changes in behaviour and psychological function. We have argued that the core changes leading to addiction occur when incentive-sensitization combines with defects in cognitive decision-making and the resulting, 'loss of inhibitory control over behaviour and poor judgment, combined with sensitization of addicts' motivational impulses to obtain and take drugs, makes for a potentially disastrous combination' (Robinson & Berridge 2003, p. 44–46). Thus, bolstered by the evidence that has accumulated over recent years, we remain confident in still concluding, 'that at its heart, addiction is a disorder of aberrant incentive motivation due to drug-induced sensitization of neural systems that attribute salience to particular stimuli. It can be triggered by drug cues as a *learned motivational response* of the brain, but it is not a disorder of aberrant learning per se. Once it exists, sensitized "wanting" may compel drug pursuit whether or not an addict has any withdrawal symptoms at all. And because incentive salience is distinct from pleasure or "liking" processes, sensitization gives impulsive drug "wanting" an enduring life of its own' (Robinson & Berridge 2003).

Acknowledgements

Research by the authors was supported by grants from the National Institute on Drug Abuse (USA).

References

Ahmed, S. H. & Cador, M. 2006 Dissociation of psychomotor sensitization from compulsive cocaine consumption. *Neuropsychopharmacology* **31**, 563–71.

Ahmed, S. H. & Koob, G. F. 1998 Transition from moderate to excessive drug intake: change in hedonic set point. *Science* **282**, 298–300.

Ahmed, S. H., Lutjens, R., van der Stap, L. D. et al. 2005 Gene expression evidence for remodeling of lateral hypothalamic circuitry in cocaine addiction. *Proc Natl Acad Sci USA* **102**, 11533–8.

Ahmed, S. H., Walker, J. R. & Koob, G. F. 2000 Persistent increase in the motivation to take heroin in rats with a history of drug escalation. *Neuropsychopharmacology* **22**, 413–21.

Anagnostaras, S. G. & Robinson, T. E. 1996 Sensitization to the psychomotor stimulant effects of amphetamine: modulation by associative learning. *Behav Neurosci* **110**, 1397–1414.

Anagnostaras, S. G., Schallert, T. & Robinson, T. E. 2002 Memory process governing amphetamine-induced psychomotor sensitization. *Neuropsychopharmacology* **26**, 703–15.

Bechara, A., Dolan, S. & Hindes, A. 2002 Decision-making and addiction (part II): myopia for the future or hypersensitivity to reward? *Neuropsychologia* **40**, 1690–705.

Ben-Shahar, O., Ahmed, S. H., Koob, G. F. & Ettenberg, A. 2004 The transition from controlled to compulsive drug use is associated with a loss of sensitization. *Brain Res* **995**, 46–54.

Berke, J. D. & Hyman, S. E. 2000 Addiction, dopamine, and the molecular mechanisms of memory. *Neuron* **25**, 515–32.

Berridge, K. C. 2001 Reward learning: Reinforcement, incentives and expectations. In *Psychology of Learning and Motivation, Vol. 40* (ed. D. L. Medin), pp. 223–78. New York: Academic Press.

Boileau, I., Dagher, A., Leyton, M. et al. 2006 Modeling sensitization to stimulants in humans: an [11C]raclopride/positron emission tomography study in healthy men. *Arch Gen Psychiatry* **63**, 1386–95.

Boileau, I., Dagher, A., Leyton, M. et al. 2007 Conditioned dopamine release in humans: a positron emission tomography [11C]raclopride study with amphetamine. *J Neurosci* **27**, 3998–4003.

Briand, L. A., Flagel, S. B., Garcia-Fuster, M. J. et al. 2008a Persistent alterations in cognitive function and prefrontal dopamine D2 receptors following extended, but not limited, access to self-administered cocaine. *Neuropsychopharmacology* **33**, 2969–80.

Briand, L. A., Flagel, S. B., Seeman, P. & Robinson, T. E. 2008b Cocaine self-administration produces a persistent increase in dopamine D2(high) receptors. *Eur Neuropsychopharm* **18**, 551–56.

Calu, D. J., Stalnaker, T. A., Franz, T. M., Singh, T., Shaham, Y. & Schoenbaum, G. 2007 Withdrawal from cocaine self-administration produces long-lasting deficits in orbitofrontal-dependent reversal learning in rats. *Learn Mem* **14**, 325–8.

Cardinal, R. N., Parkinson, J. A., Hall, J. & Everitt, B. J. 2002 Emotion and motivation: the role of the amygdala, ventral striatum, and prefrontal cortex. *Neurosci Biobehav Rev* **26**, 321–52.

Childress, A. R., Ehrman, R. N., Wang, Z. et al. 2008 Prelude to passion: limbic activation by "unseen" drug and sexual cues. *PLoS One* **3**(1): e1506. doi:10.1371/journal.pone.0001506.

Crombag, H. C., Mueller, H., Browman, K. E., Badiani, A. & Robinson, T. E. 1999 A comparison of two behavioral measures of psychomotor activation following intravenous amphetamine or cocaine: dose- and sensitization-dependent changes. *Behavioural Pharmacology* **10**, 205–13.

Dalia, A. D., Norman, M. K., Tabet, M. R., Schlueter, K. T., Tsibulsky, V. L. & Norman, A. B. 1998 Transient amelioration of the sensitization of cocaine-induced behaviors in rats by the induction of tolerance. *Brain Res* **797**, 29–34.

De Vries, T. J., Schoffelmeer, A. N., Binnekade, R., Raaso, H. & Vanderschuren, L. J. 2002 Relapse to cocaine- and heroin-seeking behavior mediated by dopamine D2 receptors is time-dependent and associated with behavioral sensitization. *Neuropsychopharmacology* **26**, 18–26.

Deroche-Gamonet, V., Belin, D. & Piazza, P. V. 2004 Evidence for addiction-like behavior in the rat. *Science* **305**, 1014–7.

Di Ciano, P. 2008 Facilitated acquisition but not persistence of responding for a cocaine-paired conditioned reinforcer following sensitization with cocaine. *Neuropsychopharmacology* **33**, 1426–31.

Duvauchelle, C. L., Ikegami, A., Asami, S., Robens, J., Kressin, K. & Castaneda, E. 2000 Effects of cocaine context on NAcc dopamine and behavioral activity after repeated intravenous cocaine administration. *Brain Res* **862**, 49–58.

Edwards, S., Whisler, K. N., Fuller, D. C., Orsulak, P. J. & Self, D. W. 2007 Addiction-related alterations in D1 and D2 dopamine receptor behavioral responses following chronic cocaine self-administration. *Neuropsychopharmacology* **32**, 354–66.

Evans, A. H., Pavese, N., Lawrence, A. D. et al. 2006 Compulsive drug use linked to sensitized ventral striatal dopamine transmission. *Ann Neurol* **59**, 852–8.

Everitt, B. J., Dickinson, A. & Robbins, T. W. 2001 The neuropsychological basis of addictive behaviour. *Brain Res Rev* **36**, 129–38.

Ferrario, C. R., Gorny, G., Crombag, H. S., Li, Y., Kolb, B. & Robinson, T. E. 2005 Neural and behavioral plasticity associated with the transition from controlled to escalated cocaine use. *Biol Psychiatry* **58**, 751–9.

Ferrario, C. R. & Robinson, T. E. 2007 Amphetamine pretreatment accelerates the subsequent escalation of cocaine self-administration behavior. *Eur Neuropsychopharmacol* **17**, 352–7.

Fiorino, D. F. & Phillips, A. G. 1999a Facilitation of sexual behavior and enhanced dopamine efflux in the nucleus accumbens of male rats after D-amphetamine-induced behavioral sensitization. *J Neurosci* **19**, 456–63.

Fiorino, D. F. & Phillips, A. G. 1999b Facilitation of sexual behavior in male rats following D-amphetamine-induced behavioral sensitization. *Psychopharmacology* **142**, 200–8.

Flagel, S. B. & Robinson, T. E. 2007 Quantifying the psychomotor activating effects of cocaine in the rat. *Behav Pharmacol* **18**, 297–302.

Fontana, D. J., Post, R. M. & Pert, A. 1993 Conditioned increases in mesolimbic dopamine overflow by stimuli associated with cocaine. *Brain Res* **629**, 31–39.

George, O., Mandyam, C. D., Wee, S. & Koob, G. F. 2008 Extended access to cocaine self-administration produces long-lasting prefrontal cortex-dependent working memory impairments. *Neuropsychopharmacology* **33**, 2474–82.

Grimm, J. W., Hope, B. T., Wise, R. A. & Shaham, Y. 2001 Neuroadaptation. Incubation of cocaine craving after withdrawal. *Nature* **412**, 141–2.

Harmer, C. J. & Phillips, G. D. 1998 Enhanced appetitive conditioning following repeated pretreatment with D-amphetamine. *Behav Pharmacol* **9**, 299–308.

Hasin, D., Hatzenbuehler, M. L., Keyes, K. & Ogburn, E. 2006 Substance use disorders: diagnostic and statistical manual of mental disorders, fourth edition (DSM-IV) and international classification of diseases, tenth edition (ICD-10). *Addiction* **101** (Suppl. 1), 59–75.

Heyne, A. & Wolffgramm, J. 1998 The development of addiction to D-amphetamine in an animal model: same principles as for alcohol and opiate. *Psychopharmacology* **140**, 510–18.

Hyman, S. E. 2005 Addiction: a disease of learning and memory. *Am J Psychiatry* **162**, 1414–22.

Hyman, S. E., Malenka, R. C. & Nestler, E. J. 2006 Neural mechanisms of addiction: the role of reward-related learning and memory. *Annu Rev Neurosci* **29**, 565–98.

Jentsch, J. D. & Taylor, J. R. 1999 Impulsivity resulting from frontostriatal dysfunction in drug abuse: implications for the control of behavior by reward-related stimuli. *Psychopharmacology* **146**, 373–90.

Kalivas, P. W. & O'Brien, C. 2008 Drug addiction as a pathology of staged neuroplasticity. *Neuropsychopharmacology* **33**, 166–80.

Kapur, S., Mizrahi, R. & Li, M. 2005 From dopamine to salience to psychosis—linking biology, pharmacology and phenomenology of psychosis. *Schizophr Res* **79**, 59–68.

Knackstedt, L. A. & Kalivas, P. W. 2007 Extended access to cocaine self-administration enhances drug-primed reinstatement but not behavioral sensitization. *J Pharmacol Exp Ther* **322**, 1103–9.

Koob, G. F. & Le Moal, M. 2006 *Neurobiology of Addiction*. London: Academic Press.

Lett, B. T. 1989 Repeated exposures intensify rather than diminish the rewarding effects of amphetamine, morphine, and cocaine. *Psychopharmacology (Berlin)* **98**, 357–62.

Leyton, M. 2007 Conditioned and sensitized responses to stimulant drugs in humans. *Prog Neuropsychopharmacol Biol Psychiatry* **31**, 1601–13.

Li, Y., Acerbo, M. J. & Robinson, T. E. 2004 The induction of behavioural sensitization is associated with cocaine-induced structural plasticity in the core (but not shell) of the nucleus accumbens. *Eur J Neurosci* **20**, 1647–54.

Mantsch, J. R., Yuferov, V., Mathieu-Kia, A. M., Ho, A. & Kreek, M. J. 2004 Effects of extended access to high versus low cocaine doses on self-administration, cocaine-induced reinstatement and brain mRNA levels in rats. *Psychopharmacology (Berl)* **175**, 26–36.

Martinez, D., Broft, A., Foltin, R. W. et al. 2004 Cocaine dependence and d2 receptor availability in the functional subdivisions of the striatum: relationship with cocaine-seeking behavior. *Neuropsychopharmacology* **29**, 1190–202.

Martinez, D., Narendran, R., Foltin, R. W. et al. 2007 Amphetamine-induced dopamine release: markedly blunted in cocaine dependence and predictive of the choice to self-administer cocaine. *Am J Psychiatry* **164**, 622–9.

Miles, F. J., Everitt, B. J. & Dickinson, A. 2003 Oral cocaine seeking by rats: action or habit? *Behav Neurosci* **117**, 927–38.

Mitchell, J. B. & Stewart, J. 1990 Facilitation of sexual behaviors in the male rat associated with intra-VTA injections of opiates. *Pharmacol Biochem Behav* **35**, 643–50.

Nelson, A. & Killcross, S. 2006 Amphetamine exposure enhances habit formation. *J Neurosci* **26**, 3805–12.

Nestler, E. J. 2001 Molecular basis of long-term plasticity underlying addiction. *Nat Rev Neurosci* **2**, 119–28.

Nocjar, C. & Panksepp, J. 2002 Chronic intermittent amphetamine pretreatment enhances future appetitive behavior for drug- and natural-reward: interaction with environmental variables. *Behav Brain Res* **128**, 189–203.

Nordquist, R. E., Voorn, P., de Mooij-van Malsen, J. G. et al. 2007 Augmented reinforcer value and accelerated habit formation after repeated amphetamine treatment. *Eur Neuropsychopharmacol* **17**, 532–40.

Paterson, N. E. & Markou, A. 2003 Increased motivation for self-administered cocaine after escalated cocaine intake. *Neuroreport* **14**, 2229–32.

Paulson, P. E. & Robinson, T. E. 1995 Amphetamine-induced time-dependent sensitization of dopamine neurotransmission in the dorsal and ventral striatum: a microdialysis study in behaving rats. *Synapse* **19**, 56–65.

Pelloux, Y., Everitt, B. J. & Dickinson, A. 2007 Compulsive drug seeking by rats under punishment: effects of drug taking history. *Psychopharmacology (Berl)* **194**, 127–37.

Pierce, R. C., Bell, K., Duffy, P. & Kalivas, P. W. 1996 Repeated cocaine augments excitatory amino acid transmission in the nucleus accumbens only in rats having developed behavioral sensitization. *J Neurosci* **16**, 1550–60.

Porrino, L. J., Smith, H. R., Nader, M. A. & Beveridge, T. J. 2007 The effects of cocaine: a shifting target over the course of addiction. *Prog Neuropsychopharmacol Biol Psychiatry* **31**, 1593–600.

Post, R. 1980 Intermittent versus continuous stimulation: effect of time interval on the development of sensitization or tolerance. *Life Sci* **26**, 1275–82.

Post, R. M. & Rose, H. 1976 Increasing effects of repetitive cocaine administration in the rat. *Nature* **260**, 731–2.

Robinson, T. E. & Becker, J. B. 1986 Enduring changes in brain and behavior produced by chronic amphetamine administration: a review and evaluation of animal models of amphetamine psychosis. *Brain Res Rev* **11**, 157–98.

Robinson, T. E. & Berridge, K. C. 1993 The neural basis of drug craving: an incentive-sensitization theory of addiction. *Brain Res Rev* **18**, 247–91.

Robinson, T. E. & Berridge, K. C. 2000 The psychology and neurobiology of addiction: an incentive-sensitization view. *Addiction* **95** (Suppl. 2), S91–S117.

Robinson, T. E. & Berridge, K. C. 2003 Addiction. *Annu Rev Psychol* **54**, 25–53.

Robinson, T. E., Browman, K. E., Crombag, H. S. & Badiani, A. 1998 Modulation of the induction or expression of psychostimulant sensitization by the circumstances surrounding drug administration. *Neurosci Biobehav Rev* **22**, 347–54.

Rogers, R. D., Everitt, B. J., Baldacchino, A. et al. 1999 Dissociable deficits in the decision-making cognition of chronic amphetamine abusers, opiate abusers, patients with focal damage to prefrontal cortex, and tryptophan-depleted normal volunteers: evidence for monoaminergic mechanisms. *Neuropsychopharmacology* **20**, 322–39.

Rogers, R. D. & Robbins, T. W. 2001 Investigating the neurocognitive deficits associated with chronic drug misuse. *Curr Opin Neurobiol* **11**, 250–7.

Schoenbaum, G. & Shaham, Y. 2008 The role of orbitofrontal cortex in drug addiction: a review of preclinical studies. *Biol Psychiatry* **63**, 256–62.

Seeman, P., McCormick, P. N. & Kapur, S. 2007 Increased dopamine D2(High) receptors in amphetamine-sensitized rats, measured by the agonist [(3)H](+)PHNO. *Synapse* **61**, 263–7.

Seeman, P., Tallerico, T., Ko, F., Tenn, C. & Kapur, S. 2002 Amphetamine-sensitized animals show a marked increase in dopamine D2 high receptors occupied by endogenous dopamine, even in the absence of acute challenges. *Synapse* **46**, 235–9.

Seeman, P., Weinshenker, D., Quirion, R. et al. 2005 Dopamine supersensitivity correlates with D2High states, implying many paths to psychosis. *Proc Natl Acad Sci USA* **102**, 3513–18.

Segal, D. S. 1975 Behavioral and neurochemical correlates of repeated D-amphetamine administration. *Adv Biochem Psychopharmacol* **13**, 247–62.

Stewart, J. & Vezina, P. 1991 Extinction procedures abolish conditioned stimulus control but spare sensitized responding to amphetamine. *Behav Pharmacol* **2**, 65–71.

Strakowski, S. M. & Sax, K. W. 1998 Progressive behavioral response to repeated D-amphetamine challenge: further evidence for sensitization in humans. *Biol Psychiatry* **44**, 1171–7.

Strakowski, S. M., Sax, K. W., Setters, M. J. & Keck, P. E., Jr. 1996 Enhanced response to repeated D-amphetamine challenge: evidence for behavioral sensitization in humans. *Biol Psychiatry* **40**, 872–80.

Taylor, J. R. & Horger, B. A. 1999 Enhanced responding for conditioned reward produced by intra-accumbens amphetamine is potentiated after cocaine sensitization. *Psychopharmacology* **142**, 31–40.

Tiffany, S. T. 1990 A cognitive model of drug urges and drug-use behavior: role of automatic and nonautomatic processes. *Psychol Rev* **97**, 147–68.

Tindell, A. J., Berridge, K. C., Zhang, J., Pecina, S. & Aldridge, J. W. 2005 Ventral pallidal neurons code incentive motivation: amplification by mesolimbic sensitization and amphetamine. *Eur J Neurosci* **22**, 2617–34.

Ujike, H., Akiyama, K. & Otsuki, S. 1990 D-2 but not D-1 dopamine agonists produce augmented behavioral response in rats after subchronic treatment with methamphetamine or cocaine. *Psychopharmacology (Berl)* **102**, 459–64.

Uslaner, J. M., Acerbo, M. J., Jones, S. A. & Robinson, T. E. 2006 The attribution of incentive salience to a stimulus that signals an intravenous injection of cocaine. *Behav Brain Res* **169**, 320–4.

Vanderschuren, L. J. & Everitt, B. J. 2004 Drug seeking becomes compulsive after prolonged cocaine self-administration. *Science* **305**, 1017–19.

Vezina, P. 2004 Sensitization of midbrain dopamine neuron reactivity and the self-administration of psychomotor stimulant drugs. *Neurosci Biobehav Rev* **27**, 827–39.

Volkow, N. D., Fowler, J. S., Wang, G. J. & Swanson, J. M. 2004 Dopamine in drug abuse and addiction: results from imaging studies and treatment implications. *Mol Psychiatry* **9**, 557–69.

Volkow, N. D., Fowler, J. S., Wolf, A. P. et al. 1990 Effects of chronic cocaine abuse on postsynaptic dopamine receptors. *Am J Psychiatry* **147**, 719–24.

Volkow, N. D., Wang, G. J., Fowler, J. S. et al. 1997 Decreased striatal dopaminergic responsiveness in detoxified cocaine-dependent subjects. *Nature* **386**, 830–3.

Ward, S. J., Lack, C., Morgan, D. & Roberts, D. C. 2006 Discrete-trials heroin self-administration produces sensitization to the reinforcing effects of cocaine in rats. *Psychopharmacology (Berl)* **185**, 150–9.

Wiers, R. W. & Stacy, A. W. (ed.) 2006 *Handbook of Implicit Cognition and Addiction*. London: Sage.

Wise, R. A. & Bozarth, M. A. 1987 A psychomotor stimulant theory of addiction. *Psychol Rev* **94**, 469–92.

Wolffgramm, J. & Heyne, A. 1995 From controlled drug intake to loss of control: the irreversible development of drug addiction in the rat. *Behav Brain Res* **70**, 77–94.

Wyvell, C. L. & Berridge, K. C. 2001 Incentive sensitization by previous amphetamine exposure: increased cue-triggered 'wanting' for sucrose reward. *J Neurosci* **21**, 7831–40.

5

The neurobiology of relapse

*Jane Stewart**

Relapse, the resumption of drug taking after periods of abstinence, remains the major problem for the treatment of addiction. Even when drugs are unavailable for long periods or when users are successful in curbing their drug use for extended periods, individuals remain vulnerable to events that precipitate relapse. Behavioural studies in humans and laboratory animals show that drug-related stimuli, drugs themselves, and stressors are powerful events for the precipitation of relapse. Molecular, neurochemical, and anatomical studies have identified lasting neural changes that arise from mere exposure to drugs and other enduring changes that arise from learning about the relation between drug-related stimuli and drug effects. Chronic drug exposure increases sensitivity of some systems of the brain to the effects of drugs and stressful events. These changes, combined with those underlying conditioning and learning, perpetuate vulnerability to drug-related stimuli. Circuits of the brain involved are those of the mesocorticolimbic dopaminergic system and its glutamatergic connections, and the corticotropin-releasing factor and noradrenergic systems of the limbic brain. This paper will review advances in our understanding of how these systems mediate the effects of events that precipitate relapse and of how lasting changes in these systems can perpetuate vulnerability to relapse.

Key Words: Relapse to drug seeking, drug-related stimuli, stress, dopamine, glutamate, CRF, noradrenaline.

In the context of drug addiction, relapse refers to the reinitiation of drug seeking and drug taking after abstinence. The following are the central questions that are being addressed by researchers in the field of drug addiction: What are the primary triggers for relapse? Which systems of the brain mediate the effects of these triggers? What maintains the vulnerability to these triggers in individuals even after drugs have been unavailable for long periods of time or when users are successful in curbing their own drug use for extended periods? Is it a set of physiological changes brought about by being exposed to the effects of drugs, per se? Is it drug-related memories that can be reactivated by drug-related cues and thoughts? Does it arise from something within individuals that make them initially vulnerable to the effects of drugs of abuse and which simply remains or is exaggerated after termination of drug taking? No doubt, factors such as these all contribute. In fact, exposure to a drug can initiate neurochemical changes with enduring molecular and anatomical consequences that affect subsequent responses to events that induce relapse; drugs that are abused activate appetitive motivational systems of the brain, inducing behaviours and emotions that very rapidly become associated with stimuli and events in the environment where they are experienced; and drug effects can be different in different individuals and differentially experienced by them.

5.1 Primary triggers for relapse

Studies carried out in humans and laboratory animals have demonstrated that craving (Childress et al. 1992; de Wit 1996; Duncan et al. 2007; Jaffe et al. 1989; Leyton et al.

* jane.stewart@concordia.ca

2002,2005; Sinha et al. 2000; Wikler 1973; Wikler & Pescor 1967) and the reinitiation of drug seeking (See 2002; Shaham et al. 2000a; Shalev et al. 2002; Spealman et al. 2004; Stewart 2004; Weiss 2005) can be induced by re-exposure to cues previously associated with drug exposure, by acute exposure to stressors and by re-exposure to the drug itself. In experimental studies in humans, various means are used to present to drug users events that are suspected of triggering relapse and subjective ratings are used to assess drug craving or wanting. Such methods are now being complemented by brain imaging techniques to assess regions of the brain that are differentially activated by these triggering events. In laboratory animals trained to self-administer drugs such as cocaine or heroin and then subjected to a period of extinction training (when associated drug cues or responses are no longer followed by drug injections) or simply to the passage of time, the presentation of cues that have been explicitly paired with drug delivery, brief exposure of a stressor, or an experimenter-delivered injection of the drug, all result in an increase in increased drug-seeking behaviours. Clearly, under non-laboratory conditions, the reinitiation of drug seeking after abstinence occurs before exposure to the drug itself and is instigated by environmental cues and stressors. It is well recognized, however, that re-exposure to the drug spurs on further drug seeking; thus, it is important to study in an experimental setting how the action of the drug, itself, increases subsequent drug seeking.

In the reinstatement model of relapse (de Wit & Stewart 1981; Epstein et al. 2006; Spealman et al. 2004; Stewart 2004), animals are trained to self-administer a drug by pressing one of two levers and are then exposed to a period when the drug is no longer available. During this abstinence period, animals may simply be left in their home cages (Fuchs et al. 2006; Grimm et al. 2001), or they may be free to try to obtain drug in the testing chambers (a period of extinction training). In extinction training, the sight of the lever and stimuli previously associated with drug delivery are usually present; in the case of tests for cue-induced reinstatement, however, the cues previously associated with drug delivery are absent. When animals reduce responding to very low levels during tests for extinction, tests for reinstatement can begin. During these tests for reinitiation of drug seeking, animals are given access to the levers, but drugs remains unavailable. It is on this background of renewed drug seeking, or reinstatement, that we are able to begin a search for pharmacological and neurochemical manipulations that can block or attenuate such behaviour. Using this procedure, the periods of self-administration training, abstinence, extinction, and reinstatement can be separated by days and weeks allowing for the study of factors such as the extent and amount of initial exposure to drug-taking and the effect of the passage of time since last exposure on the susceptibility to relapse.

5.2 How might drugs and stressors initiate reinstatement or relapse in experienced drug users

The observation that a brief exposure to stress or an abused drug reinstates drug-seeking behaviour implies a change in the motivational state of the animal that alters responses to stimuli in its environment. Traditionally, the term motivation is invoked by the observation that a particular goal-directed behaviour, such as food seeking, occurs at some times and not others, with more or less vigour and persistence. The ease with which behaviour is engaged by environmental stimuli, its persistence, and the energy expended to obtain the goal all appears to depend on internal changes that alter stimulus effectiveness and readiness to act.

On the basis of our studies showing that a priming injection of previously self-administered drug in experienced drug users can reinstate drug seeking, we have argued that the priming injection acts to renew the significance or salience of the learned stimulus–drug associations. Such drug-related stimuli gain conditioned incentive value, drawing the animal to approach the lever and to engage in lever pressing (Stewart 1992; Stewart et al. 1984). Thus, after extinction, a priming injection of the previously self-administered drug (and presumably exposure to stress) can be said to renew the salience of the drug-associated lever and surrounding stimuli. We have used the conditioned place preference (CPP) procedure to explore this hypothesis directly.

In this procedure, a particular stimulus complex, or environment, is paired with the effects of the drug, without the animal having to learn to make a response to obtain the drug, and a second environment is explicitly paired with the absence of the drug. On the test trial, the animal is allowed, while in a drug-free state, to move freely between the area previously paired with drug and the unpaired environment. If the animal stays longer in the presence of stimuli previously paired with the drug (the conditioned cues), these stimuli can be said to have acquired secondary or conditioned incentive properties through pairings with the incentive effects of the drug (see also Uslaner et al. 2006).

Using this procedure, we have tested the idea that a priming injection of the drug used to develop the CPP, given after an extinction training, acts to restore the salience or attractiveness of the environment previously paired with drug. It has been found that following the extinction of the CPP by repeatedly pairing both compartments with saline or by giving repeated tests in the absence of drug, the former preference for the 'drug-paired' compartment can be completely reinstated by giving a single injection of the drug before the test (Mueller et al. 2002; Mueller & Stewart 2000; Parker & McDonald 2000).

Results from a study on stress-induced reinstatement lend further support to this idea (Liu & Weiss 2002). Rats were trained to lever press to obtain access to a 10% ethanol solution; ethanol reinforced responses were accompanied by onset of a light stimulus that served as a conditioned stimulus paired with ethanol. After extinction training, given in the absence of both ethanol and the light, lever pressing was reinstated by response-contingent presentations of the conditioned light cue or by brief exposure to intermittent footshock stress. Animals tested with the conditioned light cue present after footshock stress showed greatly enhanced responding compared to animals tested with either the light cues or stress alone. Interestingly, it was found as well that, although the effects were additive, different neurochemical systems contributed to the overall effect. The effect of footshock stress was blocked by intraventricular (ICV) infusions of a corticotropin-releasing factor (CRF) receptor antagonist, whereas the effect of conditioned ethanol cues was blocked by injections of the opioid receptor antagonist naltrexone. It required injections of both antagonists to block the enhanced reinstatement effect induced by the footshock/conditioned cue combination. These data suggest that the stress state induced by prior exposure to footshock enhances the salience and effectiveness of the drug-related cues to engage the animal in drug-seeking behaviour.

Another more direct approach to this question was taken in an experiment in which rats were given pairings of a compound stimulus with passive intravenous infusions of cocaine (0, 0.5, or 1.0 mg/kg/infusion). After training, rats were allowed to lever press for the conditioned stimulus under extinction conditions, and the amount of pressing was shown to be dependent on the training dose. After extinction, a single priming injection of cocaine (20 mg/kg i.p.) or exposure to footshock stress reinstated lever pressing for the conditioned stimulus, in a training dose-dependent manner, even though the rats had never been trained to administer cocaine (Goddard & Leri 2006). Again, these data support the view that both a priming drug injection and exposure to stress induce reinstatement by restoring the incentive salience or value of the conditioned drug-related cues that previously activated appetitive behaviour. These ideas have been studied in cocaine-dependent men. Using fMRI, it was shown that the activation by cocaine-associated cues of brain regions associated with reward processing and attention was enhanced in the presence of stress (Duncan et al. 2007).

5.3 Primary neural pathways mediating relapse

Studies carried out in a number of laboratories have provided evidence that the brain systems mediating the effects of conditioned stimuli, priming injections of drugs, and stress on the reinitiation of drug seeking are to some degree dissociable (Erb et al. 2001; McFarland & Kalivas 2001; Shaham et al. 2000a; Shalev et al. 2002; Stewart 2000), although common pathways beginning to be identified (McFarland et al. 2004; McFarland & Kalivas 2001; Rodaros et al. 2007; Saal et al. 2003; See 2002; Stewart 2004; Wang et al. 2005; Weiss 2005). Below, I will review briefly evidence concerning the role of different brain systems, and regions and transmitters in cue-, drug-, and stress-induced reinstatement.

5.4 Drug-induced reinstatement

The reinstatement of drug craving or seeking by priming injections of the abused or training drug, drugs of a similar class, or drug that activate pathways in common with the training drug is a robust phenomenon in humans and laboratory animals. As expected, specific receptor antagonists for drugs such as opioids and nicotine or, in the case of cocaine and amphetamines, dopamine receptor antagonists will block the effects of priming injections. Furthermore, and inasmuch as most, if not all, addictive drugs activate the mesocorticolimbic pathways of the brain, it is not surprising that, in general, dopaminergic receptor agonists induce reinstatement of drug seeking in experienced users, whereas antagonists attenuate or block drug-induced reinstatement. A sketch of the circuits identified and the primary neurotransmitters implicated in drug-induced reinstatement is shown in Fig. 5.1. These include dopaminergic projections from the ventral tegmental area (VTA) to the nucleus accumbens (NAc), medial prefrontal cortex (mPFC), and glutamatergic inputs to VTA from mPFC, peduncular pontine and laterodorsal tegmental nuclei (PPT/LDT), and from the mPFC to the NAc. There is evidence that dopaminergic receptor antagonists attenuate drug-induced reinstatement more effectively when given into the shell region of the NAc (Anderson et al. 2003, 2006; Schmidt et al. 2006), although there is some evidence that they are effective in the core as well (Bachtell et al. 2005). Evidence that dopamine in the shell is effective in inducing reinstatement is consistent with previous work showing the importance of the shell in stimulant drug-induced enhancement of responding in the presence of conditioned stimuli (Parkinson et al. 1999). Interestingly, however, reversible inactivation of either core or shell blocks drug-induced reinstatement (McFarland & Kalivas 2001), suggesting, as we will see below, that increases in dopamine in the shell facilitate the effectiveness of cues acting through the core.

A great number of studies have shown the importance of glutamatergic projections in this circuitry contributing to reinstatement. Though studies have found effects of glutamate agonists and antagonists in tests for drug-induced reinstatement (Cornish & Kalivas 2000), it is

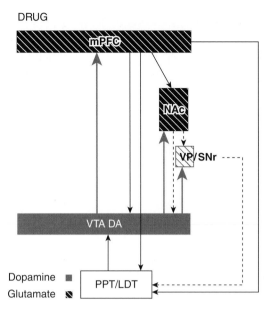

Fig. 5.1 Diagram showing the primary circuits and neurotransmitters implicated in drug-induced rein-statement. VTA (ventral tegmental area), cell body regions of mesocortiolimbic dopaminergic (DA) pathway, NAc (nucleus accumbens), mPFC (medial prefrontal cortex), VP/SNr (ventral pallidum/substantia nigra reticulata), and PPT/LDT (peduncular pontine and laterodorsal tegmental nuclei).

not clear to what extent these effects are important to the mediation of the drug effects, per se, or to the mediation of the effects of drug-related cues in drug-induced reinstatement (see section on cue- and context-induced reinstatement that follows).

5.4 Cue- and context-induced reinstatement

Contexts or environments where drug are used can serve as conditioned stimuli (cues), eliciting expectations, thoughts, neural and neurochemical responses, emotional and motivational responses, and behavioural responses such as approach. Discrete stimuli such as odours, visual stimuli, people, music, etc. can have similar effects. Although these stimuli are paired with the effects of drugs whenever they are self-administered, their effectiveness can best be studied using classical conditioning procedures where environments or discrete stimuli are explicitly paired with injections of a drug. Discrete stimuli paired either with passive infusions (classical conditioning) or with response-contingent presentation of a drug (instrumental learning) can come to serve as conditioned reinforcers, maintaining behavioural responses such as lever pressing in the absence of drugs. Finally, cues that predict the availability/nonavailability of drugs (discriminative stimuli) can differentially control the occurrence of drug-seeking/-taking behaviours.

The neural systems involved in mediating cue-induced reinstatement have been studied using a number of different methods, including systemic injections of receptor antagonists, intracranial infusions of receptor agonists and antagonists and reversible or non-reversible lesions of specific regions. A sketch of the circuits identified and the primary neurotransmitters implicated in cue-induced reinstatement is shown in Fig. 5.2. The principal regions

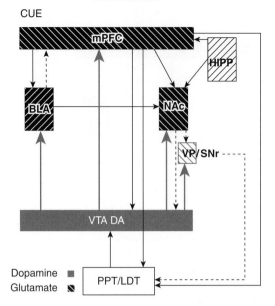

Fig. 5.2 Diagram showing the primary circuits and neurotransmitters implicated in cue-induced reinstatement. VTA (ventral tegmental area), cell body regions of mesocortiolimbic dopaminergic (DA) pathway, NAc (nucleus accumbens), mPFC (medial prefrontal cortex), VP/SNr (ventral pallidum/substantia nigra reticulata), PPT/LDT (peduncular pontine and laterodorsal tegmental nuclei), BLA (basolateral amygdala), and HIPP (hippocampus).

associated with cue- and context-induced reinstatement are the basolateral amygdala (BLA), the hippocampus (HIPP), the mPFC, the NAc core, the dopaminergic inputs to BLA, mPFC, and NAc from the VTA and glutamatergic inputs to VTA and from BLA and PFC to the NAc (Bossert et al. 2004, 2006; Fuchs et al. 2007; Fuchs & See 2002; Ito et al. 2000; See 2002; Weiss 2005). In a recent study, an attempt was made using reversible inactivation to assess the role of the NAc core and shell and dorsal striatum in a number of behaviours controlled by a conditioned reinforcer (Di Ciano et al. 2008). Cue-induced reinstatement of responding was dependent on the NAc core, as were all other conditioned-stimulus controlled behaviours studied (see also Di Ciano & Everitt 2001, 2004), again suggesting a special role for the circuits involving the NAc core in cue-induced reinstatement and relapse.

Recently Kalivas and colleagues have argued for a key role for glutamate projections from the PFC to the core of the NAc in the precipitation of relapse to drug seeking in general (Kalivas 2004; Kalivas & McFarland 2003), serving as the final common pathway for all events that induce relapse. Glutamatergic agonists given into the NAc induce reinstatement (Cornish & Kalivas 2000), whereas antagonists (Backstrom & Hyytia 2007) and mGLU 2/3 receptor agonists, which reduce glutamate release, given systemically or into NAc (Bossert et al. 2006) block cue-induced reinstatement. There is also evidence that mGLU 2/3 receptor agonists given into the VTA block both cue-induced reinstatement of heroin seeking (Bossert et al. 2004) and cue- and nicotine-induced reinstatement of nicotine (Liechti et al. 2007), suggesting that glutamatergic activation of dopaminergic neurons may play an important role in both cue and drug seeking especially when the drugs have their effects by activating dopaminergic neurons. In a recent study, it was shown that the initiation of self-administration in cocaine-trained rats was accompanied by a sharp transient release of glutamate in the VTA.

It was further demonstrated that this was a conditioned response associated with drug-related cues and that it disappeared after extinction training (You et al. 2007). These finding seem to suggest that drug-related cues normally activate glutamate release in the VTA, where they would serve to activate the VTA dopaminergic system. Thus, cue-induced reinstatement probably involves activation of glutamatergic receptors in both NAc and VTA.

5.5 Stress-induced reinstatement

In our initial work on stress-induced reinstatement, rats were trained to self-administer heroin intravenously and were then given extinction training. Subsequently over a four-day period, animals were given tests for reinstatement in a counterbalanced order, after an injection of saline, after an injection of heroin (drug priming), after an injection of morphine followed by the opioid receptor antagonist, naltrexone (precipated withdrawal), and after 10 min of intermittent footshock (acute stress). Both heroin and footshock reinstated heroin seeking; precipitated withdrawal did not. The effects of heroin and foodshock were seen again in tests made 4–6 weeks later (Shaham & Stewart 1995).

In cocaine-trained rats, footshock stress was as effective in inducing relapse as it was in rats trained to self-administer heroin (Erb et al. 1996). Similar effects were found in other laboratories in rats trained to self-administer nicotine (Buczek et al. 1999) and ethanol (Lê et al. 1998), but interestingly not in rats trained to lever press for food (Ahmed & Koob 1997) or sucrose solutions (Buczek et al. 1999). These findings show that exposure to stress effectively reinstates drug seeking in animals experienced in the self-administration of drugs of abuse from several different pharmacological classes. In a search for the hormonal and neurochemical systems involved in stress-induced relapse, we found early that stress-induced corticosterone release was not responsible for the effect in either cocaine- or heroin-trained rats (Erb et al. 1998; Shaham et al. 1997; see also Shalev et al. 2003). This latter finding led us to explore the role of CRF systems of the brain. Infusions of CRF given ICV or into the bed nucleus of the stria terminalis (BNST) induce reinstatement in the absence of an external stressor, whereas infusions into the CRF containing regions of the amygdala, central nucleus of the amygdala (CeA), have no effect. Infusions of CRF receptor antagonists block footshock-induced reinstatement when given ICV (Erb et al. 1998; Shaham et al. 1997) or into the ventrolateral BNST, but have no effect in the amygdala (Erb & Stewart 1999). Similar effects for central CRF systems have been found for rats trained to self-administer alcohol (Lê et al. 2000; Liu & Weiss 2002); see Fig. 5.3.

We next studied the role of central noradrenergic systems in stress-induced relapse. We and others found that systemic injections of agents that reduce cell firing and release of noradrenaline in the brain (Aghajanian & VanderMaelen 1982; Carter 1997), such as the alpha-2 adrenoceptor agonists clonidine and lofexidine, block stress-induced reinstatement in cocaine- (Erb et al. 2000), in heroin- (Shaham et al. 2000b), and in alcohol-trained rats (Lê et al. 2005). Interestingly, in both rats and monkeys, the alpha-2 antagonist, yohimbine, induces reinstatement, acting like a stressor (Gass & Olive 2007; Lee et al. 2004; Shepard et al. 2004). The two major noradrenergic systems of the brain arise from the locus coeruleus, origin of noradrenergic projections to cortex, HIPP, and other forebrain structures, and from the lateral tegmental nuclei (LTN) projecting via the ventral bundle to the CeA, the septum, and the BNST (Aston-Jones et al. 1999). Using infusions of clonidine or ST-91 (a charged analog of clonidine with reduced lipophilic properties) and selective 6-hydroxdopamine lesions, we determined that the ventral noradrenergic bundle neurons

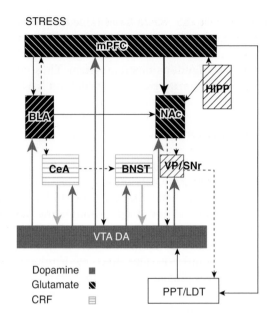

Fig. 5.3 Diagram showing the primary circuits and neurotransmitters implicated in stress-induced reinstatement. VTA (ventral tegmental area), cell body regions of mesocortiolimbic dopaminergic (DA) pathway, NAc (nucleus accumbens), mPFC (medial prefrontal cortex), VP/SNr (ventral pallidum/substantia nigra reticulata), PPT/LDT (peduncular pontine and laterodorsal tegmental nuclei), BLA (basolateral amygdala), HIPP (hippocampus), CeA (central nucleus of the amygdala), BNST (bed nucleus of the stria terminalis), and CRF (corticotropin-releasing hormone).

were of primary importance in stress-induced reinstatement (Shaham et al. 2000b). These findings, combined with those showing the importance of extra-hypothalamic CRF activity in stress-induced reinstatement, led us to study the role of noradrenergic activity in the BNST and CeA region in stress-induced reinstatement. We found a dose-dependent reduction of stress-induced reinstatement after infusions of a cocktail of the beta-1 and beta-2 receptor antagonists, betaxolol, and ICI 181,555 into the BNST and a complete blockade of stress-induced reinstatement after infusions into the CeA at all doses tested. The same treatments did not block cocaine-induced reinstatement at either site (Leri et al. 2002).

These data suggest that the mediation of the effects of footshock on reinstatement of drug seeking is via the release of noradrenaline in the amygdala and BNST. Through effects at beta noradrenergic receptors, noradrenaline may activate CRF-containing cells in both regions. Some of these CRF-neurons may project from the CeA to the BNST and others are intrinsic to the BNST itself. This idea, of course, does not rule out other actions of noradrenaline in these regions, but it does suggest that the critical event for the initiation of reinstatement induced by stress is the release of CRF in the BNST. Interference in this circuit has no effect on cocaine-induced relapse. These findings that the drug-induced relapse was not affected by manipulations that affected the CRF or noradrenergic systems of the brain led us to conclude that the brain systems mediating stress-induced relapse could be dissociated from those mediating drug-induced relapse. Furthermore, we had found in an early study that stress-induced reinstatement of heroin seeking was relatively unaffected by systemic injections of dopaminergic D1 or D2 receptor antagonists; only sustained treatment with a mixed antagonist was able to block stress-induced heroin seeking (Shaham & Stewart 1996). However, the role of the dopaminergic system in stress-induced relapse was shown in subsequent studies to include the mPFC. We found that infusions of a D1 receptor antagonist, SCH23390, into the prelimbic region (PL) block footshock-induced reinstatement, but not cocaine-induced reinstatement, whereas a D2 receptor antagonist alone had no effect. Neither TTX nor SCH23390 infusions had any effect on lever pressing for sucrose (Capriles et al. 2003). Similarly, placed mPFC infusions of the D1/D2 antagonist, fluphenaxine, blocked footshock-induced reinstatement, and interestingly, reversible inactivation of PL by TTX infusions blocked both footshock (McFarland et al. 2004) and cocaine-induced reinstatement (McFarland & Kalivas 2001). These findings combined with that showing that inactivation of the shell or core blocks stress-induced reinstatement (McFarland et al. 2004) establishes a role for the dopaminergic system in stress-induced, as well as in cue- and drug-induced reinstatement. In addition, these findings taken together with those discussed above for cue-induced reinstatement confirm the idea that PL region of the mPFC serves as a common pathway for cue, drug, and footshock stress-induced reinstatement of drug seeking. Sketches of the circuits identified and the primary neurotransmitters implicated in stress-induced are shown in Figs. 5.3 and 5.4.

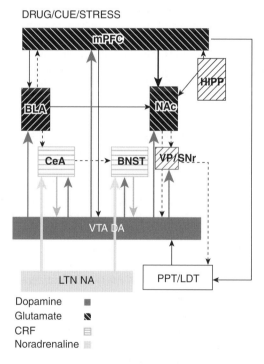

Fig. 5.4 Diagram showing the primary circuits and neurotransmitters implicated in reinstatement by drugs, cues, and stressors. VTA (ventral tegmental area), cell body regions of mesocortiolimbic dopaminergic (DA) pathway, NAc (nucleus accumbens), mPFC (medial prefrontal cortex), VP/SNr (ventral pallidum/substantia nigra reticulata), PPT/LDT (peduncular pontine and laterodorsal tegmental nuclei), BLA (basolateral amygdala), HIPP (hippocampus), CeA (central nucleus of the amygdala), BNST (bed nucleus of the stria terminalis), CRF (corticotropin-releasing hormone), LTN (lateral tegmental nuclei), and NA (noradrenaline).

In an earlier section, we saw how drugs and stressors might have their effects on relapse by renewing the effectiveness of cues previously paired with drugs. It is clear that such cues acquire through learning the ability to instigate appetitive, drug-seeking behaviours. Another issue is how the activation of the CRF systems, found to be critical for stress-induced relapse, gain access to those systems that mediate these learned appetitive behaviours such as drug seeking.

CRF systems are known to be activated in response to stressors and to mediate a wide variety of physiological and behavioural responses to stress including fear and anxiety (Davis 2006; Schulkin et al. 2005; also see Merali et al. 2004). In addition, CRF has been shown to be activated by feeding (Merali et al. 1998) to facilitate locomotor activity (Kalivas et al. 1987; Cador et al. 1993; Kalivas et al. 1987) and responses to positive incentive stimuli (Pecina et al. 2006), responses involved in appetitive behaviour. Although much is known about the role of CRF systems in aversive behaviours, less is known about the pathways through which activation of CRF systems facilitates appetitive behaviour.

In a recent study on the role of CRF in drug seeking, it was found that CRF is released directly in the VTA during footshock stress and that, in cocaine-experienced rats, infusions of CRF induce reinstatement and infusions of a CRF receptor antagonist into the VTA block stress-induced reinstatement of drug seeking (Wang et al. 2005). These findings point to an interaction between CRF-containing cell groups and the dopaminergic neurons in the VTA, providing a possible pathway for stress activation of CRF to modulate appetitive behaviour. Interestingly, it was found in earlier studies that prior exposure to stress facilitates glutamatergic synaptic transmission in dopaminergic neurons in the VTA in a manner similar to prior exposure to drugs of abuse (Saal et al. 2003). Furthermore, it was found that CRF applied directly to a VTA slice preparation had a similar effect (Ungless et al. 2003; see also Wanat et al. 2008). Little is known, however, about the sources of CRF-containing fibres in the VTA. An understanding of the sources of the CRF innervation of the VTA would help to explain the role of stress and CRF in the modulation of appetitive behaviours. We recently found using a fluorescent retrograde tracer and fluorescence immunocytochemistry for CRF that the VTA region receives CRF projections from the oval nucleus of the bed nucleus of the stria terminalis (BNSTov), the CeA, and paraventricular nucleus of the hypothalamus (Rodaros et al. 2007), pointing to a means whereby activation of CRF systems of these brain regions by stressors could facilitate the activity within the mesocorticolimbic dopaminergic system and, thus, appetitive behaviour. A final summary sketch of all the circuits identified and the primary neurotransmitters implicated reinstatement is shown in Fig. 5.4.

5.6 Sources of plasticity within pathways mediating relapse

The major sources of plasticity within pathways mediating relapse derive from exposure to the pharmacological effects of the drugs, themselves, and from conditioning and learning associated with drugs.

The idea that long-term changes within specific circuitry might alter the motivational effects of drugs has received considerable attention within the field of drug abuse (see for example Nestler et al. 2001; Piazza et al. 1990; Robinson & Berridge 2000). The circuitry best studied and found to undergo lasting changes as a result of repeated exposure to stimulant drugs is the mesocorticolimbic dopaminergic system and its targets in striatum, amygdala, and mPFC. Stimulant and opioid drugs induce increases in extracellular dopamine in all of these regions, as well as in the BNST (see Di Chiara et al. 1999).

Repeated exposure to stimulant drugs, such as amphetamine and cocaine, results in enhancement of their behavioural activating effects. This phenomenon, known as behavioural sensitization, develops over time and has been observed months and even years after termination of drug treatment (Castner & Goldman-Rakic 1999; Paulson et al. 1991). Behavioural sensitization is accompanied by increased responsiveness of the mesolimbic dopaminergic system to drugs (see Kalivas & Stewart 1991; Robinson & Becker 1986). It has been found in numerous experiments that the increase in extracellular dopamine in striatal terminal regions after acute systemic injections of amphetamine or cocaine is enhanced following repeated exposure to these drugs (e.g. Heidbreder et al. 1996; Paulson & Robinson 1995). This enhancement in dopaminergic function develops gradually after termination of drug treatment and is long-lasting (Heidbreder et al. 1996; Kalivas & Duffy 1993; Kolta et al. 1985; Paulson et al. 1991;Paulson & Robinson 1995; Robinson et al. 1988; Vezina 1993; Wolf et al. 1993). Enhancement of function appears to result from a series of changes within the dopaminergic system and its targets that occur over time after termination of drug treatment. Electrophysiological studies have shown that initially there is reduced D2 dopamine autoreceptor sensitivity that results in reduced suppression of dopamine cell firing by dopamine and other agonists lasting about one week; this is followed by a period of enhanced sensitivity of D1 dopamine receptors on NAc neurons lasting about one month; after about 10–20 days depending on the pre-treatment regimen, there are increased extra-cellular levels of dopamine in NAcc in response to drug challenge (Henry et al. 1989, 1991; Wolf et al. 1994). Importantly, it has been found that in addition to behavioural sensitization (Kalivas et al. 1988; Vezina 1993; Vezina & Stewart 1990), these changes in dopaminergic function and their time course can be mimicked by direct application of amphetamine in the VTA (Hu et al. 2002), demonstrating that processes initiated in the cell body region of dopamine neurons are responsible for sensitized functioning within the system. The relevance of such drug-induced sensitization within the mesolimbic dopaminergic system to the motivational effects of drugs and drug-related stimuli has been pointed out by several investigators over the years (Piazza & LeMoal 1996; Piazza et al. 1990; Vezina 2004; Vezina et al. 2002). For a recent set of reviews on sensitization, see Vezina (2007).

The long-lasting changes induced by stimulant drugs suggest structural modifications in neuronal circuitry and, in fact, studies have shown selective and persistent changes in transcription factors known to be involved in neuroplasticity (Chen et al. 1995; Nestler et al. 2001, 1999), drug-induced changes in synaptic facilitation, and long-term potentiation of dopaminergic neurons in the VTA (Bonci & Williams 1996; Borgland et al. 2004; Liu et al. 2006; Ungless et al. 2001), long-term depression and potentiation in NAc (Kourrich et al. 2007; Thomas et al. 2001), and structural changes in VTA, NAc, and mPFC neurons following repeated exposure to these drugs (Hu et al. 2002; Mueller et al. 2006; Robinson & Kolb 1997; Sarti et al. 2007). The fact that many of the important long-lasting changes are enhanced by the passage of time after termination of drug exposure and involve structural changes in neurons suggests that neurotrophic factors are involved.

5.7 Neurotrophic factors in drug-induced sensitization

In a set of studies done to determine whether the neurotrophic and neuroprotective factor, basic fibroblast growth factor (bFGF or FGF-2), plays a role in the development of enduring changes in dopaminergic functioning seen after repeated exposure to amphetamine, we found that amphetamine induces increases in bFGF expression in astrocytes in the cell body region of the midbrain dopaminergic neurons. These increases are seen early after termination of drug treatment and last for at least one month (Flores et al. 1998). We found as well that, as is the case for the development of behavioural sensitization to amphetamine (see Wolf 1998), the induction of bFGF by amphetamine is prevented by the co-administration of glutamate antagonists (Flores et al. 1998) and, importantly, that inactivation of bFGF in the VTA prevents the development of behavioural sensitization to amphetamine (Flores et al. 2000). These data led us to propose that repeated exposure to stimulant drugs increases the demands on dopaminergic cell functioning, and by stimulating glutamate release recruits neurotrophic and neuroprotective substances such as bFGF. This sequence of events could provide a mechanism for the initiation and maintenance of the long-lasting neuronal adaptations that underlie sensitized responding to further drug exposure (Flores & Stewart 2000; see also Belluardo et al. 1998; Fumagalli et al. 2006; Mueller et al. 2006).

5.8 Brain-derived neurotrophic factor (BDNF)

Recent studies have pointed to a major role for the neurotrophic factor, brain-derived neurotrophic factor (BDNF) in the long-lasting changes in brain, and behaviour induced by drugs of abuse (Berglind et al. 2007; Graham et al. 2007; Grimm et al. 2003; Liu et al. 2006; Lu et al. 2004; Thomas et al. 2008). In earlier studies of the effects of BDNF on dopaminergic functioning, it was found that following continuous local infusion of BDNF into the cell body and terminal regions of midbrain dopaminergic neurons, the firing rate of these neurons increases (Shen et al. 1994) and the behavioural activating effects of cocaine and the motivational effects of conditioned reinforcers are enhanced (Horger et al. 1999). These studies suggested that BDNF can induce long-lasting changes in the sensitivity of this pathway to stimulus inputs arising from motivationally significant stimuli. Support for this view comes from a study showing that the potentiation of excitatory synapses at dopaminergic neurons in the VTA after withdrawal from cocaine is dependent on BDNF TrkB receptor signalling (Pu et al. 2006). These findings led the authors to suggest that BDNF release during cocaine exposure may initiate effects at synapses that are expressed long after withdrawal of cocaine.

Increases in BDNF expression were explored in previous studies aimed at determining the basis for the time-dependent enhancement of cue-induced reinstatement in rats, days and months after termination of cocaine self-administration (Grimm et al. 2001). This phenomenon, referred to as 'an incubation effect', was found to be accompanied by increased expression of BDNF in VTA NAc and amygdala over time (Grimm et al. 2003). In another study, the incubation effect was shown to be further enhanced by a single infusion of BDNF into the VTA given shortly after the last cocaine session, an effect that appears to be mediated by the mitogen-activated protein kinase (MAPK) pathway (Lu et al. 2004). More recent evidence comes from a study in which it was found that if BDNF was infused into the NAc of rats immediately following daily cocaine self-administration sessions, reinstatement of cocaine seeking was greatly enhanced after presentations of drug-associated cues, priming injections of cocaine, or footshock stress. Importantly, these effects were blocked by co-infusions of an antibody to BDNF (Graham et al. 2007).

Time-dependent effects have been found for stress-induced reinstatement of both heroin (Shalev et al. 2001) and cocaine seeking (Sorge & Stewart 2005). It is likely that a number of systems are involved in these changes over time, including dopaminergic, CRF (Orozco-Cabal et al. 2008), and noradrenergic systems (Beveridge et al. 2005; Dumont & Williams 2004; Leri et al. 2002).

5.9 Drug-induced plasticity in glutamatergic function

As discussed above, there is evidence that BDNF plays a role in the facilitation of NMDA receptor-mediated glutamatergic transmission at dopaminergic neurons in the VTA after termination of cocaine exposure (Pu et al. 2006). Interestingly, this effect was seen 10–15 days after cocaine exposure, but not 1 day after, suggestive of processes taking place over time after termination of cocaine exposure. Exactly how this increased sensitivity to glutamate is mediated is not understood, but increases in NMDAR1 subunits have been reported in VTA for up to 90 days after termination of cocaine (Lu et al. 2003). Blockade of glutamate receptors in VTA decreases cocaine-induced reinstatement of cocaine seeking (Sun et al. 2005a), and intra-VTA infusions of a group II metabotropic glutamate receptor agonist thought to act by reducing glutamate release, blocks cue-induced reinstatement in heroin-trained rats (Bossert et al. 2004). Furthermore, there is evidence that glutamate receptors on dopaminergic neurons play a role in the persistence of drug seeking (Engblom et al. 2008). In a study discussed above, it was shown that, after termination of cocaine self-administration, CRF released in the VTA during exposure to stress causes glutamate release, an effect not seen in cocaine naïve rats. Furthermore, it was found that stress-induced reinstatement could be blocked by a glutamate receptor antagonist (Wang et al. 2005). This study provides another example of long-lasting facilitation of glutamatergic activity in the VTA resulting from exposure to cocaine, in this case via changes in the effectiveness of a peptide, CRF. It is likely, in my view, that in the future, changes of a similar kind will be found following exposure to drug within those brains already identified as playing critical roles in reinstatement induced by various triggers.

Another region of the mesolimbic dopaminergic system and its terminal regions where changes in glutamatergic functioning have already been found to play a critical role in reinstatement of drug seeking is the NAc core, as discussed in an earlier section. Marked increases in glutamate release in the NAc in response to drugs or stress have been found after extinction in rats trained to self-administer cocaine for heroin. Simple exposure to drugs does not seem to be sufficient to induce this effect, again suggesting, as discussed in an earlier section, that learning about drug-associated cues may be critical (McFarland et al. 2003, 2004). These researchers have argued that this enhanced release of glutamate arises from activation of mPFC inputs to the NAc, and it will be remembered that inactivation of this input blocks reinstatement by cues, drugs, and stressors. There is other evidence that there are changes in glutamate receptors in the NAc after cocaine exposure that would make cells more sensitive to glutamatergic input (Boudreau & Wolf 2005; Gao et al. 2006; Sun et al. 2005b). Interestingly, reported increases in cell-surface glutamatergic AMPA receptors are not seen immediately after discontinuation of cocaine (they were in fact decreased), but are seen after 14 days (Boudreau et al. 2007; Conrad et al. 2008), temporal changes that parallel changes in sensitivity to glutamatergic input to NAc neurons seen in electrophysiological studies (Kourrich et al. 2007).

It has been proposed that drug-induced changes in cystine–glutamate exchange in the NAc, which would induce changes in glutamatergic tone in the NAc, may underlie these lasting changes in glutamatergic function in this region (Baker et al. 2002, 2003). It is considered that the reduced tone affects presynaptic mGlu receptors causing dysregulation of glutamatergic function (Moran et al. 2005). Restoration of cystine–glutamate exchange has been shown to block both cocaine-induced reinstatement of cocaine seeking (Baker et al. 2003) and cue- and heroin-induced reinstatement of heroin seeking (Zhou & Kalivas 2007). Interestingly, chronic treatment with the partial opioid agonist, buprenorphine, which blocks drug-induced reinstatement of both heroin and cocaine seeking and reduces responding to drug-paired cues, increases basal levels of both dopamine and glutamate in the NAc, suggesting that it may have its 'therapeutic' effect by stabilizing dysregulated transmitter function following termination of drug taking (Placenza et al. 2007, 2008; Sorge et al. 2005; Sorge & Stewart 2006). In addition, as mentioned above, a group II mGluR agonist given into the NAc blocks cue-induced reinstatement of heroin seeking and given systemically, cue- and stress-induced ethanol seeking (Zhao et al. 2006). Together, these data lend strong support to the idea that long-lasting dysregulation of glutamatergic function involving the mPFC and NAc contributes importantly to sensitivity to triggers for, and thus vulnerability to, relapse.

5.10 Summary

Experience with drug self-administration promotes long-lasting changes in systems of the brain mediating the effects of events that trigger relapse to drug seeking. These lasting changes are induced, in part, by mere pharmacological effects of exposure to these drugs and, in part, through conditioning and learning. Circuits of the brain involved in relapse are those of the mesocorticolimbic dopaminergic system and its glutamatergic inputs, and the CRF and noradrenergic systems of the limbic brain. We have seen that exposure to drugs changes sensitivity to subsequent exposure to drugs and to the effects of stressors. Many neurochemical and molecular mechanisms have been found to underlie drug-induced plasticity. These changes develop with repeated exposure and are progressive, time-dependent, and enduring. Environmental stimuli that acquire secondary or conditioned incentive properties through pairings with the incentive effects of drugs become powerful instigators of drug seeking and, in the absence of extinction training, maintain this capacity in spite of long-term abstinence from drugs. After extinction training, when the capacity of these conditioned stimuli to induce relapse is diminished or absent, exposure to a stressor or to the drug, itself, is able to enhance the salience of these conditioned stimuli leading to the reinitiation (reinstatement) of drug-seeking behaviours. Although a number of manipulations have been found to block or attenuate reinstatement by cues, drugs or stressors, few, if any, are yet sufficiently broad in their effects to serve as effective treatments.

Acknowledgements

This work was supported by grants from the Canadian Institutes of Health Research (CIHR) and Le Fonds de la recherche en santé du Québec (FRSQ).

References

Aghajanian, G. K. & VanderMaelen, C. P. 1982 Alpha 2-adrenoceptor-mediated hyperpolarization of locus coeruleus neurons: intracellular studies in vivo. *Science* **215**, 1394–6.
Ahmed, S. H. & Koob, G. F. 1997 Cocaine- but not food-seeking behavior is reinstated by stress after extinction. *Psychopharmacology* **132**, 289–95.
Anderson, S. M., Bari, A. A. & Pierce, R. C. 2003 Administration of the D1-like dopamine receptor antagonist SCH-23390 into the medial nucleus accumbens shell attenuates cocaine priming-induced reinstatement of drug-seeking behavior in rats. *Psychopharmacology (Berl)* **168**, 132–8.

Anderson, S. M., Schmidt, H. D. & Pierce, R. C. 2006 Administration of the D2 dopamine receptor antagonist sulpiride into the shell, but not the core, of the nucleus accumbens attenuates cocaine priming-induced reinstatement of drug seeking. *Neuropsychopharmacology* **31**, 1452–61.

Aston-Jones, G., Delfs, J. M., Druhan, J. & Zhu, Y. 1999 The bed nucleus of the stria terminalis. A target site for noradrenergic actions in opiate withdrawal. *Ann N Y Acad Sci* **877**, 486–98.

Bachtell, R. K., Whisler, K., Karanian, D. & Self, D. W. 2005 Effects of intra-nucleus accumbens shell administration of dopamine agonists and antagonists on cocaine-taking and cocaine-seeking behaviors in the rat. *Psychopharmacology (Berl)* **183**, 41–53.

Backstrom, P. & Hyytia, P. 2007 Involvement of AMPA/kainate, NMDA, and mGlu5 receptors in the nucleus accumbens core in cue-induced reinstatement of cocaine seeking in rats. *Psychopharmacology (Berl)* **192**, 571–80.

Baker, D. A., McFarland, K., Lake, R. W. et al. 2003 Neuroadaptations in cystine-glutamate exchange underlie cocaine relapse. *Nat Neurosci* **6**, 743–9.

Baker, D. A., Shen, H. & Kalivas, P. W. 2002 Cystine/glutamate exchange serves as the source for extracellular glutamate: modifications by repeated cocaine administration. *Amino Acids* **23**, 161–2.

Belluardo, N., Blum, M., Mudo, G., Andbjer, B. & Fuxe, K. 1998 Acute intermittent nicotine treatment produces regional increases of basic fibroblast growth factor messenger RNA and protein in the tel- and diencephalon of the rat. *Neuroscience* **83**, 723–40.

Berglind, W. J., See, R. E., Fuchs, R. A. et al. 2007 A BDNF infusion into the medial prefrontal cortex suppresses cocaine seeking in rats. *Eur J Neurosci* **26**, 757–66.

Beveridge, T. J., Smith, H. R., Nader, M. A. & Porrino, L. J. 2005 Effects of chronic cocaine self-administration on norepinephrine transporters in the nonhuman primate brain. *Psychopharmacology (Berl)* **180**, 781–8.

Bonci, A. & Williams, J. T. 1996 A common mechanism mediates long-term changes in synaptic transmission after chronic cocaine and morphine. *Neuron* **16**, 631–639.

Borgland, S. L., Malenka, R. C. & Bonci, A. 2004 Acute and chronic cocaine-induced potentiation of synaptic strength in the ventral tegmental area: electrophysiological and behavioral correlates in individual rats. *J Neurosci* **24**, 7482–90.

Bossert, J. M., Gray, S. M., Lu, L. & Shaham, Y. 2006 Activation of group II metabotropic glutamate receptors in the nucleus accumbens shell attenuates context-induced relapse to heroin seeking. *Neuropsychopharmacology* **31**, 2197–209.

Bossert, J. M., Liu, S. Y., Lu, L. & Shaham, Y. 2004 A role of ventral tegmental area glutamate in contextual cue-induced relapse to heroin seeking. *J Neurosci* **24**, 10726–30.

Boudreau, A. C., Reimers, J. M., Milovanovic, M. & Wolf, M. E. 2007 Cell surface AMPA receptors in the rat nucleus accumbens increase during cocaine withdrawal but internalize after cocaine challenge in association with altered activation of mitogen-activated protein kinases. *J Neurosci* **27**, 10621–35.

Boudreau, A. C. & Wolf, M. E. 2005 Behavioral sensitization to cocaine is associated with increased AMPA receptor surface expression in the nucleus accumbens. *J Neurosci* **25**, 9144–51.

Buczek, Y., Le, A. D., Stewart, J. & Shaham, Y. 1999 Stress reinstates nicotine seeking but not sucrose solution seeking in rats. *Psychopharmacology* **144**, 183–8.

Cador, M., Cole, B. J., Koob, G. F., Stinus, L. & Le Moal, M. 1993 Central administration of corticotropin releasing factor induces long-term sensitization to D-amphetamine. *Brain Research* **606**, 181–6.

Capriles, N., Rodaros, D., Sorge, R. E. & Stewart, J. 2003 A role for the prefrontal cortex in stress- and cocaine-induced reinstatement of cocaine seeking in rats. *Psychopharmacology (Berl)* **168**, 66–74.

Carter, A. J. 1997 Hippocampal noradrenaline release in awake, freely moving rats is regulated by alpha-2 adrenoceptors but not by adenosine receptors. *J Pharmacol Exp Ther* **281**, 648–54.

Castner, S. A. & Goldman-Rakic, P. S. 1999 Long-lasting psychotomimetic consequences of repeated low-dose amphetamine exposure in rhesus monkeys. *Neuropsychopharmacology* **20**, 10–28.

Chen, J., Nye, H. E., Kelz, M. B., Hiroi, N., Nakabeppu, Y., Hope, B. T. & Nestler, E. J. 1995 Regulation of delta FosB and FosB-like proteins by electroconvulsive seizure and cocaine treatments. *Mol Pharmacol* **48**, 880–9.

Childress, A. R., Ehrman, R., Rohsenow, D. J., Robbins, S. J. & O'Brien, C. P. 1992 Classically conditioned factors in drug dependence. In *Substance Abuse: A Comprehensive Textbook* (eds. J. W. Lowinson, P. Luiz, R. B. Millman & G. Langard), pp. 56–69. Baltimore: Williams and Wilkins.

Conrad, K. L., Tseng, K. Y., Uejima, J. L. et al. 2008 Formation of accumbens GluR2-lacking AMPA receptors mediates incubation of cocaine craving. *Nature* **454**, 118–21.

Cornish, J. L. & Kalivas, P. W. 2000 Glutamate transmission in the nucleus accumbens mediates relapse in cocaine addiction. *J Neurosci* **20**, RC89.

Davis, M. 2006 Neural systems involved in fear and anxiety measured with fear-potentiated startle. *Am Psychol* **61**, 741–56.

de Wit, H. 1996 Priming effects with drugs and other reinforcers. *Exp Clin Psychopharmacol* **4**, 5–10.

de Wit, H. & Stewart, J. 1981 Reinstatement of cocaine-reinforced responding in the rat. *Psychopharmacology* **75**, 134–43.

Di Chiara, G., Tanda, G., Bassareo, V. et al. 1999 Drug addiction as a disorder of associative learning. Role of nucleus accumbens shell/extended amygdala dopamine. *Ann N Y Acad Sci* **877**, 461–85.

Di Ciano, P. & Everitt, B. J. 2001 Dissociable effects of antagonism of NMDA and AMPA/KA receptors in the nucleus accumbens core and shell on cocaine-seeking behavior. *Neuropsychopharmacology* **25**, 341–60.

Di Ciano, P. & Everitt, B. J. 2004 Direct interactions between the basolateral amygdala and nucleus accumbens core underlie cocaine-seeking behavior by rats. *J Neurosci* **24**, 7167–73.

Di Ciano, P., Robbins, T. W. & Everitt, B. J. 2008 Differential effects of nucleus accumbens core, shell, or dorsal striatal inactivations on the persistence, reacquisition, or reinstatement of responding for a drug-paired conditioned reinforcer. *Neuropsychopharmacology* **33**, 1413–25.

Dumont, E. C. & Williams, J. T. 2004 Noradrenaline triggers GABAA inhibition of bed nucleus of the stria terminalis neurons projecting to the ventral tegmental area. *J Neurosci* **24**, 8198–204.

Duncan, E., Boshoven, W., Harenski, K. et al. 2007 An fMRI study of the interaction of stress and cocaine cues on cocaine craving in cocaine-dependent men. *Am J Addict* **16**, 174–82.

Engblom, D., Bilbao, A., Sanchis-Segura, C. et al. 2008 Glutamate receptors on dopamine neurons control the persistence of cocaine seeking. *Neuron* **59**, 497–508.

Epstein, D. H., Preston, K. L., Stewart, J. & Shaham, Y. 2006 Toward a model of drug relapse: an assessment of the validity of the reinstatement procedure. *Psychopharmacology (Berl)* **189**, 1–16.

Erb, S., Hitchcott, P. K., Rajabi, H., Mueller, D., Shaham, Y. & Stewart, J. 2000 Alpha-2 adrenergic receptor agonists block stress-induced reinstatement of cocaine seeking. *Neuropsychopharmacology* **23**, 138–50.

Erb, S., Shaham, Y. & Stewart, J. 1996 Stress reinstates cocaine-seeking behavior after prolonged extinction and a drug-free period. *Psychopharmacology* **128**, 408–12.

Erb, S., Shaham, Y. & Stewart, J. 1998 The role of corticotropin-releasing factor and corticosterone in stress- and cocaine-induced relapse to cocaine seeking in rats. *J Neurosci* **18**, 5529–36.

Erb, S., Shaham, Y. & Stewart, J. 2001 Stress-induced relapse to drug seeking in the rat: role of the bed nucleus of the stria terminalis and amygdala. *Stress* **4**, 289–303.

Erb, S. & Stewart, J. 1999 A role for the bed nucleus of the stria terminalis, but not the amygdala, in the effects of corticotropin-releasing factor on stress-induced reinstatement of cocaine seeking. *J Neurosci* **19**, RC35, 1–6.

Flores, C., Rodaros, D. & Stewart, J. 1998 Long-lasting induction of astrocytic basic fibroblast growth factor by repeated injections of amphetamine: blockade by concurrent treatment with a glutamate antagonist. *J Neurosci* **18**, 9547–55.

Flores, C., Samaha, A. N. & Stewart, J. 2000 Requirement of endogenous basic fibroblast growth factor for sensitization to amphetamine. *J Neurosci* **20**, RC55.

Flores, C. & Stewart, J. 2000 Basic fibroblast growth factor as a mediator of the effects of glutamate in the development of long-lasting sensitization to stimulant drugs: studies in the rat. *Psychopharmacology* **151**, 152–65.

Fuchs, R. A., Branham, R. K. & See, R. E. 2006 Different neural substrates mediate cocaine seeking after abstinence versus extinction training: a critical role for the dorsolateral caudate-putamen. *J Neurosci* **26**, 3584–8.

Fuchs, R. A., Eaddy, J. L., Su, Z. I. & Bell, G. H. 2007 Interactions of the basolateral amygdala with the dorsal hippocampus and dorsomedial prefrontal cortex regulate drug context-induced reinstatement of cocaine-seeking in rats. *Eur J Neurosci* **26**, 487–98.

Fuchs, R. A. & See, R. E. 2002 Basolateral amygdala inactivation abolishes conditioned stimulus- and heroin-induced reinstatement of extinguished heroin-seeking behavior in rats. *Psychopharmacology (Berl)* **160**, 425–33.

Fumagalli, F., Pasquale, L., Racagni, G. & Riva, M. A. 2006 Dynamic regulation of fibroblast growth factor 2 (FGF-2) gene expression in the rat brain following single and repeated cocaine administration. *J Neurochem* **96**, 996–1004.

Gao, C., Sun, X. & Wolf, M. E. 2006 Activation of D1 dopamine receptors increases surface expression of AMPA receptors and facilitates their synaptic incorporation in cultured hippocampal neurons. *J Neurochem* **98**, 1664–77.

Gass, J. T. & Olive, M. F. 2007 Reinstatement of ethanol-seeking behavior following intravenous self-administration in Wistar rats. *Alcohol Clin Exp Res* **31**, 1441–5.

Goddard, B. & Leri, F. 2006 Reinstatement of conditioned reinforcing properties of cocaine-conditioned stimuli. *Pharmacol Biochem Behav* **83**, 540–6.

Graham, D. L., Edwards, S., Bachtell, R. K., DiLeone, R. J., Rios, M. & Self, D. W. 2007 Dynamic BDNF activity in nucleus accumbens with cocaine use increases self-administration and relapse. *Nat Neurosci* **10**, 1029–37.

Grimm, J. W., Hope, B., Wise, R. A. & Shaham, Y. 2001 Incubation of cocaine craving after withdrawal. *Nature* **412**, 141–2.

Grimm, J. W., Lu, L., Hayashi, T., Hope, B. T., Su, T. P. & Shaham, Y. 2003 Time-dependent increases in brain-derived neurotrophic factor protein levels within the mesolimbic dopamine system after withdrawal from cocaine: implications for incubation of cocaine craving. *J Neurosci* **23**, 742–7.

Heidbreder, C. A., Thompson, A. C. & Shippenberg, T. S. 1996 Role of extracellular dopamine in the initiation and long-term expression of behavioral sensitization to cocaine. *J Pharmacol Exp Ther* **278**, 490–502.

Henry, D. J., Greene, M. A. & White, F. J. 1989 Electrophysiological effects of cocaine in the mesoaccumbens dopamine system: repeated administration. *J Pharmacol Exp Ther* **251**, 833–9.

Henry, D. J. & White, F. J. 1991 Repeated cocaine administration causes persistent enhancement of D1 dopamine receptor sensitivity within the rat nucleus accumbens. *J Pharmacol Exp Ther* **258**, 882–90.

Horger, B. A., Iyasere, C. A., Berhow, M. T., Messer, C. J., Nestler, E. J. & Taylor, J. R. 1999 Enhancement of locomotor activity and conditioned reward to cocaine by brain-derived neurotrophic factor. *J Neurosci* **19**, 4110–22.

Hu, X. T., Koeltzow, T. E., Cooper, D. C., Robertson, G. S., White, F. J. & Vezina, P. 2002 Repeated ventral tegmental area amphetamine administration alters dopamine D1 receptor signaling in the nucleus accumbens. *Synapse* **45**, 159–70.

Ito, R., Dalley, J. W., Howes, S. R., Robbins, T. W. & Everitt, B. J. 2000 Dissociation in conditioned dopamine release in the nucleus accumbens core and shell in response to cocaine cues and during cocaine-seeking behavior in rats. *J Neurosci* **20**, 7489–95.

Jaffe, J. H., Cascell, N. G., Kumor, K. M. & Sherer, M. A. 1989 Cocaine-induced cocaine craving. *Psychopharmacology* **97**, 59–64.

Kalivas, P. W. 2004 Glutamate systems in cocaine addiction. *Curr Opin Pharmacol* **4**, 23–9.

Kalivas, P. W. & Duffy, P. 1993 Time course of extracellular dopamine and behavioral sensitization to cocaine I. Dopamine axon terminals. *J Neurosci* **13**, 266–75.

Kalivas, P. W., Duffy, P., DuMars, L. A. & Skinner, C. 1988 Behavioral and neurochemical effects of acute and daily cocaine administration in rats. *J Pharmacol Exp Ther* **245**, 485–92.

Kalivas, P. W., Duffy, P. & Latimer, G. 1987 Neurochemical and behavioral effects of corticotropin-releasing factor in the ventral tegmental area of the rat. *J Pharmacol Exp Ther* **242**, 757–63.

Kalivas, P. W. & McFarland, K. 2003 Brain circuitry and the reinstatement of cocaine-seeking behavior. *Psychopharmacology (Berl)* **168**, 44–56.

Kalivas, P. W. & Stewart, J. 1991 Dopamine transmission in the initiation and expression of drug- and stress-induced sensitization of motor activity. *Brain Res Rev* **16**, 223–44.

Kolta, M. G., Shreve, P., De Souza, V. & Uretsky, N. J. 1985 Time course of the development of the enhanced behavioral and biochemical responses to amphetamine after pretreatment with amphetamine. *Neuropharmacology* **24**, 823–9.

Kourrich, S., Rothwell, P. E., Klug, J. R. & Thomas, M. J. 2007 Cocaine experience controls bidirectional synaptic plasticity in the nucleus accumbens. *J Neurosci* **27**, 7921–8.

Lê, A. D., Harding, S., Juzytsch, W., Funk, D. & Shaham, Y. 2005 Role of alpha-2 adrenoceptors in stress-induced reinstatement of alcohol seeking and alcohol self-administration in rats. *Psychopharmacology (Berl)* **179**, 366–73.

Lê, A. D., Harding, S., Juzytsch, W., Watchus, J., Shalev, U. & Shaham, Y. 2000 The role of corticotrophin-releasing factor in stress-induced relapse to alcohol-seeking behavior in rats. *Psychopharmacology* **150**, 317–24.

Lê, A. D., Quan, B., Juzytsch, W., Fletcher, P. J., Joharchi, N. & Shaham, Y. 1998 Reinstatement of alcohol-seeking by priming injections of alcohol and exposure to stress in rats. *Psychopharmacology* **135**, 169–74.

Lee, B., Tiefenbacher, S., Platt, D. M. & Spealman, R. D. 2004 Pharmacological blockade of alpha(2)-adrenoceptors induces reinstatement of cocaine-seeking behavior in squirrel monkeys. *Neuropsychopharmacology* **29**, 686–93.

Leri, F., Flores, J., Rodaros, D. & Stewart, J. 2002 Blockade of stress-induced, but not cocaine-induced reinstatement, by infusion of noradrenergic antagonists into the bed nucleus of the stria terminalis or the central nucleus of the amygdala. *J Neurosci* **22**, 5713–18.

Leyton, M., Boileau, I., Benkelfat, C., Diksic, M., Baker, G. & Dagher, A. 2002 Amphetamine-induced increases in extracellular dopamine, drug wanting, and novelty seeking. A PET/[11C]raclopride study in healthy men. *Neuropsychopharmacology* **27**, 1027–35.

Leyton, M., Casey, K. F., Delaney, J. S., Kolivakis, T. & Benkelfat, C. 2005 Cocaine craving, euphoria, and self-administration: a preliminary study of the effect of catecholamine precursor depletion. *Behav Neurosci* **119**, 1619–27.

Liechti, M. E., Lhuillier, L., Kaupmann, K. & Markou, A. 2007 Metabotropic glutamate 2/3 receptors in the ventral tegmental area and the nucleus accumbens shell are involved in behaviors relating to nicotine dependence. *J Neurosci* **27**, 9077–85.

Liu, Q. R., Lu, L., Zhu, X. G., Gong, J. P., Shaham, Y. & Uhl, G. R. 2006 Rodent BDNF genes, novel promoters, novel splice variants, and regulation by cocaine. *Brain Res* **1067**, 1–12.

Liu, X. & Weiss, F. 2002 Additive effect of stress and drug cues on reinstatement of ethanol seeking: exacerbation by history of dependence and role of concurrent activation of corticotropin-releasing factor and opioid mechanisms. *J Neurosci* **22**, 7856–61.

Lu, L., Dempsey, J., Liu, S. Y., Bossert, J. M. & Shaham, Y. 2004 A single infusion of brain-derived neurotrophic factor into the ventral tegmental area induces long-lasting potentiation of cocaine seeking after withdrawal. *J Neurosci* **24**, 1604–11.

Lu, L., Grimm, J. W., Shaham, Y. & Hope, B. T. 2003 Molecular neuroadaptations in the accumbens and ventral tegmental area during the first 90 days of forced abstinence from cocaine self-administration in rats. *J Neurochem* **85**, 1604–13.

McFarland, K., Davidge, S. B., Lapish, C. C. & Kalivas, P. W. 2004 Limbic and motor circuitry underlying footshock-induced reinstatement of cocaine-seeking behavior. *J Neurosci* **24**, 1551–60.

McFarland, K. & Kalivas, P. W. 2001 The circuitry mediating cocaine-induced reinstatement of drug-seeking behavior. *J Neurosci* **21**, 8655–63.

McFarland, K., Lapish, C. C. & Kalivas, P. W. 2003 Prefrontal glutamate release into the core of the nucleus accumbens mediates cocaine-induced reinstatement of drug-seeking behavior. *J Neurosci* **23**, 3531–7.

Merali, Z., Khan, S., Michaud, D. S., Shippy, S. A. & Anisman, H. 2004 Does amygdaloid corticotropin-releasing hormone (CRH) mediate anxiety-like behaviors? Dissociation of anxiogenic effects and CRH release. *Eur J Neurosci* **20**, 229–39.

Merali, Z., McIntosh, J., Kent, P., Michaud, D. & Anisman, H. 1998 Aversive and appetitive events evoke the release of corticotropin-releasing hormone and bombesin-like peptides at the central nucleus of the amygdala. *J Neurosci* **18**, 4758–66.

Moran, M. M., McFarland, K., Melendez, R. I., Kalivas, P. W. & Seamans, J. K. 2005 Cystine/ glutamate exchange regulates metabotropic glutamate receptor presynaptic inhibition of excitatory transmission and vulnerability to cocaine seeking. *J Neurosci* **25**, 6389–93.

Mueller, D., Chapman, C. A. & Stewart, J. 2006 Amphetamine induces dendritic growth in ventral tegmental area dopaminergic neurons in vivo via basic fibroblast growth factor. *Neuroscience* **137**, 727–35.

Mueller, D., Perdikaris, D. & Stewart, J. 2002 Persistence and drug-induced reinstatement of a morphine-induced conditioned place preference. *Behav Brain Res* **136**, 389–97.

Mueller, D. & Stewart, J. 2000 Cocaine-induced conditioned place preference: reinstatement by priming injections of cocaine after extinction. *Behav Brain Res* **115**, 39–47.

Nestler, E. J. 2001 Molecular basis of long-term plasticity underlying addiction. *Nat. Rev. Neurosci.* **2**, 119–28.

Nestler, E. J., Barrot, M. & Self, D. W. 2001 DeltaFosB: a sustained molecular switch for addiction. *Proc Natl Acad Sci USA* **98**, 11042–6.

Nestler, E. J., Kelz, M. B. & Chen, J. 1999 DeltaFosB: a molecular mediator of long-term neural and behavioral plasticity. *Brain Res.* **835**, 10–17.

Orozco-Cabal, L., Liu, J., Pollandt, S., Schmidt, K., Shinnick-Gallagher, P. & Gallagher, J. P. 2008 Dopamine and corticotropin-releasing factor synergistically alter basolateral amygdala-to-medial prefrontal cortex synaptic transmission: functional switch after chronic cocaine administration. *J Neurosci* **28**, 529–42.

Parker, L. A. & McDonald, R. V. 2000 Reinstatement of both a conditioned place preference and a conditioned place aversion with drug primes. *Pharmacol Biochem Behav* **66**, 559–61.

Parkinson, J. A., Olmstead, M. C., Burns, L. H., Robbins, T. W. & Everitt, B. J. 1999 Dissociation in effects of lesions of the nucleus accumbens core and shell on appetitive pavlovian approach behavior and the potentiation of conditioned reinforcement and locomotor activity by D-amphetamine. *J Neurosci* **19**, 2401–11.

Paulson, P. E., Camp, D. M. & Robinson, T. E. 1991 Time course of transient behavioral depression and persistent behavioral sensitization in relation to regional brain monoamine concentrations during amphetamine withdrawal in rats. *Psychopharmacology* **103**, 480–92.

Paulson, P. E. & Robinson, T. E. 1995 Amphetamine-induced time-dependent sensitization of dopamine neurotransmission in the dorsal and ventral striatum: a microdialysis study in behaving rats. *Synapse* **19**, 56–65.

Pecina, S., Schulkin, J. & Berridge, K. C. 2006 Nucleus accumbens corticotropin-releasing factor increases cue-triggered motivation for sucrose reward: paradoxical positive incentive effects in stress? *BMC Biol* **4**, 8.

Piazza, P.-V. & LeMoal, M. 1996 Pathophysiological basis of vulnerability to drug abuse: interaction between stress, glucocorticoids and dopaminergic neurons. *Ann Rev Pharmacol Toxicol* **36**, 359–378.

Piazza, P. V., Deminere, J. M., Le Moal, M. & Simon, H. 1990 Stress- and pharmacologically-induced behavioral sensitization increases vulnerability to acquisition of amphetamine self-administration. *Brain Res* **514**, 22–6.

Placenza, F. M., Rajabi, H. & Stewart, J. 2007 Levels of nucleus accumbens dopamine and glutamate in cocaine- sensitized and non-sensitized rats are altered by chronic buprenorphine treatment. *Abstracts Society for Neuroscience*.

Placenza, F. M., Rajabi, H. & Stewart, J. 2008 Effects of chronic buprenorphine treatment on levels of nucleus accumbens glutamate and on the expression of cocaine-induced behavioral sensitization in rats. *Psychopharmacology*, **200**, 347–55.

Pu, L., Liu, Q. S. & Poo, M. M. 2006 BDNF-dependent synaptic sensitization in midbrain dopamine neurons after cocaine withdrawal. *Nat Neurosci* **9**, 605–7.

Robinson, T. E. & Becker, J. B. 1986 Enduring changes in brain and behavior produced by chronic amphetamine administration: a review and evaluation of animal models of amphetamine psychosis. *Brain Res Rev* **396**, 157–98.

Robinson, T. E. & Berridge, K. C. 2000 The psychology and neurobiology of addiction: an incentive-sensitization view. *Addiction* **95**, S91–S117.

Robinson, T. E., Jurson, P. A., Bennett, J. A. & Bentgen, K. M. 1988 Persistent sensitization of dopamine neurotransmission in ventral striatum nucleus accumbens produced by prior experience with +-amphetamine: a microdialysis study in freely moving rats. *Brain Res* **462**, 211–22.

Rodaros, D., Caruana, D. A., Amir, S. & Stewart, J. 2007 Corticotropin-releasing factor projections from limbic forebrain and paraventricular nucleus of the hypothalamus to the region of the ventral tegmental area. *Neuroscience* , **150**, 8–13.

Saal, D., Dong, Y., Bonci, A. & Malenka, R. C. 2003 Drugs of abuse and stress trigger a common synaptic adaptation in dopamine neurons. *Neuron* **37**, 577–82.

Schmidt, H. D., Anderson, S. M. & Pierce, R. C. 2006 Stimulation of D1-like or D2 dopamine receptors in the shell, but not the core, of the nucleus accumbens reinstates cocaine-seeking behaviour in the rat. *Eur J Neurosci* **23**, 219–28.

Schulkin, J., Morgan, M. A. & Rosen, J. B. 2005 A neuroendocrine mechanism for sustaining fear. *Trends Neurosci* **28**, 629–35.

See, R. E. 2002 Neural substrates of conditioned-cued relapse to drug-seeking behavior. *Pharmacol Biochem Behav* **71**, 517–29.

Shaham, Y., Erb, S. & Stewart, J. 2000a Stress-induced relapse to heroin and cocaine seeking in rats: a review. *Brain Res Rev* **33**, 13–33.

Shaham, Y., Funk, D., Erb, S., Brown, T. J., Walker, C.-D. & Stewart, J. 1997 Corticotropin-releasing factor, but not corticosterone, is involved in stress-induced relapse to heroin-seeking in rats. *J Neurosci* **17**, 2605–14.

Shaham, Y., Highfield, D., Delfs, J., Leung, S. & Stewart, J. 2000b Clonidine blocks stress-induced reinstatement of heroin seeking in rats: an effect independent of locus coeruleus noradrenergic neurons. *Eur J Neurosci* **12**, 292–302.

Shaham, Y. & Stewart, J. 1995 Stress reinstates heroin-seeking in drug-free animals: an effect mimicking heroin, not withdrawal. *Psychopharmacology (Berl)* **119**, 334–41.

Shaham, Y. & Stewart, J. 1996 Effects of opioid and dopamine receptor antagonists on relapse induced by stress and re-exposure to heroin in rats. *Psychopharmacology (Berl)* **125**, 385–91.

Shalev, U., Grimm, J. W. & Shaham, Y. 2002 Neurobiology of relapse to heroin and cocaine seeking: a review. *Pharmacol Rev* **54**, 1–42.

Shalev, U., Hope, B., Clements, A., Morales, M. & Shaham, Y. 2001 Time-dependent changes in extinction behavior and stress-induced reinstatement of drug seeking following withdrawal from heroin in rats. *Psychopharmacology* **156**, 98–107.

Shalev, U., Marinelli, M., Baumann, M. H., Piazza, P. V. & Shaham, Y. 2003 The role of corticosterone in food deprivation-induced reinstatement of cocaine seeking in the rat. *Psychopharmacology (Berl)* **168**, 170–6.

Shen, R.-Y., Altar, C. A. & Chiodo, L. A. 1994 Brain-derived neurotrophic factor increases the electrical activity of pars compacta dopamine neurons in vivo. *Proc Natl Acad Sci USA* **91**, 8920–4.

Shepard, J. D., Bossert, J. M., Liu, S. Y. & Shaham, Y. 2004 The anxiogenic drug yohimbine reinstates methamphetamine seeking in a rat model of drug relapse. *Biol Psychiatry* **55**, 1082–9.

Sinha, R., Fuse, T., Aubin, L. R. & O'Malley, S. S. 2000 Psychological stress, drug-related cues and cocaine craving. *Psychopharmacology (Berl)* **152**, 140–8.

Sorge, R. E., Rajabi, H. & Stewart, J. 2005 Rats maintained chronically on buprenorphine show reduced heroin and cocaine seeking in tests of extinction and drug-induced reinstatement. *Neuropsychopharmacology*, **30**, 1681–92.

Sorge, R. E. & Stewart, J. 2005 The contribution of drug history and time since termination of drug taking to footshock stress-induced cocaine seeking in rats. *Psychopharmacology (Berl)* **183**, 210–17.

Sorge, R. E. & Stewart, J. 2006 The effects of chronic buprenorphine on intake of heroin and cocaine in rats and its effects on nucleus accumbens dopamine levels during self-administration. *Psychopharmacology (Berl)* **188**, 28–41.

Spealman, R. D., Lee, B., Tiefenbacher, S., Platt, D. M., Rowlett, J. K. & Khroyan, T. V. 2004 Triggers of relapse: nonhuman primate models of reinstated cocaine seeking. *Nebr Symp Motiv* **50**, 57–84.

Stewart, J. 1992 Neurobiology of conditioning to drugs of abuse. In *The Neurobiology of Drug and Alcohol Addiction. Annals of the New York Academy of Sciences*, Vol. 654 (eds. P. W. Kalivas & H. H. Samson), pp. 335–46. New York: New York Academy of Sciences.

Stewart, J. 2000 Pathways to relapse: the neurobiology of drug- and stress-induced relapse to drug taking. *J Psychiatry Neurosci* **25**, 125–36.

Stewart, J. 2004 Pathways to relapse: factors controlling the reinitiation of drug seeking after abstinence. *Nebr Symp Motiv* **50**, 197–234.

Stewart, J., de Wit, H. & Eikelboom, R. 1984 Role of unconditioned and conditioned drug effects in the self-administration of opiates and stimulants. *Psychological Review* **91**, 251–268.

Sun, W., Akins, C. K., Mattingly, A. E. & Rebec, G. V. 2005a Ionotropic glutamate receptors in the ventral tegmental area regulate cocaine-seeking behavior in rats. *Neuropsychopharmacology* **30**, 2073–81.

Sun, X., Zhao, Y. & Wolf, M. E. 2005b Dopamine receptor stimulation modulates AMPA receptor synaptic insertion in prefrontal cortex neurons. *J Neurosci* **25**, 7342–51.

Thomas, M. J., Kalivas, P. W. & Shaham, Y. 2008 Neuroplasticity in the mesolimbic dopamine system and cocaine addiction. *Br J Pharmacol* **154**, 327–42.

Ungless, M. A., Singh, V., Crowder, T. L., Yaka, R., Ron, D. & Bonci, A. 2003 Corticotropin-releasing factor requires CRF binding protein to potentiate NMDA receptors via CRF receptor 2 in dopamine neurons. *Neuron* **39**, 401–7.

Ungless, M. A., Whistler, J. L., Malenka, R. C. & Bonci, A. 2001 Single cocaine exposure in vivo induces long-term potentiation in dopamine neurons. *Nature* **411**, 583–7

Uslaner, J. M., Acerbo, M. J., Jones, S. A. & Robinson, T. E. 2006 The attribution of incentive salience to a stimulus that signals an intravenous injection of cocaine. *Behav Brain Res* **169**, 320–4.

Vezina, P. 1993 Amphetamine injected into the ventral tegmental area sensitizes the nucleus accumbens dopaminergic response to systemic amphetamine: an in vivo microdialysis study in the rat. *Brain Res* **605**, 332–7.

Vezina, P. 2004 Sensitization of midbrain dopamine neuron reactivity and the self-administration of psychomotor stimulant drugs. *Neurosci Biobehav Rev* **27**, 827–39.

Vezina, P. (ed.) 2007 Sensitization, drug addiction and psychophathology in animals and humans. *Prog Neuro-Psychopharmacol Biol Psychiatry*, 31, 1553–5.

Vezina, P., Lorrain, D. S., Arnold, G. M., Austin, J. D. & Suto, N. 2002 Sensitization of midbrain dopamine neuron reactivity promotes the pursuit of amphetamine. *J Neurosci* **22**, 4654–62.

Vezina, P. & Stewart, J. 1990 Amphetamine administered to the ventral tegmental area but not to the nucleus accumbens sensitizes rats to systemic morphine: lack of conditioned effects. *Brain Res* **516**, 99–106.

Wanat, M. J., Hopf, F. W., Stuber, G. D., Phillips, P. E. & Bonci, A. 2008 Corticotropin-releasing factor increases mouse ventral tegmental area dopamine neuron firing through a protein kinase C-dependent enhancement of Ih. *J Physiol* **586**, 2157–70.

Wang, B., Shaham, Y., Zitzman, D., Azari, S., Wise, R. A. & You, Z. B. 2005 Cocaine experience establishes control of midbrain glutamate and dopamine by corticotropin-releasing factor: a role in stress-induced relapse to drug seeking. *J Neurosci* **25**, 5389–96.

Weiss, F. 2005 Neurobiology of craving, conditioned reward and relapse. *Curr Opin Pharmacol* **5**, 9–19.

Wikler, A. 1973 Dynamics of drug dependence, implication of a conditioning theory for research and treatment. *Arch Gen Psychiatry* **28**, 611–16.

Wikler, A. & Pescor, F. T. 1967 Classical conditioning of a morphine abstinence phenomenon, reinforcement of opioid-drinking behavior and 'relapse' in morphine-addicted rats. *Psychopharmacologia* **20**, 255–84.

Wolf, M. E. 1998 The role of excitatory amino acids in behavioral sensitization to psychomotor stimulants. *Prog Neurobiol* **54**, 679–720.

Wolf, M. E., White, F. J. & Hu, X. T. 1994 MK-801 prevents alterations in the mesoaccumbens dopamine system associated with behavioral sensitization to amphetamine. *J Neurosci* **14**, 1735–45.

Wolf, M. E., White, F. J., Nassar, R. N., Brooderson, R. J. & Khansa, M. R. 1993 Differential development of autoreceptor supersensitivity and enhanced dopamine release during amphetamine sensitization. *J Pharmacol Exp Therap* **264**, 249–55.

You, Z. B., Wang, B., Zitzman, D., Azari, S. & Wise, R. A. 2007 A role for conditioned ventral tegmental glutamate release in cocaine seeking. *J Neurosci* **27**, 10546–55.

Zhao, Y., Dayas, C. V., Aujla, H., Baptista, M. A., Martin-Fardon, R. & Weiss, F. 2006 Activation of group II metabotropic glutamate receptors attenuates both stress and cue-induced ethanol-seeking and modulates c-fos expression in the hippocampus and amygdala. *J Neurosci* **26**, 9967–74.

Zhou, W. & Kalivas, P. W. 2007 *N*-acetylcysteine reduces extinction responding and induces enduring reductions in cue- and heroin-induced drug-seeking. *Biol Psychiatry* **63**, 338–40.

Part 2

Extending the Concept of Addiction

6

Neurobiology of nicotine dependence

*Athina Markou**

Nicotine is a psychoactive ingredient in tobacco that significantly contributes to the harmful tobacco smoking habit. Nicotine dependence is more prevalent than dependence on any other substance. Preclinical research in animal models of the various aspects of nicotine dependence suggests a critical role of glutamate, γ-aminobutyric acid (GABA), acetylcholine, and dopamine neurotransmitter interactions in the ventral tegmental area and possibly other brain sites, such as the central nucleus of the amygdala and the prefrontal cortex, in the effects of nicotine. Specifically, decreasing glutamate transmission or increasing GABA transmission with pharmacological manipulations decreased the rewarding effects of nicotine and cue-induced reinstatement of nicotine seeking. Furthermore, early nicotine withdrawal is characterized by decreased function of presynaptic inhibitory metabotropic glutamate 2/3 receptors and increased expression of postsynaptic glutamate receptor subunits in limbic and frontal brain sites, while protracted abstinence may be associated with increased glutamate response to stimuli associated with nicotine administration. Finally, adaptations in nicotinic acetylcholine receptor function are also involved in nicotine dependence. These neuroadaptations probably develop to counteract the decreased glutamate and cholinergic transmission that is hypothesized to characterize early nicotine withdrawal. In conclusion, glutamate, GABA, and cholinergic transmission in limbic and frontal brain sites are critically involved in nicotine dependence.

Key Words: Nicotine; dependence; withdrawal; glutamate; γ-aminobutyric acid; reinstatement.

6.1 Tobacco, nicotine, and neuronal nicotinic acetylcholine receptors

Nicotine is one of the main psychoactive ingredients in tobacco that contributes to the harmful tobacco smoking habit (Stolerman & Jarvis 1995; Royal College of Physicians of London 2000), leading to high morbidity and mortality throughout the world (Murray & Lopez 1997). Nicotine dependence is more prevalent than dependence on any other substance of abuse (Anthony et al. 1994). Unfortunately, quit rates remain low despite the availability of several pharmacological treatments aimed at cessation of tobacco smoking (Haas et al. 2004). This article will summarize our current knowledge of the neurobiology of nicotine dependence, with emphasis on the glutamate and γ-aminobutyric acid (GABA) neurotransmitter systems. Although other ingredients in tobacco smoke and metabolites, such as monoamine oxidase inhibitors and nornicotine, are recognized to contribute to tobacco addiction (DeNoble & Mele 1983; Crooks & Dwoskin 1997; Bardo et al. 1999; Belluzzi et al. 2005; Guillem et al. 2006), most neurobiological research has focused on delineating the neurobiology of nicotine dependence as a first step towards discovering the neurosubstrates of tobacco addiction.

Nicotine is an alkaloid that acts as an agonist at brain and peripheral nicotinic acetylcholine receptors (nAChRs). Neuronal nAChRs are ligand-gated ion channels comprising five membrane-spanning subunits that combine to form a functional receptor (Changeux & Taly 2008) and include nine isoforms of the neuronal α-subunit (α 2–α10) and three isoforms of

* amarkou@ucsd. edu

the neuronal β-subunit (β2–β4). These subunits combine with a stoichiometry of two α- and three β-, or five α7-subunits to form nAChRs with distinct pharmacologic and kinetic properties. Acetylcholine is the endogenous neurotransmitter that binds and activates nAChRs. Many nAChRs are situated on presynaptic terminals and modulate neurotransmitter release (Wonnacott 1997). Nevertheless, nAChRs also are located at somatodendritic, axonal, and postsynaptic sites. Owing to the wide distribution of nAChRs, administration of nicotine stimulates the release of most neurotransmitters throughout the brain (McGehee & Role 1995). Therefore, as discussed below, various transmitter systems are probably involved in the rewarding effects of nicotine and the adaptations that occur in response to chronic nicotine exposure that gives rise to dependence and withdrawal responses.

6.2 Behavioural effects of acute nicotine and nicotine withdrawal

In humans, acute nicotine administration produces positive effects, including mild euphoria and mildly enhanced cognition. Such subjective positive effects support reliable intravenous nicotine self-administration behaviour in a variety of species, including rats, mice, non-human primates, and humans (e.g. Markou & Paterson 2001; for a review, see Picciotto & Corrigall 2002). Persistent nicotine use leads to tolerance that is mediated by neuroadaptations occurring in response to chronic nicotine exposure. Thus, within hours upon cessation of nicotine exposure, a nicotine withdrawal syndrome emerges characterized by depressed mood, irritability, mild cognitive deficits, and physiological symptoms (Shiffman et al. 2004).

The avoidance of these withdrawal syndromes, as well as the positive subjective effects of nicotine, motivates nicotine use (Kenny & Markou 2001). In addition, similar to other psychomotor stimulants, nicotine enhances the reward value of other stimuli (Harrison et al. 2002). Owing to the relatively mild euphorigenic properties of nicotine, the contribution of the reward-enhancing effects to maintaining dependence is hypothesized to be greater for nicotine than other drugs of abuse (Chaudhri et al. 2006; Kenny & Markou 2006). Finally, learning processes also contribute to nicotine dependence. Environmental stimuli predictively associated with either the positive subjective effects of nicotine or the induction of nicotine withdrawal motivate nicotine seeking and eventually drug consumption (Paterson et al. 2004; Kenny et al. 2006).

In rats, nicotine withdrawal is characterized by both increases in somatic signs of withdrawal and affective changes analogous to the effects observed in humans. These affective changes include increased anxiety-like behaviour and reward deficits. A method that is used to assess the effects of stress in rats is the light-potentiated startle procedure. In this procedure, baseline startle responding to a loud startling stimulus in the dark is compared with startle responding when the chamber is brightly lit. Bright illumination is aversive for rats and potentiates the startle response, reflecting increased reactivity to a noxious environmental stimulus under stressful conditions. Hence, this procedure allows comparisons of withdrawal effects on startle reactivity between relatively neutral and stressful contexts. Spontaneous withdrawal from chronic nicotine exposure enhanced light-potentiated startle compared with control vehicle-treated rats, while baseline startle reactivity remained unaffected (Jonkman et al. 2007). These results suggest that spontaneous nicotine withdrawal selectively potentiates responses to anxiogenic stimuli but does not by itself produce a strong anxiogenic-like effect.

A procedure that assesses brain reward function and potentially depression-like reward deficits characterizing nicotine withdrawal is the intracranial self-stimulation (ICSS) procedure. Brief electrical stimulation of brain reward sites, commonly applied along the medial forebrain bundle, is extremely rewarding. Rats will readily perform an operant task to self-stimulate specific brain reward sites. Nicotine enhances the reward value of such electrical stimulation, resulting in the rats requiring lower current intensities than under baseline conditions to perceive the stimulation as rewarding after the administration of nicotine (Harrison et al. 2002). By contrast, withdrawal from chronic nicotine exposure results in elevations in brain reward thresholds, reflecting a reward deficit and indicating that the rats require higher current intensities to perceive the stimulation as rewarding (Epping-Jordan et al. 1998). Similar reward deficits are seen when nAChR antagonists are administered to rats that are chronically treated with nicotine, while the same doses of the nAChR antagonists have no effect in control vehicle-treated rats (Epping-Jordan et al. 1998; Watkins et al. 2000). Such reward deficits can also be associated through classical conditioning processes to environmental stimuli and come to elicit a conditioned nicotine withdrawal state. Pairing of environmental stimuli, such as a flashing light, with the effects of the nAChR antagonist dihydro-β-erythroidine (DHβE) in nicotine-dependent rats resulted in the presentation of the light alone leading to small, but statistically significant and reliable, elevations in brain reward thresholds (Kenny & Markou 2006; Fig. 6.1). Such effects were not seen in rats that

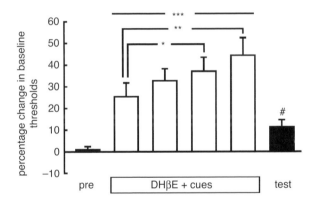

Fig. 6.1 Reward thresholds in nicotine-dependent rats treated with nAChR antagonist+cues. Conditioned nicotine withdrawal decreased the activity of brain reward systems. Rats trained in the ICSS procedure were prepared with subcutaneous osmotic minipumps containing nicotine (3.16 mg kg^{-1} per day base) or saline. Several days were allowed to elapse so that nicotine dependence would develop in the nicotine-treated rats. Then, all rats were treated with the nAChR antagonist DHβE and allowed to perform in the ICSS procedure again while a flashing light was on for the duration of the ICSS session. In this graph, only data from rats that were nicotine dependent and were treated with DHβE paired with the flashing lights are presented ($n = 8$). The results indicated a gradual increase in nAChR antagonist-precipitated nicotine withdrawal with repeated pairings of the cue flashing lights with DHβE administration. On the test day, rats were injected with saline and presented with the cue lights. The presentation of the cue light alone was sufficient to induce a small but statistically significant elevation in brain reward thresholds, similar in direction but smaller in magnitude than nicotine withdrawal precipitated by administration of the nAChR antagonist. Data from three control groups, including a group that was not nicotine dependent and did not experience explicit pairings of the cue lights with the nAChR antagonist injection, did not show such conditioned effects. Data are shown as percent change from baseline ICSS thresholds (+ s.e.m.) in paired rats on the preconditioning day (pre), during the cue/injection pairings (DHβE + cues), and on the test day when rats were presented with the cues and injected with saline. ***$p < 0.001$, **$p < 0.01$, *$p < 0.05$, compared with thresholds obtained on the preconditioning day (*post hoc* test after significant one-way analysis of variance); $^{#}p < 0.05$, compared with preconditioning day (paired *t*-test). Adapted from Kenny & Markou (2005).

had equal exposure to the light, nicotine, and the nAChR antagonist but without explicit pairings of the effects of the nAChR antagonist and the cue lights. These findings are highly relevant to the learning mechanisms that contribute to the maintenance of drug dependence because they indicate that environmental stimuli predictively paired with drug withdrawal may lead to a conditioned drug withdrawal state (Kenny & Markou 2006) that can motivate increased drug use (Kenny et al. 2006).

6.3 Neurosubstrates of nicotine reward, dependence, and withdrawal

In the midbrain of mammals, interconnected brain structures are referred to as the meso-corticolimbic brain system. This system has been shown to be critically involved in the effects of several drugs of abuse. A component of this system is the dopaminergic projection from the ventral tegmental area (VTA) to the nucleus accumbens, amygdala, and frontal cortex. The activity of these VTA dopamine neurons is regulated by the release of the excitatory neurotransmitter glutamate that is released from projections originating from several sites, including the nucleus accumbens and the frontal cortex. Other inputs that also regulate mesolimbic system activity are GABA inhibitory interneurons located within the VTA and the nucleus accumbens, and cholinergic projections from brainstem nuclei to the VTA. The latter projections release the endogenous neurotransmitter acetylcholine that acts on excitatory nAChRs located on glutamate and GABA neuronal terminals in the VTA (Fig. 6.2). Extensive research findings demonstrate a critical role of glutamate–GABA–dopamine–acetylcholine interactions, particularly in the VTA (a brain region that has been studied extensively), in several behavioural and affective responses to nicotine. Nevertheless, other brain sites not researched as extensively as the VTA are likely to also contribute to nicotine dependence.

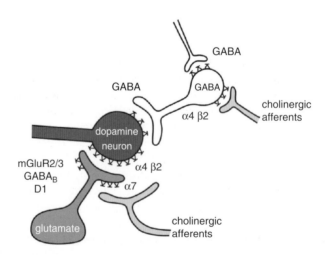

Fig. 6.2 Nicotine-acetylcholine-glutamate-GABA-dopamine interactions in the VTA. Schematic depicting neurotransmitter interactions in the VTA, which are hypothesized to be critically involved in mediating various effects of nicotine with relevance to nicotine dependence and withdrawal. Neuroadaptations have been shown to develop to several of these receptor and transmitter systems with the development of nicotine dependence. Adapted from Mansvelder & McGehee (2002); see text for details.

Exogenously administered nicotine increases dopamine transmission by direct stimulation of nAChRs, primarily α4β2-containing and α7 homomeric nAChRs within the VTA. Nicotine stimulates nAChRs on glutamatergic terminals that release glutamate, an excitatory neurotransmitter, which results in increased dopamine release in the nucleus accumbens and the frontal cortex. Nicotine also excites nAChRs on GABA-releasing terminals. Thus, the levels of GABA, an inhibitory neurotransmitter, are increased by nicotine as well. However, the interplay between the quick desensitization of nAChRs on the GABA neuron and the higher doses of nicotine required to desensitize the α7 homomeric nAChRs on the glutamate neuron results in a greater overall increase in dopamine levels (Fig. 6.2). Interestingly, nAChRs in the VTA play a more important role than those in the nucleus accumbens in the effects of nicotine on the release of nucleus accumbens dopamine (Nisell et al. 1997). Consistent with these neurochemical data, behavioural data indicated that injections of the competitive nAChR antagonist DHβE into the VTA but not into the nucleus accumbens (Corrigall et al. 1994), or lesions of the mesolimbic dopaminergic projections from the VTA to the nucleus accumbens (Corrigall et al. 1992), or cholinergic lesions of the brainstem pedunculopontine nucleus that projects to the VTA (Lança et al. 2000), or systemic administration of dopamine receptor antagonists (Corrigall & Coen 1991) decreased intravenous nicotine self-administration in rats. In terms of nAChR subtypes, studies suggest an involvement of α4β2-containing nAChR subtypes in both the nicotine-induced release of dopamine and nicotine reinforcement (Picciotto et al. 1998). In addition, mutant mice with hypersensitive α4-containing nAChRs show a 50-fold increase in sensitivity to the reinforcing effects of nicotine measured by a conditioned place preference procedure (Tapper et al. 2004). The role of α7 homomeric receptors in the reinforcing effects of nicotine remains unclear, with conflicting data provided by studies in mutant mice lacking the α7 receptor and rats injected with the relatively selective α7 nAChR antagonist methyllycaconitine (Markou & Paterson 2001; Besson et al. 2007).

6.3.1 Glutamate

Glutamate is the major excitatory neurotransmitter in the brain, which plays a critical role in the acute and long-term effects of nicotine. The actions of glutamate are regulated by ionotropic and metabotropic glutamate (mGlu) receptors. Ionotropic glutamate receptors are primarily located postsynaptically, are glutamate-gated ion channels that when activated increase cellular excitability, and comprise the following receptor subtypes: N-methyl-D-aspartate (NMDA), α-amino-3-hydroxy-5-methyl-4-isoxazole-propionate (AMPA), and kainate. Eight mammalian mGlu receptor subtypes have been identified and classified into three groups (I, II, and III) based on sequence homology, signal transduction pathways and pharmacological selectivity (for review, Kenny & Markou 2004). Group I (mGlu1 and mGlu5) receptors are predominately located postsynaptically where they couple to G_q-proteins to activate phospholipase C. In addition, group I receptors couple to intracellular Homer proteins that play an important role in trafficking mGlu receptors in and out of the synapses and functionally connect metabotropic to ionotropic glutamate receptors. Group II (mGlu2 and mGlu3) receptors are primarily found presynaptically and also on glial cells and couple to $G_{i/o}$ proteins to negatively regulate adenylyl cyclase activity. Group III (mGlu4, mGlu6, mGlu7, and mGlu8) receptors are predominately presynaptic autoreceptors coupled to $G_{i/o}$-proteins to decrease adenylyl cyclase activity. Thus, mGlu receptors are slow acting and modulate glutamate transmission. They are also widely, but differentially, expressed in the brain. Hence, these receptors offer unique opportunities to alter in pharmacologically subtle ways glutamate transmission, and thus affect motivated behaviour and affective processes without producing gross undesirable or toxic side effects (Markou 2007).

As discussed above, nicotine increases glutamate release by agonist actions at excitatory presynaptic nAChRs on glutamatergic terminals in various brain sites, including the VTA, nucleus accumbens, prefrontal cortex, and hippocampus (for reviews, see Mansvelder & McGehee 2002; Kenny & Markou 2004). Furthermore, glutamatergic afferents project from areas such as the frontal cortex, amygdala, and hippocampus to brain sites that contain dopaminergic cell bodies or terminals, such as the VTA and the nucleus accumbens (for a review, see Kenny & Markou 2004). Indeed, experimenter-administered nicotine has been shown to increase glutamate levels in the VTA (Fu et al. 2000), which presumably acts at metabotropic and ionotropic glutamate receptors on postsynaptic dopamine neurons and increases their bursting activity and neurotransmitter release. Considerable evidence suggests that these actions partly mediate the reinforcing effects of acute nicotine.

Specifically, the blockade of postsynaptic mGlu5 receptors with 2-methyl-6-(phenylethynyl)-pyridine (MPEP) decreased intravenous nicotine self-administration in rats and mice (Paterson et al. 2003) and also decreased the motivation to self-administer nicotine assessed by the progressive-ratio schedule of reinforcement (Paterson & Markou 2005). Furthermore, the blockade of postsynaptic NMDA receptors either globally via systemic administration of an NMDA receptor antagonist or via injections of the NMDA receptor antagonist directly into the VTA or the central nucleus of the amygdala decreased intravenous nicotine self-administration in rats (Kenny et al. 2009). The effects of mGlu5 and NMDA receptor antagonists on intravenous nicotine self-administration are both seen at doses that have no effects on responding for food reinforcement under similar schedules of reinforcement or reinforcement schedules that equate overall rates of responding for nicotine and food. The effects of the glutamate compounds on nicotine self-administration are likely to be mediated by attenuation of nicotine-stimulated glutamate transmission in the mesolimbic system via the blockade of postsynaptic mGlu5 or NMDA receptors. Finally, the administration of LY379268, an mGlu2/3 receptor agonist, systemically or directly into the posterior VTA or the nucleus accumbens shell, dose-dependently decreased nicotine self-administration at doses that had no effect on responding for food. Considering that mGlu2/3 receptors are located presynaptically and negatively modulate glutamate release, the latter data are consistent with the NMDA and mGlu5 receptor data that indicate that decreasing glutamate transmission blocks the rewarding effects of nicotine, thus leading to decreases in nicotine self-administration. Unfortunately, however, rapid tolerance occurred to the LY379268-induced decreases in nicotine self-administration, possibly attributable to the rapid adaptations in function that these receptors have been shown to exhibit (see below). This potential tolerance is unfortunate and may limit the potential usefulness of mGlu2/3 receptors as targets for the treatment of nicotine dependence. Medications for smoking cessation, therefore, would need to be administered chronically to humans to aid in smoking cessation. The chronic effects of repeatedly administering other glutamate compounds that have been shown to decrease nicotine self-administration in rats have not yet been investigated.

As discussed previously, in addition to the primary rewarding effects of nicotine, it also enhances the reward value of other rewarding stimuli (Harrison et al. 2002). Nicotine enhances the reward value of brain stimulation reward so that rats require lower current intensities than under baseline conditions to perceive the stimulation as rewarding (Harrison et al. 2002). Similarly to the primary rewarding effects of nicotine, the reward-enhancing effects of nicotine were also blocked by the administration of an mGlu5 receptor antagonist or an mGlu2/3 receptor agonist, compounds that both decrease glutamate transmission

(Harrison et al. 2002). However, this 'blockade' of the reward-enhancing effects of nicotine may be a 'non-specific effect'. The effects of nicotine and glutamatergic compounds are additive. That is, nicotine enhances brain reward function, and the glutamate compounds decrease brain reward function, resulting in an apparent blockade of the reward-enhancing effects of nicotine. Although these effects appear to be pharmacologically additive coupled with the ability of these compounds to decrease nicotine self-administration, these additive effects on nicotine-induced enhancement of reward may be clinically relevant. These compounds may block the ability of tobacco smoking to enhance the reward value of environmental stimuli and thus remove a source of motivation to smoke tobacco.

With chronic exposure to nicotine and the development of nicotine dependence, adaptations in glutamate neurotransmission occur, which are likely to mediate the behavioural signs of nicotine withdrawal. In a series of studies, we investigated adaptations in glutamate receptors that may mediate the deficits in brain reward function measured by elevations in ICSS thresholds associated with nicotine withdrawal in rats. The mGlu2/3 receptor agonist LY314582 precipitated withdrawal-like elevations in ICSS thresholds, a sensitive measure of reward function, in nicotine-dependent but not in control rats. LY314582 did not affect response latencies, a measure of performance in the ICSS paradigm. These effects were seen either when LY314582 was injected systemically or when microinfused directly into the VTA (Kenny et al. 2003). These behavioural data suggest that altered function/number of mGlu2/3 receptors, particularly in the VTA, after chronic exposure to nicotine renders them more sensitive to the effects of an agonist. This interpretation is corroborated by recent findings demonstrating that 24 hours after the last daily intravenous nicotine self-administration session, mGlu2/3 receptor function was downregulated, demonstrated by decreased coupling of mGlu2/3 receptors to G-proteins in the $[^{35}S]$GTPγS-binding assay in all brain sites assessed, including the VTA, prefrontal cortex, nucleus accumbens, amygdala, hippocampus, and hypothalamus (Fig. 6.3). Because mGlu2/3 receptors mainly function as inhibitory autoreceptors to control glutamate release, this decrease in mGlu2/3 receptor function indicates impaired negative feedback control on glutamatergic terminals, possibly to counteract the decreased glutamate transmission that probably characterizes early nicotine withdrawal. Consistent with this interpretation, a single injection of the Glu2/3 receptor antagonist LY341495 attenuated the threshold elevations observed in rats undergoing spontaneous nicotine withdrawal (Kenny et al. 2003).

To further explore whether alterations in mGlu2/3 receptor function contribute to nicotine withdrawal by decreasing glutamatergic transmission, we examined whether direct blockade of postsynaptic glutamate receptors precipitated withdrawal-like reward deficits in nicotine-dependent rats. Indeed, the AMPA/kainate receptor antagonist NBQX precipitated withdrawal-like threshold elevations in nicotine-dependent but not in control rats, indicating that decreased glutamate neurotransmission through these receptors contributes to the reward deficits associated with nicotine withdrawal. This conclusion is corroborated by findings showing that 24 hours after nicotine self-administration, increased postsynaptic expression levels of the following were observed: (i) NMDA receptor NR2A subunit in the VTA, (ii) NR1, NR2A and NR2B subunits in the central nucleus of the amygdala, (iii) AMPA receptor GluR1 and GluR2 subunits in the central nucleus of the amygdale, and (iv) GluR1 subunit in the nucleus accumbens (Kenny et al. 2009). Additionally, decreased expression levels of the NR2A, NR2B and Glu2 subunits were observed in the prefrontal cortex, and these effects were similar to those seen previously in rat brains immediately after prolonged nicotine self-administration sessions (Wang et al. 2007). This increased expression of ionotropic glutamate receptor subunits may reflect compensatory changes in the glutamatergic system

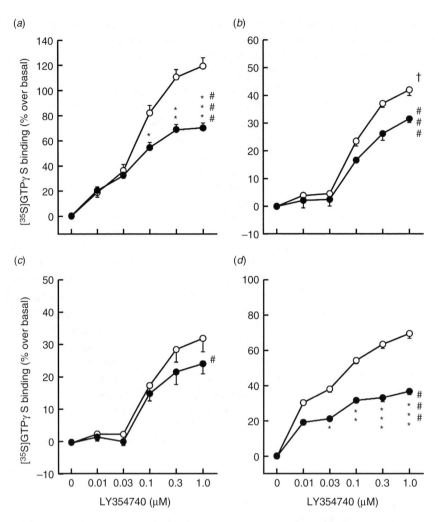

Fig. 6.3 Effects of 24-hour withdrawal from nicotine or food self-administration on functional coupling of mGlu2/3 receptors to G-proteins. Stimulation of [^{35}S]GTPγS binding by the mGlu2/3 receptor agonist LY354740 was significantly decreased in rats self-administering nicotine (filled circles) compared with animals responding for food (open circles), suggesting mGlu2/3 receptor downregulation in all assessed brain areas (LY354740 × reward interactions, [#]$p < 0.05$, [###]$p < 0.001$, [*]$p < 0.05$, [**]$p < 0.01$, [***]$p < 0.001$, difference from food). Data are expressed as mean ± s.e.m., $n=6$. Adapted from Liechti et al. (2007). (*a*) Prefrontal cortex, (*b*) nucleus accumbens, (*c*) VTA, (*d*) amygdala.

to counteract the effects of decreased glutamate transmission associated with the nicotine withdrawal state. Interestingly, the opposite effects (i.e. decreases rather than increases) in the expression of postsynaptic glutamate receptor subunits were seen in the prefrontal cortex in these same subjects, indicating that different brain sites may mediate different aspects of nicotine dependence. For example, increased activity of glutamatergic projections from the prefrontal cortex to the nucleus accumbens has been shown to play an important role in cocaine seeking (Moran et al. 2005), and the same appears to be true for nicotine (Liechti et al. 2007). Thus, increased glutamate neurotransmission appears to occur during nicotine self-administration and perhaps during nicotine seeking, while decreased glutamate transmission occurs during early nicotine withdrawal that probably mediates the reward deficits, and perhaps other behavioural effects, associated with nicotine withdrawal and low nicotine seeking. Interestingly, however, MPEP or dizocilpine, antagonists at mGlu5 and NMDA receptors, respectively, did not precipitate reward deficits in nicotine-dependent rats. Overall, these data demonstrate that mGlu2/3 receptors play an important role in generating the reward deficits associated with nicotine withdrawal, in part by decreasing glutamate transmission at AMPA/kainate receptors (Markou 2007). Nevertheless, although antagonists at mGlu5 receptors decrease the rewarding effects of nicotine self-administration (Paterson et al. 2003; see above) and block cue-induced reinstatement (Bespalov et al. 2005; see below), these receptors do not appear to show adaptations in function/number with the development of nicotine dependence.

Finally, glutamate appears to play an important role in the reinstatement of nicotine-seeking behaviour seen during protracted abstinence. Systemic administration of the mGlu5 receptor antagonist MPEP (Bespalov et al. 2005) or the mGlu2/3 receptor agonist LY379268 (Liechti et al. 2007) decreased cue-induced reinstatement of nicotine seeking in rats. In the case of MPEP, no effects on cue-induced reinstatement of food were observed. In the case of LY379268, similar doses decreased cue-induced reinstatement of either nicotine or food seeking, suggesting that stimulatory actions at presynaptic inhibitory mGlu2/3 receptors have general effects on the motivational impact of conditioned reinforcers. Thus, protracted abstinence may be associated with an enhanced glutamate response to environmental stimuli that have motivational significance, and this response may be blocked by compounds that directly (e.g. antagonists at postsynaptic glutamate receptors) or indirectly (agonists at presynaptic inhibitory glutamate receptors) diminish the glutamate response to the stimuli (Moran et al. 2005).

6.3.2 γ-Aminobutyric acid

GABA is the major inhibitory transmitter in the brain and another transmitter system critically involved in the reinforcing effects of acute nicotine administration. GABAergic afferents to the VTA from the pedunculopontine tegmental nucleus, ventral pallidum, and nucleus accumbens, as well as GABA interneurons within the VTA and medium spiny GABA neurons in the nucleus accumbens, inhibit dopaminergic mesocorticolimbic activity (Klitenick et al. 1992). As discussed previously and depicted in Fig. 6.1, complex interactions occur between the GABA, dopaminergic and glutamatergic systems in the VTA (Mansvelder & McGehee 2002). Increased GABAergic transmission abolishes both the nicotine-induced dopamine increases in the nucleus accumbens and the reinforcing effects of nicotine (Dewey et al. 1999; Brebner et al. 2002). γ-Vinyl GABA (GVG; also referred to as vigabatrin) is an irreversible inhibitor of GABA transaminase, the primary enzyme involved in GABA metabolism. Thus, administration of GVG increases GABA levels, and accordingly decreases nicotine self-administration (Paterson & Markou 2002) and abolishes both the acquisition and the expression of conditioned place preference (Dewey et al. 1998). GVG administration also dose-dependently lowered nicotine-induced increases in nucleus accumbens dopamine in both naive and chronically nicotine-treated rats and blocked nicotine-induced increases in striatal dopamine in primates as measured by positron emission tomography (Brebner et al. 2002).

The use of receptor-selective agonists suggests the involvement of $GABA_B$ receptors in these effects. Two receptors bind the endogenous neurotransmitter GABA: $GABA_A$ ionotropic receptors and $GABA_B$ metabotropic receptors. Both $GABA_A$ and $GABA_B$ receptors are inhibitory and both are found presynaptically and postsynaptically. Systemic injections or microinjections of baclofen or CGP44532 [(3-amino-2[S]-hydroxypro-pyl)-methylphosphonic acid], two $GABA_B$ receptor agonists, into the nucleus accumbens shell, VTA or pedunculopontine tegmental nucleus that sends cholinergic, GABAergic and glutamatergic projections to the VTA (but not injections into the caudate-putamen) decreased the reinforcing effects of nicotine (Shoaib et al. 1998; Corrigall et al. 2000, 2001; Fattore et al. 2002; Paterson et al. 2004; Fig. 6.4a). These decreases in nicotine self-administration persisted even after chronic administration of CGP44532 for 14 days, indicating little tolerance to this effect of the $GABA_B$ receptor agonist with this length of treatment (Paterson et al. 2005b). The issue of tolerance is important because drug therapies currently need to be administered chronically to humans for smoking cessation. However, in studies of rats, GVG and $GABA_B$ receptor agonists also decreased responding for food, although at higher doses than the threshold doses for inducing decreases in nicotine self-administration (Paterson & Markou 2002; Paterson et al. 2004, 2005b; Fig. 6.4a). These effects on responding for food may reflect nonspecific performance effects of the GABAergic compounds or specific effects on food intake. The latter possibility is intriguing because abstinence-associated weight gain is often a concern for smokers, especially women, who wish to quit smoking cigarettes. Finally, the $GABA_B$

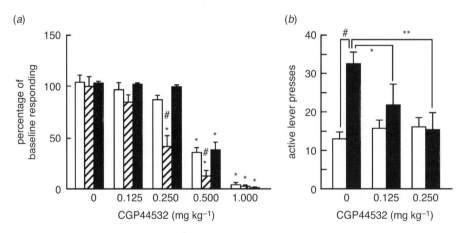

Fig. 6.4 Acute administration of the $GABA_B$ receptor agonist CGP44532 decreased nicotine self-administration and cue-induced reinstatement of nicotine seeking. a: Primary rewarding effects: nicotine was available for self-administration at either of two doses (0.01 or 0.03 mg kg^{-1} per infusion base). Rats were trained to respond for nicotine or food under a fixed-ratio 5, timeout 20 s schedule of reinforcement. CGP44532 administration decreased both nicotine and food self-administration but affected nicotine self-administration at doses lower than those that decreased food self-administration. Data are expressed as percentage of baseline responding (mean+s.e.m.). *$p < 0.05$, difference from vehicle pretreatment condition. #$p < 0.05$, difference from the group that responded for food and received the same CGP44532 dose. Adapted from Paterson et al. (2004). Open bars, 0.03 mgkg^{-1} per infusions of nicotine (n= 10); hatched bars, 0.01 mgkg^{-1} per infusions of nicotine (n = 8); filled bars, food (n = 12). b: CGP44532 administration blocked cue-induced reinstatement of nicotine seeking in rats. A within-subjects design was used in which all rats (n = 8) received all doses of CGP44532. Between drug treatments, rats were returned to extinction conditions. *$p < 0.05$, **$p < 0.01$, difference from saline pretreatment. #$p < 0.05$, difference between the test day and the preceding 3-day baseline. Data are expressed as mean number of lever presses +s.e.m. Adapted from Paterson et al. (2005b). Open bars, extinction conditions (n = 8); filled bars, conditioned stimulus presentation.

receptor agonist CGP44532 also blocked cue-induced reinstatement of nicotine-seeking behaviour (Fig. 6.4b). Thus, increased GABA transmission through $GABA_B$ receptor activation blocks the reinforcing effects of nicotine.

Nonetheless, $GABA_B$ receptor agonists have undesirable side effects, including disruption of performance on the rotarod test, a measure of locomotor impairment (Cryan et al. 2004), and decreased responding for non-drug rewards, such as food and electrical brain stimulation (Macey et al. 2001; Paterson et al. 2005a; Slattery et al. 2005). Interestingly, $GABA_B$ receptor-positive allosteric modulator compounds, such as GS39783 and the more recently synthesized BHF177, are likely to have more subtle effects than $GABA_B$ receptor agonists, due to their modulatory, rather than full agonist, properties at the receptors (Guery et al. 2007). Accordingly, such compounds do not impair performance in the rotarod test when administered alone (Cryan et al. 2004). In a series of recent studies, we demonstrated that several $GABA_B$ receptor positive allosteric modulators decreased nicotine self-administration, decreased breakpoints for nicotine under a progressive-ratio schedule of reinforcement and blocked the reward-enhancing effects of nicotine (Paterson et al. 2008). These effects were seen at a range of doses that did not affect behaviours reinforced by food. Thus, $GABA_B$ receptor-positive allosteric modulators may decrease the rewarding and reward-enhancing effects of nicotine with a better side effect profile than full $GABA_B$ receptor agonists.

6.3.3 Adaptations in nAChR function

Chronic nicotine administration leads to an interesting paradoxical change in the function of nAChRs, which consists of receptor desensitization leading to receptor upregulation (Marks et al. 1983; Schwartz & Kellar 1983; Changeux et al. 1984; Wonnacott 1990; Flores et al. 1997; Perry et al. 1999; Mansvelder et al. 2002). Complex theoretical speculations have been put forth about the role of nAChR desensitization and upregulation in the subjective effects of acute nicotine and in the development and maintenance of nicotine dependence (Marks et al. 1992; Dani & Heinemann 1996; Buisson & Bertrand 2002; Quick & Lester 2002). Long-term exposure to nicotine induces an increase in the number (Wonnacott 1990; Marks et al. 1992; Buisson & Bertrand 2001) and function (Rowell & Wonnacott 1990) of nAChRs. Nevertheless, this finding is not consistently demonstrated; others have observed a decrease in nAChR number (Gentry et al. 2003) and function (Marks et al. 1993) with chronic exposure to nicotine. Most studies reporting changes in nAChR number and function have been conducted in *in vitro* experimental designs, and the functional significance of these changes *in vivo* is unknown (Buisson & Bertrand 2002) and needs to be explored (Kellar et al. 1999). Behavioural findings are most readily explained by decreased number and/or function of nAChRs with the development of nicotine dependence that counteract the continuous agonist actions of nicotine on the receptors. Specifically, administration of a variety of nAChR antagonists induces withdrawal-like changes in rats exposed to nicotine at doses that have no effect in saline-treated subjects (Epping-Jordan et al. 1998; Watkins et al. 2000; Markou & Paterson 2001; Skjei & Markou 2003). Furthermore, different subtypes of nAChRs desensitize and upregulate at different rates, which may explain the seemingly opposite effects seen in some studies (Kellar et al. 1999; Buisson & Bertrand 2002; Levin 2002; Mansvelder et al. 2002). For example, Mansvelder & McGehee (2002) have shown rapid desensitization of the α4β2 nAChR located on GABAergic terminals and no changes in α7 nAChR function located on glutamatergic terminals in the VTA. Behaviourally, we observe the net effect of these complex adaptations in different receptor types and brain sites. Thus, adaptations in nAChR number and function probably contribute to the various aspects of nicotine dependence and the difficulty in achieving and sustaining nicotine abstinence.

6.4 Conclusions

Ample evidence indicates that cholinergic–glutamatergic–GABAergic–dopaminergic inter-actions in limbic brain sites, such as the VTA (Fig. 6.2), are critically involved in the primary rewarding effects of nicotine, and possibly the reward-enhancing effects of nicotine. Although many investigations have been conducted that focus on the VTA, it should be emphasized that other brain sites, such as the central nucleus of the amygdala and the frontal cortex, are probably involved in the behavioural effects of nicotine with relevance to dependence. Nicotine-induced changes in these brain sites have started to be investigated, as well as how manipulations of these brain sites may impact on the effects of nicotine (e.g. Liechti et al. 2007; Wang et al. 2007; Kenny et al. 2009). Accordingly, compounds that decrease glutamate transmission either through presynaptic or postsynaptic action, or enhance GABA function through $GABA_B$ receptors, decrease the primary rewarding effects of nicotine, the motivation to self-administer nicotine and the reward-enhancing effects of nicotine, as well as the motivational impact of stimuli previously associated with nicotine administration. Furthermore, neurochemical and behavioural evidence demonstrates pro-found changes in glutamate transmission in limbic brain sites, such as the VTA, nucleus accumbens, amygdala and frontal cortex, which are likely to be critically involved in the development of dependence and the expression of affective signs of nicotine withdrawal upon cessation of drug administration. As anticipated, the changes in nAChR receptor number and function are also observed with the development of nicotine dependence, with different receptors showing differential changes in response to chronic nicotine exposure. By contrast, no evidence has shown adaptations in GABA function with the development of nicotine dependence, although this system is critically involved in the acute effects of nicotine. Thus, compounds that modulate glutamate and/or GABA transmission are likely to have therapeutic potential for treating various aspects of nicotine dependence and withdrawal.

This work was supported by research grants (R01)DA11946, (R01)DA023209 and (U01) MH69062 from the National Institutes of Health, USA. The author thanks Mike Arends for outstanding editorial assistance.

References

Anthony, J. C., Warner, L. A. & Kessler, R. C. 1994 Comparative epidemiology of dependence on tobacco, alcohol, controlled substances, and inhalants: basic findings from the National Comorbidity Survey. *Exp. Clin. Psychopharmacol.* **2**, 244–268. (doi:10.1037/1064–1297.2.3.244)

Bardo, M. T., Green, T. A., Crooks, P. A. & Dwoskin, L. P. 1999 Nornicotine is self-administered intravenously by rats. *Psychopharmacologia* **146**, 290–296. (doi:10.1007/ s002130051119)

Belluzzi, J. D., Wang, R. & Leslie, F. M. 2005 Acetaldehyde enhances acquisition of nicotine self-administration in adolescent rats. *Neuropschopharmacology* **30**, 705–712. (doi:10.1038/sj.npp. 1300586)

Bespalov, A. Y., Dravolina, O. A., Sukhanov, I., Zakharova, E., Blokhina, E., Zvartau, E., Danysz, W., van Heeke, G. & Markou, A. 2005 Metabotropic glutamate receptor (mGluR5) antagonist MPEP attenuated cue- and schedule-induced reinstatement of nicotine self-administration behavior in rats. *Neuropharmacology* **49**(Suppl. 1), 167–178. (doi:10.1016/j.neuropharm.2005.06.007)

Besson, M. et al. 2007 Long-term effects of chronic nicotine exposure on brain nicotinic receptors. *Proc. NatlAcad. Sci. USA* **104**, 8155–8160. (doi:10.1073/pnas.0702698104)

Brebner, K., Childress, A. R. & Roberts, D. C. 2002 A potential role for GABA$_B$ agonists in the treatment of psychostimulant addiction. *Alcohol Alcohol.* **37**, 478–484.

Buisson, B. & Bertrand, D. 2001 Chronic exposure to nicotine upregulates the human $\alpha 4\beta 2$ nicotinic acetyl-choline receptor function. *J. Neurosci.* **21**, 1819–1829.

Buisson, B. & Bertrand, D. 2002 Nicotine addiction: the possible role of functional upregulation. *Trends Pharmacol. Sci.* **23**, 130–136. (doi:10.1016/S0165–6147(00)01979–9)

Changeux, J.-P. & Taly, A. 2008 Nicotinic receptors, allosteric proteins and medicine. *Trends Mol. Med.* 14, 93–102. (doi:10.1016/j.molmed.2008.01.001)

Changeux, J.-P., Devillers-Thiery, A. & Chemouilli, P. 1984 Acetylcholine receptor: an allosteric protein. *Science* **225**, 1335–1345. (doi:10.1126/science.6382611)

Chaudhri, N., Caggiula, A. R., Donny, E. C., Palmatier, M. I., Liu, X. & Sved, A. F. 2006 Complex interactions between nicotine and nonpharmacological stimuli reveal multiple roles for nicotine in reinforcement. *Psychopharmacology* **184**, 353–366. (doi:10.1007/s00213–005–0178–1)

Corrigall, W. A. & Coen, K. M. 1991 Selective dopamine antagonists reduce nicotine self-administration. *Psychopharmacology* **104**, 171–176. (doi:10.1007/BF02244174)

Corrigall, W. A., Franklin, K. B. J., Coen, K. M. & Clarke, P. B. S. 1992 The mesolimbic dopaminergic system is implicated in the reinforcing effects of nicotine. *Psychopharmacology* **107**, 285–289. (doi:10.1007/BF02245149)

Corrigall, W. A., Coen, K. M. & Adamson, K. L. 1994 Self-administered nicotine activates the mesolimbic dopamine system through the ventral tegmental area. *Brain Res.* **653**, 278–284. (doi:10.1016/0006–8993(94)90401–4)

Corrigall, W. A., Coen, K. M., Adamson, K. L., Chow, B. L. C. & Zhang, J. 2000 Response of nicotine self-administration in the rat to manipulations of mu-opioid and γ-aminobu-tyric acid receptors in the ventral tegmental area. *Psychopharmacology* **149**,107–114. (doi:10.1007/s002139900355)

Corrigall, W. A., Coen, K. M., Zhang, J. & Adamson, K. L. 2001 GABA mechanisms in the pedunculopontine tegmental nucleus influence particular aspects of nicotine self-administration selectively in the rat. *Psychopharmacology* **158**, 190–197. (doi:10.1007/s002130100869)

Crooks, P. A. & Dwoskin, L. P. 1997 Contribution of CNS nicotine metabolites to the neuropharmacological effects of nicotine and tobacco smoking. *Biochem. Pharmacol.* **54**, 743–753. (doi:10.1016/S0006–2952(97)00117–2)

Cryan, J. F. et al. 2004 Behavioral characterization of the novel GABA$_B$ receptor-positive modulator GS39783 (N,N^1-dicyclopentyl-2-methylsulfanyl-5-nitro-pyrimidine-4,6-diamine): anxiolytic-like activity without side effects associated with baclofen or benzodiazepines. *J. Pharmacol. Exp. Ther.* **310**, 952–963. (doi:10.1124/ jpet.104.066753)

Dani, J. A. & Heinemann, S. 1996 Molecular and cellular aspects of nicotine abuse. *Neuron* **16**, 905–908. (doi:10. 1016/S0896–6273(00)80112–9)

DeNoble, V. J. & Mele, P. C. 1983 Behavioral pharmacology annual report. Philip Morris collection. Bates no. 1003060364/0441. See http://legacy.library.ucsf.edu/tid/ wot74e00.

Dewey, S. L. et al. 1998 A novel strategy for the treatment of cocaine addiction. *Synapse* **30**, 119–129. (doi:10.1002/ (SICI)1098–2396(199810)30:2 > 119::AID–SYN1 > 3. 0. CO;2–F)

Dewey, S. L., Brodie, J. D., Gerasimov, M., Horan, B., Gardner, E. L. & Ashby Jr, C. R. 1999 A pharmacologic strategy for the treatment of nicotine addiction. *Synapse* **31**, 76–86. (doi:10.1002/ (SICI)1098–2396(199901)31: 1 < 76::AID–SYN10 > 3.0.CO;2–Y)

Epping-Jordan, M. P., Watkins, S. S., Koob, G. F. & Markou, A. 1998 Dramatic decreases in brain reward function during nicotine withdrawal. *Nature* **393**, 76–79. (doi:10. 1038/30001)

Fattore, L., Cossu, G., Martellotta, M. C. & Fratta, W. 2002 Baclofen antagonizes intravenous self-administration of nicotine in mice and rats. *Alcohol Alcohol.* **37**, 495–498.

Flores, C. M., Davila-Garcia, M. I., Ulrich, Y. M. & Kellar, K. J. 1997 Differential regulation of neuronal nicotinic receptor binding sites following chronic nicotine administration. *J. Neurochem.* **69**, 2216–2219.

Fu, Y., Matta, S. G., Gao, W., Brower, V. G. & Sharp, B. M. 2000 Systemic nicotine stimulates dopamine release in nucleus accumbens: re-evaluation of the role of N-methyl-D-aspartate receptors in
the ventral tegmental area. *J. Pharmacol. Exp. Ther.* **294**, 458–465.

Gentry, C. L., Wilkins Jr, L. H. & Lukas, R. J. 2003 Effects of prolonged nicotinic ligand exposure on
function of heterologously expressed, human α4β2– and α4 β4–nicotinic acetylcholine receptors.
J. Pharmacol. Exp. Ther. **304**, 206–216. (doi:10.1124/jpet.102.041756)

Guery, S., Floersheim, P., Kaupmann, K. & Froestl, W. 2007 Syntheses and optimization of new
GS39783 analogues as positive allosteric modulators of GABA$_B$ receptors. *Bioorg. Med. Chem.
Lett.* **17**, 6206–6211. (doi:10.1016/j.bmcl. 2007.09.023)

Guillem, K., Vouillac, C., Azar, M. R., Parsons, L. H., Koob, G. F., Cador, M. & Stinus, L. 2006
Monoamine oxidase A rather than monoamine oxidase B inhibition increases nicotine reinforcement in rats. *Eur. J. Neurosci.* **24**, 3532–3540. (doi:10.1111/j.1460–9568.2006.05217.x)

Haas, A. L., Munoz, R. F., Humfleet, G. L., Reus, V. I. & Hall, S. M. 2004 Influences of mood, depression history, and treatment modality on outcomes in smoking cessation. *J. Consult. Clin. Psychol.*
72, 563–570. (doi:10.1037/ 0022–006X.72.4.563)

Harrison, A. A., Gasparini, F. & Markou, A. 2002 Nicotine potentiation of brain stimulation reward
reversed by DHβE and SCH 23390, but not by eticlopride, LY 314582 or MPEP in rats.
Psychopharmacology **160**, 56–66. (doi:10.1007/s00213–001–0953–6)

Jonkman, S., Risbrough, V. B., Geyer, M. A. & Markou, A. 2007 Spontaneous nicotine withdrawal
potentiates the effects of stress in rats. *Neuropsychopharmacology* **33**, 2131–2138. (doi:10.1038/
sj.npp. 1301607)

Kellar, K. J., Dáviía-Garcia, M. I. & Xiao, Y. 1999 Pharmacology of neuronal nicotinic acetylcholine
receptors: effect of acute and chronic nicotine. *Nicotine Tob. Res.* 1(Suppl. 1), S117–S120; discussion S139–S140. (doi:10.1080/14622299050011921)

Kenny, P. J. & Markou, A. 2001 Neurobiology of the nicotine withdrawal syndrome. *Pharmacol.
Biochem. Behav.* **70**, 531–549. (doi:10.1016/S0091–3057(01)00651–7)

Kenny, P. J. & Markou, A. 2004 The ups and downs of addiction: role of metabotropic glutamate
receptors. *Trends Pharmacol. Sci.* **25**, 265–272. (doi:10.1016/j.tips. 2004.03.009)

Kenny, P. J. & Markou, A. 2005 Conditioned nicotine withdrawal profoundly decreases the activity of
brain reward systems. *J. Neurosci.* **29**, 6208–6212. (doi:10.1523/ JNEUROSCI.4785–04.2005)

Kenny, P. J. & Markou, A. 2006 Nicotine self-administration acutely activates brain reward systems
and induces a long-lasting increase in reward sensitivity. *Neuropsychopharmacology* **31**,
1203–1211.

Kenny, P. J., Gasparini, F. & Markou, A. 2003 Group II metabotropic and α-amino–3–hydroxy–5–
methyl-4-isoxa-zole propionate (AMPA)/kainate glutamate receptors regulate the deficit in brain
reward function associated with nicotine withdrawal in rats. *J. Pharmacol. Exp. Ther.* **306**, 1068–1076.
(doi:10.1124/jpet.103.052027)

Kenny, P. J., Chen, S. A., Kitamura, O., Markou, A. & Koob, G. F. 2006 Conditioned withdrawal
drives heroin consumption and decreases reward sensitivity. *J. Neurosci.* **26**, 5894–5900. (doi:10.1523/
JNEUROSCI.0740–06.2006)

Kenny, P. J., Chartoff, E., Roberto, M., Carlezon Jr, W. A. & Markou, A. 2009. NMDA receptors regulate nicotine-enhanced brain reward function and intravenous nicotine self-administration: role of
the ventral tegmental area and central nucleus of the amygdala. *Neuropsychopharmacology* **34**,
266–281.

Klitenick, M. A., DeWitte, P. & Kalivas, P. W. 1992 Regulation of somatodendritic dopamine release
in the ventral tegmental area by opioids and GABA: an *in vivo* microdialysis study. *J. Neurosci.* **12**,
2623–2632.

Lanca, A. J., Adamson, K. L., Coen, K. M., Chow, B. L. C. & Corrigall, W. A. 2000 The pedunculopontine tegmental nucleus and the role of cholinergic neurons in nicotine self-administration in the
rat: a correlative neuroanatomi-cal and behavioral study. *Neuroscience* **96**, 735–742. (doi:10.1016/
S0306–4522(99)00607–7)

Levin, E. D. 2002 Nicotinic receptor subtypes and cognitive function. *J. Neurobiol.* **53**, 633–640.
(doi:10.1002/neu. 10151)

Liechti, M. E., Lhuillier, L., Kaupmann, K. & Markou, A. 2007 Metabotropic glutamate 2/3 receptors in the ventral tegmental area and the nucleus accumbens shell are involved in behaviors relating to nicotine dependence. *J. Neurosci.* **27**, 9077–9085. (doi: 10.1523/JNEUROSCI. 1766–07.2007)

Macey, D. J., Froestl, W., Koob, G. F. & Markou, A. 2001 Both GABA$_B$ receptor agonist and antagonists decreased brain stimulation reward in the rat. *Neuropharmacology* **40**, 676–685. (doi:10.1016/S0028–3908(00)00204–5)

Mansvelder, H. D. & McGehee, D. S. 2002 Cellular and synaptic mechanisms of nicotine addiction. *J. Neurobiol.* **53**, 606–617. (doi:10.1002/neu.10148)

Mansvelder, H. D., Keath, J. R. & McGehee, D. S. 2002 Synaptic mechanisms underlie nicotine-induced excitability of brain reward areas. *Neuron* **33**, 905–919. (doi:10.1016/ S0896–6273 (02)00625–6)

Markou, A. 2007 Metabotropic glutamate receptor antagonists: novel therapeutics for nicotine dependence and depression? *Biol. Psychiatry* **61**, 17–22. (doi:10.1016/ j.biopsych.2006.03.053)

Markou, A. & Paterson, N. E. 2001 The nicotinic antagonist methyllycaconitine has differential effects on nicotine self-administration and nicotine withdrawal in the rat. *Nicotine Tob. Res.* **3**, 361–373. (doi:10.1080/14622200110073380)

Marks, M. J., Burch, J. B. & Collins, A. C. 1983 Effects of chronic nicotine infusion on tolerance development and nicotinic receptors. *J. Pharmacol. Exp. Ther.* **226**, 817–825.

Marks, M. J., Pauly, J. R., Gross, S. D., Deneris, E. S., Hermans-Borgmeyer, I., Heinemann, S. F. & Collins, A. C. 1992 Nicotine binding and nicotinic receptor subunit RNA after chronic nicotine treatment. *J. Neurosci.* **12**, 2765–2784.

Marks, M. J., Grady, S. R. & Collins, A. C. 1993 Down-regulation of nicotinic receptor function after chronic nicotine infusion. *J. Pharmacol. Exp. Ther.* **266**, 1268–1276.

McGehee, D. S. & Role, L. W. 1995 Physiological diversity of nicotinic acetylcholine receptors expressed by vertebrate neurons. *Annu. Rev. Physiol.* **57**, 521–546. (doi:10.1146/ annurev. ph.57.030195.002513)

Moran, M. M., McFarland, K., Melendez, R. I., Kalivas, P. W. & Seamans, J. K. 2005 Cystine/glutamate exchange regulates metabotropic glutamate receptor presynaptic inhibition of excitatory transmission and vulnerability to cocaine seeking. *J. Neurosci.* **25**, 6389–6393. (doi:10.1523/ JNEUROSCI. 1007–05.2005)

Murray, C. J. & Lopez, A. D. 1997 Alternative projections of mortality and disability by cause 1990–2020: global burden of disease study. *Lancet* **349**, 1498–1504. (doi: 10. 1016/S0140–6736 (96)07492–2)

Nisell, M., Marcus, M., Nomikos, G. G. & Svensson, T. H. 1997 Differential effects of acute and chronic nicotine on dopamine output in the core and shell of the rat nucleus accumbens. *J. Neural Transm.* **104**, 1–10. (doi:10.1007/ BF01271290)

Paterson, N. E. & Markou, A. 2002 Increased GABA neurotransmission via administration of gamma-vinyl GABA decreased nicotine self-administration in the rat. *Synapse* **44**, 252–253. (doi:10.1002/syn.10073)

Paterson, N. E. & Markou, A. 2005 The metabotropic glutamate receptor 5 antagonist MPEP decreased break points for nicotine, cocaine and food in rats. *Psychopharmacology* **179**, 255–261. (doi:10.1007/s00213–004–2070–9)

Paterson, N. E., Semenova, S., Gasparini, F. & Markou, A. 2003 The mGluR5 antagonist MPEP decreased nicotine self-administration in rats and mice. *Psychopharmacology* **167**, 257–264.

Paterson, N. E., Froestl, W. & Markou, A. 2004 The GABA$_B$ receptor agonists baclofen and CGP44532 decreased nicotine self-administration in the rat. *Psychopharmacology* **172**, 179–186. (doi:10.1007/ s00213–003–1637–1)

Paterson, N. E., Bruijnzeel, A. W., Kenny, P. J., Wright, C. D., Froestl, W. & Markou, A. 2005a Prolonged nicotine exposure does not alter GABA$_B$ receptor-mediated regulation of brain reward function. *Neuropharmacology* **49**, 953–962. (doi:10.1016/j.neuropharm.2005.04.031)

Paterson, N. E., Froestl, W. & Markou, A. 2005b Repeated administration of the GABA$_B$ receptor agonist CGP44532 decreased nicotine self-administration, and acute administration decreased cue-reinstatement of nicotine-seeking in rats. *Neuropsychopharmacology* **30**, 119–128. (doi:10. 1038/sj.npp. 1300524)

Paterson, N. E., Vlachou, S., Guery, S., Kaupmann, K., Froestl, W. & Markou, A. 2008. Positive modulation of GABA$_B$ receptors decreased nicotine self-administration and counteracted nicotine-induced enhancement of brain reward function in rats. *J. Pharmacol. Exp. Ther* **326**, 306–314.

Perry, D. C., Davila-Garcia, M. I., Stockmeier, C. A. & Kellar, K. J. 1999 Increased nicotinic receptors in brains from smokers: membrane binding and autoradiography studies. *J. Pharmacol. Exp. Ther.* **289**, 1545–1552.

Picciotto, M. R. & Corrigall, W. A. 2002 Neuronal systems underlying behaviors related to nicotine addiction: neural circuits and molecular genetics. *J. Neurosci.* **22**, 3338–3341.

Picciotto, M. R., Zoli, M., Rimondini, R., Lena, C., Marubio, L. M., Pich, E. M., Fuxe, K. & Changeux, J. P. 1998 Acetylcholine receptors containing the β2 subunit are involved in the reinforcing properties of nicotine. *Nature* **391**, 173–177. (doi:10.1038/34413)

Quick, M. W. & Lester, R. A. 2002 Desensitization of neuronal nicotinic receptors. *J. Neurobiol.* **53**, 457–478. (doi:10.1002/neu.10109)

Rowell, P. P. & Wonnacott, S. 1990 Evidence for functional activity of up-regulated nicotine binding sites in rat striatal synaptosomes. *J. Neurochem.* **55**, 2105–2110. (doi:10. 1111/j.1471–4159.1990. tb05802.x)

Royal College of Physicians of London 2000 *Nicotine addiction in Britain: a report of the Tobacco Advisory Group of the Royal College of Physicians.* London, UK: Royal College of Physicians of London.

Schwartz, R. D. & Kellar, K. J. 1983 Nicotinic cholinergic receptor binding sites in the brain: regulation *in vivo. Science* **220**, 214–216. (doi: 10.1126/science.6828889)

Shiffman, S., West, R. J. & Gilbert, D. G. 2004 Recommendation for the assessment of tobacco craving and withdrawal in smoking cessation trials. *Nicotine Tob. Res.* **6**, 599–614. (doi:10.1080/146222004 10001734067)

Shoaib, M., Swanner, L. S., Beyer, C. E., Goldberg, S. R. & Schindler, C. W 1998 The GABA$_B$ agonist baclofen modifies cocaine self-administration in rats. *Behav. Pharmacol.* **9**, 195–206.

Skjei, K. L. & Markou, A. 2003 Effects of repeated withdrawal episodes, nicotine dose, and duration of nicotine exposure on the severity and duration of nicotine withdrawal in rats. *Psychopharmacology* **168**, 280–292. (doi:10.1007/s00213–003–1414–1)

Slattery, D. A., Markou, A., Froestl, W. & Cryan, J. F. 2005 The GABA$_B$ receptor–positive modulator GS39783 and the GABA$_B$ receptor agonist baclofen attenuate the reward–facilitating effects of cocaine: intracranial self-stimulation studies in the rat. *Neuropsychopharmacology* **30**, 2065–2072. (doi:10.1038/sj.npp.1300734)

Stolerman, I. P. & Jarvis, M. J. 1995 The scientific case that nicotine is addictive. *Psychopharmacology* **117**, 2–10. (doi: 10.1007/BF02245088)

Tapper, A. R. et al. 2004 Nicotine activation of α4* receptors: sufficient for reward, tolerance, and sensitization. *Science* **306**, 1029–1032. (doi: 10.1126/science. 1099420)

Wang, F., Chen, H., Steketee, J. D. & Sharp, B. M. 2007 Upregulation of ionotropic glutamate receptor subunits within specific mesocorticolimbic regions during chronic nicotine self-administration. *Neuropsychopharmacology* **32**, 103–109. (doi:10.1038/sj.npp.1301033)

Watkins, S. S., Stinus, L., Koob, G. F. & Markou, A. 2000 Reward and somatic changes during precipitated nicotine withdrawal in rats: centrally and peripherally mediated effects. *J. Pharmacol. Exp. Ther.* **292**, 1053–1064.

Wonnacott, S. 1990 The paradox of nicotinic acetylcholine receptor upregulation by nicotine. *Trends Pharmacol. Sci.* **11**, 216–219. (doi:10.1016/0165–6147(90)90242–Z)

Wonnacott, S. 1997 Presynaptic nicotinic ACh receptors. *Trends Neurosci.* **20**, 92–98. (doi: 10.1016/S0 166–2236 (96)10073–4)

7

Cognitive and emotional consequences of binge drinking: Role of amygdala and prefrontal cortex

David N. Stephens* and Theodora Duka

Binge drinking is an increasingly recognized problem within the UK. We have studied the relationship of binge drinking to cognitive and emotional functioning in young adults and have found evidence for increased impulsivity, impairments in spatial working memory, and impaired emotional learning. In human studies, because it is difficult to understand whether such behavioural changes predate, or are a consequence of binge drinking, we studied parallel behaviours in a rodent model, in which rats are exposed to intermittent episodes of alcohol consumption and withdrawal. In this model, and in parallel with our findings in human binge drinkers and alcoholic patients who have undergone multiple episodes of detoxification, we have found evidence for impairments in aversive conditioning as well as increased impulsivity. These behavioural changes are accompanied by facilitated excitatory neurotransmission and reduced plasticity (long-term potentiation (LTP)) in amygdala and hippocampus. The impaired LTP is accompanied by both impaired associative learning and inappropriate generalization of previously learned associations to irrelevant stimuli. We propose that repeated episodes of withdrawal from alcohol induce aberrant neuronal plasticity that results in altered cognitive and emotional competence.

Keywords: Alcoholism; withdrawal; conditioning; aberrant plasticity; executive function; anxiety.

7.1 Introduction

Alcohol abuse and dependence is an increasingly recognized problem of western societies. The UK, in particular, has a high incidence of binge drinking. Such patterns of abuse have major cost implications in the UK for health (£1.7 bn per annum), for crime and disorder (£12 bn per annum), as well as for lost productivity (£6.4 bn per annum) according to a recent Cabinet Office Report (Cabinet Office 2004). Binge drinking has been defined as consumption of twice the recommended daily limit of alcohol. According to UK government recommendations, this amount corresponds to 8 units (a unit equals 7.9 g alcohol) for men (equivalent to four pints of 5% beer) and six units for women (equivalent to 3 large glasses of wine). Using these definitions, men binge drink on 40% of occasions on which they consume alcohol and women on 22% of such occasions (Drummond et al. 2004), with ca. 5.9 million UK residents drinking at these levels on at least one occasion per annum. Those aged 16–24 are more likely to engage in binge drinking, with 36% of men and 27% of women in this age group reporting that they binge drink at least once a week, with some evidence that the frequency with which young women engage in binge drinking is increasing. There is emerging evidence that this pattern of drinking continues into middle age, with one in three men, and one in five women drinking twice the daily-recommended limit at least once a week. A recent American study suggests that adolescent binge drinking predicts binge drinking well into adulthood (Jefferis et al. 2005).

* d.stephens@sussex.ac.uk

In the USA, a different measure of binge-drinking has been used, the standard binge measure of consuming 5 or more drinks (a drink is defined as 14 g alcohol) in a row for men (4 or more drinks for women) per occasion (Wechsler et al. 1994). Confusion among the general public as what constitutes a 'unit' or a 'drink' has made both the UK and the US definitions of little use in offering advice on drinking behaviour, especially as the alcoholic contents of drinks has risen steadily, and so individual perception of consumption tends to underestimate actual intake. The definition of bingeing has been criticized on several grounds (Dejong 2001; Lange & Voas 2001; Perkins et al. 2001; Wechsler & Austin 1998; Wechsler & Nelson 2001), including that it ignores duration of consumption and does not map onto levels of blood alcohol concentration (BAC) that are associated with intoxication (Lange & Voas 2001). In an attempt to address these concerns, the USA National Institute on Alcohol Abuse and Alcoholism (NIAAA) approved the following definition: 'A "binge" is a pattern of drinking alcohol that brings BAC to about 0.08 g% or above. For the typical adult, this pattern corresponds to consuming 5 or more drinks (male), or 4 or more drinks (female), in about 2 hours' (NIAAA 2004). This new definition incorporates the duration of the drinking episode in addition to the quantity of alcohol consumed to define binge drinking, as well as providing a quantitative level of alcohol levels.

In our studies of binge drinking, we have used a more behavioural and potentially more conservative approach based on the Alcohol Use Questionnaire (Mehrabian & Russell 1978), which incorporates the speed of drinking, the behavioural measures 'numbers of times being drunk in the last 6 months' (with drunkenness defined as loss of coordination, nausea, and/or inability to speak clearly, or blackout), and the percentage of times getting drunk when drinking (Townshend & Duka 2002). Nevertheless, although differences in definition of binge drinking may give rise to some confusion both in the scientific literature and among the general public, it is likely that the multiple definitions tap into closely related phenomena, albeit with different sensitivity (Cranford et al. 2006).

Although definitions of binge drinking have concentrated on amounts consumed, rates of consumption, and incidence of drunkenness, we have pointed to a feature of binge drinking that is not addressed in these definitions. Thus, a characteristic marker of binge drinking behaviour is the consumption of large amounts of alcohol within a limited period followed by a period of abstinence, as opposed to regular drinking in which a person might consume similar weekly amounts of alcohol but without the extremes of alcohol intoxication and withdrawal. This pattern of cycles of alcohol intoxication followed by acute episodes of withdrawal may be analogous to a common clinical experience, in which alcoholic patients undergo cycles of alcohol abuse, followed by detoxification, a period of abstinence (that may be very short), followed by relapse, a further period of abuse, and further detoxification treatment. It has long been recognized that such repeated episodes of alcohol abuse and detoxification lead to increased risk of withdrawal-induced seizures (Ballenger & Post 1978), and more recently, we, and others, have demonstrated a wide range of cognitive deficits in such patients (Duka et al. 2004). Several of the cognitive deficits we have observed in repeatedly detoxified alcoholic patients are also to be found in young adult binge drinkers (Duka et al. 2004). In studies of alcoholic patients and of binge drinkers, it is difficult to determine whether the cognitive and behavioural differences observed are consequences of the drinking patterns or pre-date excessive consumption. However, by imposing periods of alcohol consumption and withdrawal, we have been able to model several aspects of the cognitive deficit in rodents. These experiments suggest that binge patterns of alcohol consumption in both humans and rats lead to altered function of amygdala and frontal cortices.

7.2 Evidence of altered cognitive function in binge drinkers

Alcohol itself is known to have long-term effects on prefrontal cortex function (Moselhy et al. 2001; Tarter et al. 2004), while studies of alcoholic patients who have undergone multiple withdrawals suggest that previous experience of detoxification is also associated with prefrontal cortex dysfunction (Duka et al. 2003). In a series of studies, we have compared prefrontal cortex function between binge drinkers and non-binge drinkers among heavy social drinkers who were matched for age and IQ. Binge drinkers were impaired in the vigilance task from the Gordon Diagnostic System, a task that challenges the ability to withhold a pre-potent response and is thus a measure of impulsivity. In this task, participants presented with 3 digits on a screen are asked to concentrate on the middle digit and respond only when a 9 in the middle of the digit triad (target) follows a triad of digits with 1 in the middle (alerting stimulus). Thus, participants are required to inhibit their responding following the alerting stimulus, until the target stimulus appears. Female binge drinkers were particularly impaired in this task being unable to inhibit their response to the alerting stimulus, suggesting a lack of inhibitory control from the frontal lobes (Townshend & Duka 2005). Age at which heavy drinking started also appeared to play a role in this impairment associated with the binge drinking. Previous studies have also shown impairments in cognitive function associated with heavy drinking during early adolescence (Brown et al. 2000), and early exposure to binge drinking is associated with frontal lobe damage (Crews et al. 2007).

Increased impulsivity is not always deleterious, and in the same study (Townshend & Duka 2005), we found binge drinkers to be faster on the visual search matching task, a task from the CANTAB test battery that allows a separation between choice and movement time. In this task, participants are required to search among 8 similar shapes to match one single identical shape to a target displayed simultaneously. Binge drinkers showed faster movement time, rather than thinking time, suggestive of a motor impulsivity. Such impulsivity is associated with altered functioning of prefrontal–subcortical circuits, particularly the orbitofrontal circuit (Spinella 2004).

Binge drinking was also found to be associated with impairment in a spatial working memory task from the CANTAB, which is also dependent on prefrontal function (Weissenborn & Duka 2003). We have recently replicated this finding, but in our more recent studies, we find that only female binge drinkers make more errors than their counterparts (Townshend & Duka 2005; Scaife & Dula (unpublished data)), whereas male drinkers appear not to be impaired (see Table 7.1). In our studies, although male binge drinkers are usually found to drink more alcohol overall than female binge drinkers, their binge scores are lower. Presumably, this reflects a lower tolerance of females, and so the female drinkers, although they consume less, may become drunk more often when drinking, thus achieving a higher binge score in the Alcohol Use Questionnaire. Thus, it may be less the amount of alcohol consumed than the magnitude of its effect on individuals that predict impairment of cognitive function.

In agreement with our observations, in a study that compared student social drinkers to teetotalers (Randall et al. 2004), high alcohol consumers (especially females) were worse in performing a colour STROOP task, indicating a reduced ability to inhibit a pre-potent response, an executive function controlled by prefrontal cortex. A similar conclusion, of a relationship between harmful drinking and neurocognitive deficits, was derived from Zeigler et al.'s (2005) review of articles identified in a MEDLINE search for articles addressing neurotoxic and neurocognitive effects of harmful drinking among young adolescents and college students.

Many studies have suggested that prefrontal dysfunction is a predisposing factor to heavy drinking. For instance, in young adult social drinkers, a relationship was found between

Table 7.1 Binge scores for male and female social drinkers and the number of errors they make when performing in the spatial working memory task from the CANTAB test battery.

	Non-bingers		Bingers	
	Males	**Females**	**Males**	**Females**
Study 1 (Weissenborn & Duka 2003)				
Binge score	12.4 ± 0.7	12.5 ± 1.0	35.8 ± 3.6	28.0 ± 2.6
Between Search Errors	9.6 ± 1.4[§]	14.9 ± 3.8[§]	15.2 ± 2.5	19.0 ± 3.0
Study 2 (Townshend & Duka 2005)				
Binge score	11.3 ± 0.7	10.3 ± 0.8	37.1 ± 2.9	45.5 ± 4.7
Between Search Errors	11.0 ± 1.6	8.5 ± 1.7*	6.9 ± 1.5	14.5 ± 2.4
Study 3 (Scaife & Duka (unpublished data))				
Binge score	16.6 ± 2.3	20.2 ± 1.8	56.7 ± 4.1	52.1 ± 4.5
Between Search Errors	8.8 ± 2.9	7.25 ± 1.5*	6.33 ± 1.6	14.0 ± 2.5

Binge drinkers (only females in studies 2 and 3) make more errors than non-bingers. Subjects commit this type of error when, in the process of searching through a spatial array of boxes to collect tokens hidden inside, they return to a box in which a token was previously found.
[§]Main effect of binge drinking.
*$p < 0.05$ compared to the same sex in the bingers group.

impaired executive function and both the frequency of drinking to 'get high' and 'get drunk' (Deckel et al. 1995) and the severity of drinking consequences (Giancola et al. 1996). This consideration makes it difficult to know from our own studies whether the cognitive effects we observe in binge drinkers may have been pre-morbid. Although impairment in certain cognitive tasks might be the cause of extreme drinking patterns (including binge drinking), data from animals suggest that binge patterns of consumption can induce cortical damage and aberrant plasticity, and lead to related cognitive deficits (see below). Only a prospective study investigating cognitive performance in adolescents before and after starting binge drinking would clarify these questions.

7.3 Evidence of altered emotional reactivity in binge drinkers

In addition to altered cognitive ability, binge drinking is also associated with changes in emotional competence. Increased negative emotional sensitivity has been recognized in patients following multiple detoxifications for some years (Adinoff et al. 1994; Duka et al. 2002). Related effects can be seen in binge drinkers, who also show a lowered positive mood state in their subjective ratings obtained via the Profile of Mood Scale (POMS) compared with their non-binge drinking counterparts (Townshend & Duka 2005). Deficits in emotional behaviour can also be found in laboratory settings. A recent study has examined conditioned fear in the form of a conditioned fear-potentiated startle response in bingers compared to non-bingers to a stimulus associated with an aversive event (Stephens et al. 2005; see Fig. 7.1). After several training trials, participants learned to discriminate an auditory stimulus that predicted an aversive white noise (S+) from a stimulus (S–) that was unpaired with the aversive noise. Subsequently, the ability of the S+ and S– to influence the startle response to an aversive stimulus was assessed. While social drinkers showed the anticipated potentiation of startle in the presence of the S+ relative to the S– condition, there was no differential conditioned response to the S+ and S– in bingers (Stephens et al. 2005).

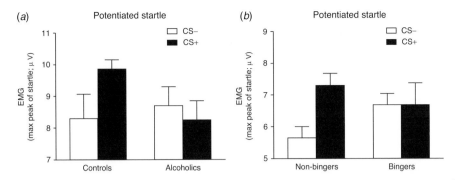

Fig. 7.1 Conditioned fear in alcoholic patients and their control counterparts (A) and in human bingeing and non-bingeing social drinkers (B); groups were matched for age, gender, and verbal IQ. Electromyographic activity of the orbicularis oculi muscle (EMG) to an aversive white noise (97 dB) in the presence of an auditory CS+ and CS– stimulus of the same intensity (63 dB) but different frequency (900 Hz or 1700 Hz). During training sessions, CS+ was followed by aversive white noise (US) and CS– by nothing. Testing took place in the presence of CS stimuli without reinforcement (test of CS effects) and also when each stimulus (CS+ and CS–) was followed by the white noise startle stimulus (test of CS-induced potentiation of startle). A group by stimulus interaction was found in the comparison between bingers and non-bingers and also between alcoholic patients and controls ($F_{2,32}$ = 6.98, $p = 0.003$ and $F_{2,48} = 4.31$, $p = 0.02$, respectively). This interaction was attributable to a higher response to the CS+ compared to the CS– in non-binger and control groups, but not in binger and alcoholic patient groups.

We have seen a similar deficit in patients with a history of multiple detoxifications (Fig. 1, see Table 7.2 for demographics). Although these deficits in learning about an aversive CS may theoretically have preceded onset of binge drinking, this possibility is made less likely by the fact that similar impairments in aversive conditioning of discrete cues are also found in rats exposed to multiple episodes of high alcohol intake and withdrawal (Stephen et al, 2001).

Further evidence of altered emotional competence following repeated detoxification is seen in the ability of alcoholic patients to interpret emotions in the facial expressions of others. Thus, when alcoholic patients were presented with a series of emotional facial expressions, they overestimated the amount of fear present if they had already undergone several detoxifications (Townshend & Duka 2003). Perception of fear in facial expressions is associated with activation of the amygdala in fMRI studies, and patients who have amygdala lesions show an impaired perception of fear in emotional facial expression (Adolphs et al. 1999; Calder et al. 2001; Morris et al. 1998). Given the similarities between the consequences of amygdala kindling and multiple alcohol detoxifications (Carrington et al. 1984; Pinel 1980; Pinel & Van Oot 1975; Pinel et al. 1975), the increased perception of fear in emotional expressions by alcoholic patients with multiple detoxifications may be the result of a facilitated neurotransmission within the amygdala (Townshend & Duka 2003). Our animal studies would support such an interpretation.

7.4 Prefrontal–amygdala interactions in alcohol abuse

Many of the behavioural impairments seen in binge drinkers can be ascribed to alterations in function of amygdala and prefrontal cortical areas (Duka et al. 2004, 2003). Recent human imaging studies indicate that activity in prefrontal cortex and amygdala are inversely correlated, suggesting prefrontal cortex may be involved in suppressing amygdala-mediated

Table 7.2 Gender distribution, age, verbal IQ, and alcohol history of the group of alcoholic patients and their control counterparts.

Variables	Controls	Alcohol patients
Gender (M/F)	8/5	8/5
Age	45 (27–63)	47 (26–66)
SADQ	1.5 (0–11)	33.8 (9–65)
Units of alcohol/week (1 unit = 8 g)	13.9 (0–53)	253 (126–354)
Starting age of drinking (years)	15.5 (14–17)	17 (14–32)
Verbal IQ	111.7	109.9

The two groups were compared in the potentiated startle response (Fig. 1). SADQ (Stockwell et al. 1983): Severity of Alcohol Dependence Questionnaire is a 20 items questionnaire for the assessment of the severity of dependence.

responses (Hariri et al. 2000). We have speculated that if repeated episodes of withdrawal impair prefrontal function, a consequence might be that such alcoholic patients may be pre-disposed to recall aversive experiences that are normally suppressed (Stephens et al. 2005).

Loss of the ability of prefrontal cortex to inhibit behaviours mediated by subcortical systems (such as amygdala) is also a major contributor to loss of control of drug taking in addicts (Volkow et al. 2003), as executive functions, such as the ability to plan and to inhibit habitual tendencies, reflect virtues that are essential for controlling excessive consumption. Thus, impairment of frontal function as a consequence of repeated detoxifications (cycles of high intake followed by periods of withdrawal) or binge drinking (which also leads to frequent high amounts of alcohol in the brain followed by withdrawal) may predispose to uncontrolled consumption and impair resistance to relapse in the abstaining alcoholic, as well as having long-term effects on the emotional behaviour.

Clinical experience, as well as animal laboratory experimental studies, indicates that repeated experience of detoxification results in profound behavioural changes associated with neurobiological changes in several brain regions. The best documented of such changes is the increased propensity to seizures experience following multiple withdrawals. This so-called kindling of convulsant activity has been suggested to reflect changes in efficiency of nervous transmission in the amygdala (Carrington et al. 1984; Pinel 1980; Pinel & Van Oot 1975; Pinel et al. 1975). The amygdala is crucially implicated in the formation of associations between discrete environmental events and aversive stimuli, and the expression of fear reactions through its projections to brainstem structures governing behavioural, autonomic, and endocrine responses to threat. It is thus of importance whether repeated periods of alcohol exposure and withdrawal also affect emotional competence and Pavlovian conditioning of emotional events.

7.5 Rodent model of binge patterns of alcohol intake

Many of the behavioural changes seen in binge drinkers can be modelled in the rodent (indeed, some of the deficits we have subsequently described in alcoholics were predicted based on our prior rat studies (Stephens et al. 2001, 2005)). Thus, the increased propensity to show seizures following several episodes of alcohol withdrawal has been routinely demonstrated (Becker & Veatch 2002). Since prior electrical kindling of the amygdala predisposes to withdrawal-induced seizures (Pinel et al. 1975), while repeated episodes of alcohol withdrawal facilitate the development of electrical kindling of the amygdala (Ulrichsen et al. 1998), facilitation of transmission in the amygdala has been viewed as an important consequence of ethanol withdrawal. In our studies, high alcohol intakes are induced in rats by providing them chronically with a 7% alcohol-containing diet that the rats receive as their sole source of nutrition for either 24 days continuously, followed by a 2 week withdrawal period before behavioural analyses (single withdrawal group), or with the treatment interrupted for 2 additional withdrawal periods, each 3 days in length, during which time the animals receive control diet (repeated withdrawal group). A third, control, group is given access to control diet for 24 days, and is pair fed to the single withdrawal group to stabilize body weight. Increasing seizure sensitivity by repeated periods of alcohol exposure and withdrawal (compared to equal alcohol intake but a single withdrawal episode) increases the degree of withdrawal-induced neuronal excitability, as measured by c-fos expression 8 h into withdrawal (about 2 h after blood ethanol levels return to undetectable levels), in several brain areas including amygdala, hippocampus, ventral striatum, periaqueductal grey (Borlikova et al. 2006b), and frontal cortical areas (Hoang & Stephens (unpublished data)).

7.6 Effects of ethanol withdrawal on amygdala function

Consistent with altered amygdala function, repeated experience of withdrawal results in impairment, several weeks after cessation of the alcohol treatment, in acquiring a conditioned emotional response, in which, in control animals, presentation of tone or flashing light conditioned stimuli (CS+), which predicted mild footshock, resulted in suppression of ongoing instrumental behaviour (Stephens et al. 2001). When the shock intensity was increased in steps over a period of 5 weeks, the repeated withdrawn rats eventually showed some evidence of behavioural suppression in response to the CS+. Whether this eventual acquisition reflected the higher shock levels or the prolonged training period is not clear. However, it is unlikely that the deficit in learning the CS-shock association reflected insensitivity to shock, as no differences were seen between repeatedly withdrawn and control rats in the acquisition of contextual fear conditioning (Borlikova et al. 2006a), which depends upon intact processing within the hippocampus (Bannerman et al. 2001; Fendt & Fanselow 1999; Selden et al. 1991), while the formation of associations between shock and discrete cues such as tones or lights is processed within the amygdala (Fanselow & LeDoux 1999; Killcross et al. 1997; Selden et al. 1991). Furthermore, if training on the conditional emotional response task took place prior to alcohol exposure and withdrawal, then the repeated withdrawal rats were not impaired in expression of the CER, suggesting that the effects of withdrawal are in learning the relationship between the CS+ and the shock, rather than in them having blunted fear responses (Ripley et al. 2003). Interestingly, however, the repeated withdrawal animals were impaired in extinguishing the CS+–shock association when the CS+ was presented repeatedly in the absence of the shock reinforcer (Ripley et al. 2003), and in a reversal experiment, in which the CS+ and CS– stimuli, trained prior to alcohol exposure, were switched and retrained following repeated alcohol withdrawal treatment. This series of experiments suggests that the repeated periods of alcohol exposure and withdrawal procedure impair the learning of new associations, but that, if the associations have been learned prior to alcohol exposure, there is no impairment in the expression of the conditioned response.

According to one model, fear conditioning depends upon information processing in amygdala; as a result of conditioning, the CS+ gains access to the lateral amygdala's outflow to the central nucleus (Fanselow & LeDoux 1999), which in turn induces activity in output pathways eliciting diverse symptoms of fear and anxiety. In keeping with this model, an acoustic signal, previously conditioned to shock, increases the number of neurones showing c-fos immunoreactivity in the central and basal nuclei of the amygdala (Beck & Fibiger 1995; Hall et al. 2001b). In keeping with those findings, high levels of c-fos expression were seen in both control and single withdrawal animals in the core and shell of the accumbens and in the basolateral and central nuclei of the amygdala after exposing the rats to a tone CS+ previously paired with shock, but c-fos was expressed in fewer neurones in the repeated withdrawal group (Stephens et al. 2005). Thus, repeated periods of alcohol exposure and withdrawal (but not simply an equivalent amount of alcohol exposure) impair the formation of associations between a tone stimulus and an aversive event, consistent with the behavioural observations (Ripley et al. 2003; Stephens et al. 2001). The deficit that occurred at the level of conditioned activation of amygdala neurones indicates that the deficit seen in CER following repeated withdrawal is because of impaired formation of the CS–shock association, rather than an inability to control the behavioural output.

These observations are commensurate with altered transmission within the amygdala following ethanol withdrawal, though there appears to be differences between the consequences of repeated ethanol exposure and withdrawal and electrical kindling. Although in the case of seizure sensitivity, there are similarities between electrical kindling of seizures and alcohol withdrawal seizures, and they cross-sensitize, in the case of fear conditioning, repeated alcohol withdrawal and electrical kindling of the basolateral amygdala have opposite effects; in contrast to repeated withdrawal, which impairs fear conditioning, electrical kindling facilitates fear conditioning to a discrete cue (Ripley et al. 2003). It should be noted, however, that although the lateral part of the amygdala plays an important role in fear conditioning as the area receives input regarding both aversive events and associated cues (Fanselow & LeDoux 1999) and then provides inputs to the central nucleus, recent studies suggest that the central nucleus may also function independently of the lateral nuclei, receiving highly processed sensory input from entorhinal cortex and related areas (see Killcross et al. 1997). It thus seems possible that the major effects of repeated withdrawal from alcohol on fear conditioning are mediated by the central amygdala, rather than the lateral aspects.

7.7 Mechanisms underlying effects of withdrawal

By what mechanism does repeated alcohol withdrawal lead to impaired fear conditioning? Long-term potentiation (LTP) has been proposed as a mechanism whereby synaptic transmission is facilitated as a result of use. In associative LTP, transmission in the pathway carrying information regarding the CS+ is facilitated as a result of it being activated contemporaneously with the pathway signalling the unconditioned stimulus (US) (Maren 2005; Sigurdsson et al. 2007). In support of this kind of mechanism underlying fear conditioning, LTP is found in the pathway from medial geniculate body to the lateral nucleus of the amygdala, which is thought to mediate conditioning of fear responses to acoustic stimuli. Tetanic stimulation of the medial geniculate body also results in a long-lasting potentiation of a field potential in the lateral amygdala elicited by a naturally transduced acoustic stimulus (Rogan & LeDoux 1995; Rogan et al. 1997). The stimulation coincidence parameters that are necessary for induction of LTP in the lateral amygdala closely resemble those required for the formation of associations between CS and US in fear conditioning experiments (Bauer et al. 2001). Taken together, these observations suggest that LTP-like mechanisms underlie amygdala-mediated fear conditioning (Blair et al. 2001). Why then should alcohol withdrawal affect such a mechanism?

Acute alcohol treatment is associated with facilitation of GABAergic inhibitory mechanisms (Roberto et al. 2004a; Samson & Harris 1992), while alcohol also acts as an antagonist of glutamatergic NMDA receptors (Samson & Harris 1992). During chronic alcohol exposure, transmission in glutamatergic systems is facilitated (to compensate for these two major actions of alcohol), both through increased NMDA receptor sensitivity (Roberto et al. 2004b) and increased glutamate turnover (Dahchour & De Witte 1999), resulting in partial tolerance to alcohol's sedative effects. Following withdrawal from alcohol, the glutamatergic system continues to be overactive (Dahchour & De Witte 1999), while NMDA receptor function remains elevated (Roberto et al. 2004b); but this overactivity is no longer balanced by alcohol's facilitatory effects on GABAergic systems

Several pieces of evidence support that intermittent exposure to ethanol and withdrawal leads to increases in glutamatergic synaptic transmission in both central (Roberto et al. 2006) and basolateral amygdala (Floyd et al. 2003; Lack et al. 2007), possibly as a consequence of increased probability of glutamate release from the presynaptic terminal (Lack et al. 2007) and increased postsynaptic NMDA-receptor function (Lack et al. 2007; Roberto et al. 2006), which may lead to alterations of postsynaptic AMPA receptor function (Lack et al. 2007). We suggest that this imbalance in the direction of glutamatergic excitatory transmission might have consequences similar to overactivation of glutamatergic synapses that occurs during LTP.

The apparent paradox of heightened seizure sensitivity, and exaggerated anxiety responses during withdrawal, but impaired fear conditioning, could then be accounted for if repeated experience of withdrawal induces synaptic plasticity, resulting in facilitated transmission in glutamatergic pathways, but reduced capacity for further plasticity necessary for learning. Information regarding discrete cues, such as the CSs in our experiments, are relayed to the lateral amygdala from sensory cortex and sensory thalamus (Pitkanen et al. 1997). LTP is found in the pathway from the external capsule to the lateral nucleus of the amygdala (Chapman et al. 1990), and high frequency stimulation of the medial geniculate input to the amygdala also results in a long-lasting potentiation of a field potential in the lateral amygdala elicited by a naturally transduced acoustic stimulus (Rogan et al. 1997).

We therefore compared the excitability and plasticity in the amygdala of rats that had undergone repeated or a single withdrawal. Field potentials in lateral amygdala increased monotonically with increased intensity of stimulation of the external capsule accessory pathway, and these input–output curves were shifted to the left in slices from rats that had undergone repeated withdrawal, consistent with increased efficiency of synaptic transmission. Such changes could in principle account for increased sensitivity to seizures following repeated withdrawal. Furthermore, such increased efficiency might imply that fear-related stimuli activating these pathways might be more effective in eliciting anxious responses following repeated periods of alcohol exposure and withdrawal, as has been reported in both humans (George et al. 1990; Krystal et al. 1997) and in some (Overstreet et al. 2002), but not all, animal models of anxiety (Borlikova et al. 2006b; Ripley et al. 2003).

As well as leftward shifts in the input–output curves, repeated withdrawal reduced the ability to support LTP in lateral amygdala response to high frequency stimulation of the external capsule. In the case of the lateral amygdala, both single withdrawal and repeated withdrawal groups showed equally reduced capacity for LTP (Stephens et al. 2005). These observations are consistent with reduced capacity for associative learning following repeated periods of alcohol exposure and withdrawal. However, while both single withdrawal and repeated withdrawal treatments gave rise to similar size reductions in LTP, in our behavioural experiments using fear conditioning, we have found the repeated withdrawal treatment to impair conditioning more than single withdrawal treatment (Ripley et al. 2003; Stephens et al. 2001). Nevertheless, these electrophysiological data provide an interesting parallel to the conditioning deficits, and the entire set of electrophysiological and behavioural data might be reconciled by suggesting that repeated withdrawal increases efficiency of synaptic connections, leading to facilitation of synaptic transmission, but reduced capacity for further plasticity. Consistent with that interpretation, several withdrawal episodes result in increased levels of c-fos expression in central amygdala relative to rats that have undergone only a single withdrawal, while in the case of another immediate early gene, zif-268, a marker of synaptic plasticity (Hall et al. 2001a), increases are seen following a single withdrawal, but not if the animals have undergone prior withdrawal experience (Borlikova et al. 2006b).

This aberrant plasticity hypothesis gives rise to an interesting prediction. Figure 7.2(A) illustrates a conventional account of conditioning. According to this model, activation of a neural system carrying information regarding a strong stimulus (such as a shock) is able to activate pathways leading to an unconditioned behavioural output (such as response suppression), while pathways carrying information regarding a weak, biologically neutral stimulus, such as a mild tone, are unable to gain access to neural pathways subserving the behavioural output. However, if the tone pathway is active at the same time as the shock pathway, then as a consequence of associative processes such as LTP, the connection between the tone pathway and the output pathway will be strengthened so that eventually the tone will itself become capable of eliciting the behavioural output, independent of the shock. Physiological accounts of such associative learning posit that it occurs as a consequence of LTP (Maren 2005). Although the exact mechanisms underlying induction and expression of LTP in amygdala remain ambiguous (Kim & Jung 2006), a conventional model holds that synapses carrying the weak signal are initially 'silent' (Liao et al. 1995), possibly because they employ only NMDA receptors that are blocked by the presence of magnesium ions in the channel, so that the glutamate released from the presynaptic terminal, although binding with NMDA receptors, is incapable of inducing depolarization events in the postsynaptic membrane. However, signalling in the US (shock) pathway synapses is postulated to be mediated by glutamate acting at AMPA receptors (Maren 2005; Sigurdsson et al. 2007) that are not subject to magnesium block. On occasions when both the tone CS and the US pathways are activated concurrently, membrane depolarization elicited by the US pathway will allow the magnesium block in neighbouring NMDA receptors (including those in the CS pathway) to be removed, allowing glutamate release in this pathway to cause postsynaptic depolarization via NMDA receptors, which will then initiate processes underlying LTP; subsequently, activation of the tone pathway will be effective in activating the behavioural output. Although the details of the mechanisms underlying amygdala LTP remain to be elucidated, we postulate that during ethanol withdrawal, enhanced glutamate release will occur in many synapses, activating processes that serve LTP (e.g. insertion of AMPA receptors into hitherto silent synapses).

Presumably, such synaptic strengthening would have at least two consequences: first, withdrawal-strengthened synapses would no longer be silent and would not be available for the formation of new associations; second, natural events activating pathways that were already strengthened by withdrawal would gain access to output pathways in the absence of conditioning. The former consequence might explain why repeatedly withdrawn rats and binge-drinking humans fail to show evidence of fear conditioning (Stephens et al. 2001, 2005). The second consequence predicts that once conditioning has occurred, then other neutral stimuli might gain access to the ouput pathways.

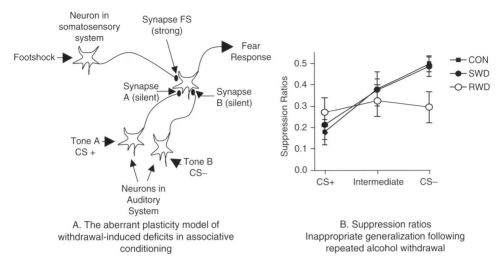

A. The aberrant plasticity model of
withdrawal-induced deficits in associative
conditioning

B. Suppression ratios
Inappropriate generalization following
repeated alcohol withdrawal

Fig. 7.2 (A) Prior to learning, activation of synapse FS as a consequence of footshock-induced activity in somatosensory systems leads to activation of an output neuron giving rise to a fear response. Activation of an auditory neurone by Tone A is unable to gain access to the output neuron subserving the fear response, as synapse A is 'silent' at this stage. During associative learning, if the neuron carrying information about Tone A (CS+) is active at the same time as the neuron carrying information regarding the footshock, then as a result of activation of the synapse FS, local depolarization will occur, allowing activity at synapse A also to induce depolarization in the postsynaptic membrane. Consequently, synapse A will be strengthened, and so activation of the tone A pathway will now gain access to the output pathway, i.e. associative conditioning has occurred. Synapse B remains silent, as it is never activated at the same time as synapse FS. However, if alcohol withdrawal, perhaps through enhanced gluatamate release, induces activation of synapse B as well as of synapse FS, then synapse B should also be strengthened, and so Tone B might now gain access to the output pathway, even though it has never been paired with footshock. Furthermore, if withdrawal-induced synaptic strengthening occurs prior to conditioning, then Synapse A will already have been strengthened and will no longer be available for conditioning. (B) Suppression ratios (a measure of conditioned fear) in repeatedly withdrawn rats (RWD), given the same exposure to alcohol, but only a single withdrawal (SWD), or rats fed a non-alcoholic control diet (CON). The rats were trained prior to alcohol treatment to associate a tone CS+ with footshock, and so the CS+ caused a suppression of behaviour (giving suppression ratio values less than 0.5). The CS− was an alternative tone signal, which did not predict shock and which therefore did not suppress behaviour (giving a suppression ratio of about 0.5). Two weeks following the final day of alcohol treatment, the rats were once again presented with the CS+, as well as the CS−, and a novel tone, intermediate between the CS+ and the CS−. SWD and control rats continued to show suppression to the CS+, but not to the CS−, with an intermediate degree of suppression to the novel tone. In contrast, the RWD rats showed equal suppression to all three tones (redrawn from Stephens et al. 2005).

We tested this idea by training rats to associate one of two tones (CS+) with shock, in a conditioned emotional response test. The other tone (CS−) was not paired with shock. After training, presentation of the CS+, but not the CS−, gave rise to a suppression of ongoing instrumental behaviour. The rats were then matched for performance and allocated to treatment groups, in which they received either ethanol diet with repeated withdrawal episodes or ethanol with only a single withdrawal episode, or control diet for approximately 4 weeks. The rats were then allowed to recover for two weeks, before being tested once again in the conditioned emotional response test. As shown in Fig. 7.2(B), both the control group and single withdrawal group behaved appropriately in showing suppression to the CS+, but not the CS−, and an intermediate suppression to a novel tone of an intermediate frequency, while the repeatedly withdrawn rats showed equal suppression to all three tones, consistent with aberrant plasticity having taken place, allowing the CS− access to the behavioural output (Stephens et al. 2005).

The results described here refer to aversive conditioning, but similar mechanisms may underlie appetitive conditioning. Thus, repeated withdrawal experience leads to deficits in aspects of appetitive conditioning, including pavlovian-to-instrumental transfer (Ripley et al. 2004). Taken together, these findings suggest a mechanism whereby chronic alcohol treatment and withdrawal may lead to a deficit in functioning of the amygdala with consequences for associative learning. Such deficits may have implications for the use of conditioning approaches to behavioural therapies for alcoholics.

7.8 Effects of ethanol withdrawal on frontal cortical function in rodents

The amygdala is connected with many brain structures, and the extent to which the effects of repeated withdrawal are due to interference with the amygdala itself, or with its connections, is not clear. Of particular interest in the study of cognitive impairments, resulting from repeated periods of alcohol exposure and withdrawal, is the connection to the prefrontal cortex and hippocampus. Although there is good evidence that repeated intermittent ethanol administration, or repeated withdrawal, results in both physiological (Stephens et al. 2005) and pathological (Obernier et al. 2002a, b) changes in the hippocampus, the limited evidence available has so far failed to demonstrate a marked impairment in behaviours, such as spatial learning (Borlikova et al. 2006a; Obernier et al. 2002b) or contextual conditioning (Borlikova et al. 2006a), that are thought to be mediated by hippocampal processes.

Borlikova et al. (2006b), however, did find a marked impairment in a negative patterning task (Bussey et al. 2000b), in which rats were required to initiate a response when either a light or a tone stimulus was presented, but to inhibit the response when both stimuli were presented simultaneously. Although this task was initially proposed as a test of the ability of rats to integrate information from different sensory modalities, and thus thought to be mediated by hippocampus (Rudy & Sutherland 1989), several studies (Bussey et al. 2000; Davidson et al. 1993; Gallagher & Holland 1992; Moreira & Bueno 2003) have not found an influence of hippocampal lesions on its performance, and it seems that deficits in performing the task may relate to an inability to withhold responding in the presence of previously rewarded cues (Blackburn & Hevenor 1996; Davidson et al. 1993; Papadimitriou & Wynne 1999; Richmond et al. 1997; Whishaw & Tomie 1991), rather than by disruption of configural association. We are therefore inclined to interpret our negative patterning data as revealing changes in responsiveness following repeated episodes of withdrawal. This kind of deficit might have more in common with alterations in frontal cortical function than hippocampus. A different rat model of binge drinking (Crews et al. 2000) reports that young adolescent rats (ca. 35 days old) show increased levels of amino cupric silver staining (indicating neuronal cell death) in the frontal areas following exposure to a binge pattern of alcohol consumption. These results would be consistent with observations in human alcoholics and binge drinkers who show impaired cognitive function in executive control tasks sensitive to dysfunction of prefrontal cortex (Duka et al. 2004, 2003; Townshend & Duka 2005; Weissenborn & Duka 2003).

There are strong interactions between amygdala and prefrontal cortex in determining behavioural output. Human imaging studies indicate that activity in prefrontal cortex and amygdala are inversely correlated, and so prefrontal cortex may be involved in suppressing amygdala-mediated fear responses (Hariri et al. 2000). Thus, withdrawal-induced changes in prefrontal cortex function might predispose alcoholics to retain fear experiences that are suppressed in normal people. Glutamatergic projections from the medial prefrontal cortex activate GABAergic interneurones in the amygdala (Grace & Rosenkranz 2002; Rosenkranz & Grace 2002), which leads to a reduction in the firing rate of neurones in the basolateral amygdala. This process is believed to be vital in the control of responsivity to conditioned stimuli, and so a decrease in activity in this inhibitory pathway may lead to overexpression of conditioned behaviours and may underlie some aspects of pathological conditions such as anxiety and drug abuse. Conversely, stimulation of infralimbic prefrontal cortex neurons results in low levels of conditioned behaviour in animals (Milad & Quirk 2002). Connections between the orbitofrontal cortex and basolateral amygdala may be vital for assessing the incentive value of cues associated with appetitive or aversive reinforcers, with neurones in these regions firing selectively to cues based on their associative strengths. Because of the time course of the acquisition of firing patterns to these cues, it has been suggested that the BLA encodes the motivational significance of the cues and then the orbitofrontal cortex uses this information to select and execute the correct behavioural strategy (Schoenbaum et al. 1999).

Exposure to repeated withdrawal results in excessive activation of several subregions of prefrontal cortex (as seen in our fos-expression studies; Hoang & Stephens (unpublished)), though whether such excessive activation would result in excitotoxicity as seen by Crews et al. (2000) in piriform and perirhinal cortices or facilitated excitatory transmission as we have seen in lateral amygdala (Stephens et al. 2005) is unclear. Behaviourally, we have found evidence that the RWD rats are impaired in suppressing prepotent responses (Borlikova et al. 2006a; Stephens et al. 2001), showing shorter latencies in initiating inappropriate responses than control rats, even when the controls fail to inhibit the response (Borlikova et al. 2006a). This impairment in suppressing a prepotent response is reminiscent of the poor performance of binge drinkers and multiple-detoxified alcoholic patients in the Gordon Diagonostic Adult Vigilance task (Duka et al. 2003; Townshend & Duka 2005).

Impaired frontal function is often associated with loss of control over drug taking. An interesting speculation is whether such changes as we have observed might predict that binge drinking itself leads to loss of control over alcohol consumption. In that context, it may be important that we (Brown et al. 1998) and others (Schulteis et al. 1996) have published evidence that in rats, previous episodes of ethanol exposure and withdrawal leads to facilitated responding for ethanol rewards, as well as to facilitated reinstatement of extinguished responding for ethanol by drug-related cues (Ciccocioppo et al. 2003).

In summary, In both human binge drinkers and in an animal model of binge patterns of alcohol intake, we have found behavioural evidence for altered function of prefrontal cortex and amygdala. Such changes may reflect aberrant plasticity induced by repeated periods of alcohol exposure and withdrawal in neuronal systems subserving conditioning, resulting in both hyperactivity of these neural systems and impaired associative learning.

Acknowledgements

The research of the authors described in this review was supported by the UK Medical Research Council. We gratefully acknowledge the contributions of our colleagues Tamzin Ripley, Julia Townshend, Gilyana Borlikova, Doris Albrecht, Ruth Weissenborn, Julie LeMerrer, Lee Hogarth, Leigh Hoang, and Jess Scaife.

References

Adinoff, B., O'Neill, K. & Ballenger, J. C. 1994 Alcohol withdrawal and limbic kindling. *Am J Addictions* **4**, 5–17.

Adolphs, R., Tranel, D., Hamann, S. et al. 1999 Recognition of facial emotion in nine individuals with bilateral amygdala damage. *Neuropsychologia* **37**, 1111–7.

Ballenger, J. C. & Post, R. M. 1978 Kindling as a model for alcohol withdrawal syndromes. *Br J Psychiatry* **133**, 1–14.

Bannerman, D. M., Yee, B. K., Lemaire, M. et al. 2001 Contextual fear conditioning is disrupted by lesions of the subcortical, but not entorhinal, connections to the hippocampus. *Exp Brain Res* **141**, 304–11.

Bauer, E. P., LeDoux, J. E. & Nader, K. 2001 Fear conditioning and LTP in the lateral amygdala are sensitive to the same stimulus contingencies. *Nat Neurosci* **4**, 687–8.

Beck, C. H. & Fibiger, H. C. 1995 Conditioned fear-induced changes in behavior and in the expression of the immediate early gene c-fos: with and without diazepam pretreatment. *J Neurosci* **15**, 709–20.

Becker, H. C. & Veatch, L. M. 2002 Effects of lorazepam treatment for multiple ethanol withdrawals in mice. *Alcohol Clin Exp Res* **26**, 371–80.

Blackburn, J. R. & Hevenor, S. J. 1996 Amphetamine disrupts negative patterning but does not produce configural association deficits on an alternative task. *Behav Brain Res* **80**, 41–9.

Blair, H. T., Schafe, G. E., Bauer, E. P., Rodrigues, S. M. & LeDoux, J. E. 2001 Synaptic plasticity in the lateral amygdala: a cellular hypothesis of fear conditioning. *Learn Mem* **8**, 229–42.

Borlikova, G. G., Elbers, N. A. & Stephens, D. N. 2006a Repeated withdrawal from ethanol spares contextual fear conditioning and spatial learning but impairs negative patterning and induces over-responding: evidence for effect on frontal cortical but not hippocampal function? *Eur J Neurosci* **24**, 205–16.

Borlikova, G. G., Le Merrer, J. & Stephens, D. N. 2006b Previous experience of ethanol withdrawal increases withdrawal-induced c-fos expression in limbic areas, but not withdrawal-induced anxiety and prevents withdrawal-induced elevations in plasma corticosterone. *Psychopharmacology (Berl)* **185**, 188–200.

Brown, G., Jackson, A. & Stephens, D. N. 1998 Effects of repeated withdrawal from chronic ethanol on oral self-administration of ethanol on a progressive ratio schedule. *Behav Pharmacol* **9**, 149–61.

Brown, S. A., Tapert, S. F., Granholm, E. & Delis, D. C. 2000 Neurocognitive functioning of adolescents: effects of protracted alcohol use. *Alcohol Clin Exp Res* **24**, 164–71.

Bussey, T. J., Dias, R., Redhead, E. S., Pearce, J. M., Muir, J. L. & Aggleton, J. P. 2000 Intact negative patterning in rats with fornix or combined perirhinal and postrhinal cortex lesions. *Exp Brain Res* **134**, 506–19.

Cabinet Office. 2004 Alcohol harm reduction strategy for England. In *Prime Minister's Strategy Unit*. London: The Stationery Office.

Calder, A. J., Lawrence, A. D. & Young, A. W. 2001 Neuropsychology of fear and loathing. *Nat Rev Neurosci* **2**, 352–63.

Carrington, C. D., Ellinwood, E. H., Jr. & Krishnan, R. R. 1984 Effects of single and repeated alcohol withdrawal on kindling. *Biol Psychiatry* **19**, 525–37.

Chapman, P. F., Kairiss, E. W., Keenan, C. L. & Brown, T. H. 1990 Long-term synaptic potentiation in the amygdala. *Synapse* **6**, 271–8.

Ciccocioppo, R., Lin, D., Martin-Fardon, R. & Weiss, F. 2003 Reinstatement of ethanol-seeking behavior by drug cues following single versus multiple ethanol intoxication in the rat: effects of naltrexone. *Psychopharmacology (Berl)* **168**, 208–15.

Cranford, J. A., McCabe, S. E. & Boyd, C. J. 2006 A new measure of binge drinking: prevalence and correlates in a probability sample of undergraduates. *Alcohol Clin Exp Res* **30**, 1896–905.

Crews, F., He, J. & Hodge, C. 2007 Adolescent cortical development: a critical period of vulnerability for addiction. *Pharmacol Biochem Behav* **86**, 189–99.

Crews, F. T., Braun, C. J., Hoplight, B., Switzer, R. C., 3rd & Knapp, D. J. 2000 Binge ethanol consumption causes differential brain damage in young adolescent rats compared with adult rats. *Alcohol Clin Exp Res* **24**, 1712–23.

Dahchour, A. & De Witte, P. 1999 Effect of repeated ethanol withdrawal on glutamate microdialysate in the hippocampus. *Alcohol Clin Exp Res* **23**, 1698–703.

Davidson, T. L., McKernan, M. G. & Jarrard, L. E. 1993 Hippocampal lesions do not impair negative patterning: a challenge to configural association theory. *Behav Neurosci* **107**, 227–34.

Deckel, A. W., Bauer, L. & Hesselbrock, V. 1995 Anterior brain dysfunctioning as a risk factor in alcoholic behaviors. *Addiction* **90**, 1323–34.

Dejong, W. 2001 Finding common ground for effective campus-based prevention. *Psychol Addict Behav* **15**, 292–6.

Drummond, C., Oyefeso, A., Phillips, T. J. et al. 2004 Alcohol needs assessment project. London: Department of Health.

Duka, T., Gentry, J., Malcolm, R. et al. 2004 Consequences of multiple withdrawals from alcohol. *Alcohol Clin Exp Res* **28**, 233–46.

Duka, T., Townshend, J. M., Collier, K. & Stephens, D. N. 2002 Kindling of withdrawal: a study of craving and anxiety after multiple detoxifications in alcoholic inpatients. *Alcohol Clin Exp Res* **26**, 785–95.

Duka, T., Townshend, J. M., Collier, K. & Stephens, D. N. 2003 Impairment in cognitive functions after multiple detoxifications in alcoholic inpatients. *Alcohol Clin Exp Res* **27**, 1563–72.

Fanselow, M. S. & LeDoux, J. E. 1999 Why we think plasticity underlying Pavlovian fear conditioning occurs in the basolateral amygdala. *Neuron* **23**, 229–32.

Fendt, M. & Fanselow, M. S. 1999 The neuroanatomical and neurochemical basis of conditioned fear. *Neurosci Biobehav Rev* **23**, 743–60.

Floyd, D. W., Jung, K. Y. & McCool, B. A. 2003 Chronic ethanol ingestion facilitates *N*-methyl-D-aspartate receptor function and expression in rat lateral/basolateral amygdala neurons. *J Pharmacol Exp Ther* **307**, 1020–9.

Gallagher, M. & Holland, P. C. 1992 Preserved configural learning and spatial learning impairment in rats with hippocampal damage. *Hippocampus* **2**, 81–8.

George, D. T., Nutt, D. J., Dwyer, B. A. & Linnoila, M. 1990 Alcoholism and panic disorder: is the comorbidity more than coincidence? *Acta Psychiatr Scand* **81**, 97–107.

Giancola, P. R., Zeichner, A., Yarnell, J. E. & Dickson, K. E. 1996 Relation between executive cognitive functioning and the adverse consequences of alcohol use in social drinkers. *Alcohol Clin Exp Res* **20**, 1094–8.

Grace, A. A. & Rosenkranz, J. A. 2002 Regulation of conditioned responses of basolateral amygdala neurons. *Physiol Behav* **77**, 489–93.

Hall, J., Thomas, K. L. & Everitt, B. J. 2001a Cellular imaging of zif268 expression in the hippocampus and amygdala during contextual and cued fear memory retrieval: selective activation of hippocampal CA1 neurons during the recall of contextual memories. *J Neurosci* **21**, 2186–93.

Hall, J., Thomas, K. L. & Everitt, B. J. 2001b Fear memory retrieval induces CREB phosphorylation and Fos expression within the amygdala. *Eur J Neurosci* **13**, 1453–8.

Hariri, A. R., Bookheimer, S. Y. & Mazziotta, J. C. 2000 Modulating emotional responses: effects of a neocortical network on the limbic system. *Neuroreport* **11**, 43–8.

Jefferis, B. J., Power, C. & Manor, O. 2005 Adolescent drinking level and adult binge drinking in a national birth cohort. *Addiction* **100**, 543–9.

Killcross, S., Robbins, T. W. & Everitt, B. J. 1997 Different types of fear-conditioned behaviour mediated by separate nuclei within amygdala. *Nature* **388**, 377–80.

Kim, J. J. & Jung, M. W. 2006 Neural circuits and mechanisms involved in Pavlovian fear conditioning: a critical review. *Neurosci Biobehav Rev* **30**, 188–202.

Krystal, J. H., Webb, E., Grillon, C. et al. 1997 Evidence of acoustic startle hyperreflexia in recently detoxified early onset male alcoholics: modulation by yohimbine and m-chlorophenylpiperazine (mCPP). *Psychopharmacology (Berl)* **131**, 207–15.

Lack, A. K., Diaz, M. R., Chappell, A., DuBois, D. W. & McCool, B. A. 2007 Chronic ethanol and withdrawal differentially modulate pre- and postsynaptic function at glutamatergic synapses in rat basolateral amygdala. *J Neurophysiol* **98**, 3185–96.

Lange, J. E. & Voas, R. B. 2001 Defining binge drinking quantities through resulting blood alcohol concentrations. *Psychol Addict Behav* **15**, 310–6.

Liao, D., Hessler, N. A. & Malinow, R. 1995 Activation of postsynaptically silent synapses during pairing-induced LTP in CA1 region of hippocampal slice. *Nature* **375**, 400–4.

Maren, S. 2005 Synaptic mechanisms of associative memory in the amygdala. *Neuron* **47**, 783–6.

Mehrabian, A. & Russell, J. A. 1978 A questionnaire measure of habitual alcohol use. *Psychol Rep* **43**, 803–6.

Milad, M. R. & Quirk, G. J. 2002 Neurons in medial prefrontal cortex signal memory for fear extinction. *Nature* **420**, 70–4.

Moreira, R. C. & Bueno, J. L. 2003 Conditional discrimination learning and negative patterning in rats with neonatal hippocampal lesion induced by ionizing radiation. *Behav Brain Res* **138**, 29–44.

Morris, J. S., Friston, K. J., Buchel, C. et al. 1998 A neuromodulatory role for the human amygdala in processing emotional facial expressions. *Brain* **121 (Pt 1)**, 47–57.

Moselhy, H. F., Georgiou, G. & Kahn, A. 2001 Frontal lobe changes in alcoholism: a review of the literature. *Alcohol Alcohol* **36**, 357–68.

NIAAA. 2004 Binge drinking defined. *NIAAA Newsletter* **3**.

Obernier, J. A., Bouldin, T. W. & Crews, F. T. 2002a Binge ethanol exposure in adult rats causes necrotic cell death. *Alcohol Clin Exp Res* **26**, 547–57.

Obernier, J. A., White, A. M., Swartzwelder, H. S. & Crews, F. T. 2002b Cognitive deficits and CNS damage after a 4-day binge ethanol exposure in rats. *Pharmacol Biochem Behav* **72**, 521–32.

Overstreet, D. H., Knapp, D. J. & Breese, G. R. 2002 Accentuated decrease in social interaction in rats subjected to repeated ethanol withdrawals. *Alcohol Clin Exp Res* **26**, 1259–68.

Papadimitriou, A. & Wynne, C. D. 1999 Preserved negative patterning and impaired spatial learning in pigeons (Columba livia) with lesions of the hippocampus. *Behav Neurosci* **113**, 683–90.

Perkins, H. W., Linkenbach, J. & Dejong, W. 2001 Estimated blood alcohol levels reached by 'binge' and 'nonbinge' drinkers: a survey of young adults in Montana. *Psychol Addict Behav* **15**, 317–20.

Pinel, J. P. 1980 Alcohol withdrawal seizures: implications of kindling. *Pharmacol Biochem Behav* **13 (Suppl 1)**, 225–31.

Pinel, J. P. & Van Oot, P. H. 1975 Generality of the kindling phenomenon: some clinical implications. *Can J Neurol Sci* **2**, 467–75.

Pinel, J. P., Van Oot, P. H. & Mucha, R. F. 1975 Intensification of the alcohol withdrawal syndrome by repeated brain stimulation. *Nature* **254**, 510–11.

Pitkanen, A., Savander, V. & LeDoux, J. E. 1997 Organization of intra-amygdaloid circuitries in the rat: an emerging framework for understanding functions of the amygdala. *Trends Neurosci* **20**, 517–23.

Randall, D. C., Elsabagh, S. M., Hartley, D. E., and File, S. E. 2004 Does drinking have effects on mood and cognition in male and female students? *PBB* **78**: 629–38.

Richmond, M. A., Nichols, B. P., Deacon, R. M. & Rawlins, J. N. 1997 Effects of scopolamine and hippocampal lesions on negative patterning discrimination performance in rats. *Behav Neurosci* **111**, 1217–27.

Ripley, T. L., Borlikova, G., Lyons, S. & Stephens, D. N. 2004 Selective deficits in appetitive conditioning as a consequence of ethanol withdrawal. *Eur J Neurosci* **19**, 415–25.

Ripley, T. L., O'Shea, M. & Stephens, D. N. 2003 Repeated withdrawal from ethanol impairs acquisition but not expression of conditioned fear. *Eur J Neurosci* **18**, 441–8.

Roberto, M., Bajo, M., Crawford, E., Madamba, S. G. & Siggins, G. R. 2006 Chronic ethanol exposure and protracted abstinence alter NMDA receptors in central amygdala. *Neuropsychopharmacology* **31**, 988–96.

Roberto, M., Madamba, S. G., Stouffer, D. G., Parsons, L. H. & Siggins, G. R. 2004a Increased GABA release in the central amygdala of ethanol-dependent rats. *J Neurosci* **24**, 10159–66.

Roberto, M., Schweitzer, P., Madamba, S. G., Stouffer, D. G., Parsons, L. H. & Siggins, G. R. 2004b Acute and chronic ethanol alter glutamatergic transmission in rat central amygdala: an in vitro and in vivo analysis. *J Neurosci* **24**, 1594–603.

Rogan, M. T. & LeDoux, J. E. 1995 LTP is accompanied by commensurate enhancement of auditory-evoked responses in a fear conditioning circuit. *Neuron* **15**, 127–36.

Rogan, M. T., Staubli, U. V. & LeDoux, J. E. 1997 Fear conditioning induces associative long-term potentiation in the amygdala. *Nature* **390**, 604–7.

Rosenkranz, J. A. & Grace, A. A. 2002 Cellular mechanisms of infralimbic and prelimbic prefrontal cortical inhibition and dopaminergic modulation of basolateral amygdala neurons in vivo. *J Neurosci* **22**, 324–37.

Rudy, J. W. & Sutherland, R. J. 1989 The hippocampal formation is necessary for rats to learn and remember configural discriminations. *Behav Brain Res* **34**, 97–109.

Samson, H. H. & Harris, R. A. 1992 Neurobiology of alcohol abuse. *Trends Pharmacol Sci* **13**, 206–11.

Schoenbaum, G., Chiba, A. A. & Gallagher, M. 1999 Neural encoding in orbitofrontal cortex and basolateral amygdala during olfactory discrimination learning. *J Neurosci* **19**, 1876–84.

Schulteis, G., Hyytia, P., Heinrichs, S. C. & Koob, G. F. 1996 Effects of chronic ethanol exposure on oral self-administration of ethanol or saccharin by Wistar rats. *Alcohol Clin Exp Res* **20**, 164–71.

Selden, N. R., Everitt, B. J., Jarrard, L. E. & Robbins, T. W. 1991 Complementary roles for the amygdala and hippocampus in aversive conditioning to explicit and contextual cues. *Neuroscience* **42**, 335–50.

Sigurdsson, T., Doyere, V., Cain, C. K. & LeDoux, J. E. 2007 Long-term potentiation in the amygdala: a cellular mechanism of fear learning and memory. *Neuropharmacology* **52**, 215–27.

Spinella, M. 2004 Neurobehavioral correlates of impulsivity: evidence of prefrontal involvement. *Int J Neurosci* **114**, 95–104.

Stephens, D. N., Brown, G., Duka, T. & Ripley, T. L. 2001 Impaired fear conditioning but enhanced seizure sensitivity in rats given repeated experience of withdrawal from alcohol. *Eur J Neurosci* **14**, 2023–31.

Stephens, D. N., Ripley, T. L., Borlikova, G. et al. 2005 Repeated ethanol exposure and withdrawal impairs human fear conditioning and depresses long-term potentiation in rat amygdala and hippocampus. *Biol Psychiatry* **58**, 392–400.

Stockwell, T., Murphy, D., and Hodgson, R. 1983 The severity of alcohol dependence questionnaire: it's not selectivity & validity. *Br J Addict* **78**: 145–55.

Tarter, R. E., Kirisci, L., Habeych, M., Reynolds, M. & Vanyukov, M. 2004 Neurobehavior disinhibition in childhood predisposes boys to substance use disorder by young adulthood: direct and mediated etiologic pathways. *Drug Alcohol Depend* **73**, 121–32.

Townshend, J. M. & Duka, T. 2002 Patterns of alcohol drinking in a population of young social drinkers: a comparison of questionnaire and diary measures. *Alcohol Alcohol* **37**, 187–92.

Townshend, J. M. & Duka, T. 2003 Mixed emotions: alcoholics' impairments in the recognition of specific emotional facial expressions. *Neuropsychologia* **41**, 773–82.

Townshend, J. M. & Duka, T. 2005 Binge drinking, cognitive performance and mood in a population of young social drinkers. *Alcohol Clin Exp Res* **29**, 317–25.

Ulrichsen, J., Woldbye, D. P., Madsen, T. M. et al. 1998 Electrical amygdala kindling in alcohol-withdrawal kindled rats. *Alcohol Alcohol* **33**, 244–54.

Volkow, N. D., Fowler, J. S. & Wang, G. J. 2003 The addicted human brain: insights from imaging studies. *J Clin Invest* **111**, 1444–51.

Wechsler, H. & Austin, S. B. 1998 Binge drinking: the five/four measure. *J Stud Alcohol* **59**, 122–4.

Wechsler, H., Davenport, A., Dowdall, G., Moeykens, B. & Castillo, S. 1994 Health and behavioral consequences of binge drinking in college. A national survey of students at 140 campuses. *Jama* **272**, 1672–7.

Wechsler, H. & Nelson, T. F. 2001 Binge drinking and the American college student: what's five drinks? *Psychol Addict Behav* **15**, 287–91.

Weissenborn, R. & Duka, T. 2003 Acute alcohol effects on cognitive function in social drinkers: their relationship to drinking habits. *Psychopharmacology (Berl)* **165**, 306–12.

Whishaw, I. Q. & Tomie, J. A. 1991 Acquisition and retention by hippocampal rats of simple, conditional, and configural tasks using tactile and olfactory cues: implications for hippocampal function. *Behav Neurosci* **105**, 787–97.

Zeigler, D. W., Wang, C. C., Yoast, R. A. et al. 2005 The neurocognitive effects of alcohol on adolescents and college students. *Prev Med* **40**, 23–32.

8

The neurobiology of pathological gambling and drug addiction: An overview and new findings

*Marc N. Potenza**

Gambling is a prevalent recreational behaviour amongst adults across cultures. Approximately 5% of adults have been estimated to experience problems with gambling. The most severe form of gambling, pathological gambling (PG), is recognized as a mental health condition. Two alternate non-mutually-exclusive conceptualizations of PG have considered it as an obsessive–compulsive–spectrum disorder and a 'behavioural' addiction. The most appropriate conceptualization of PG has important theoretical and practical implications. Data suggest a closer relationship between PG and substance use disorders than exists between PG and obsessive–compulsive disorder. This article will review data on the neurobiology of PG, consider its conceptualization as a 'behavioural' addiction, discuss impulsivity as an underlying construct, and present new brain imaging findings investigating the neural correlates of craving states in PG as compared to those in cocaine dependence. Implications for prevention and treatment strategies will be discussed.

Key Words: Gambling; addiction; impulsivity; impulse control disorder; brain imaging; fMRI.

8.1 Introduction

Technological advances in multiple domains (genetics, brain imaging) have facilitated an improved understanding of many behaviours and mental health disorders. Until recently, relatively little research has examined gambling and disorders characterized by excessive gambling (Eber & Shaffer 2000). Newly developed techniques like functional brain imaging are providing new insights into gambling behaviours, and data generated from these studies are helping to address theoretical and practical questions about gambling.

8.2 Recreational, problem, and pathological gambling

Gambling can be defined as placing something of value at risk in the hopes of gaining something of greater value (Potenza et al. 2006). A majority of adults gamble, and most do so without encountering significant problems. Nonetheless, gambling problems amongst adults have been estimated as high as 5%, with certain groups (young adults, people with mental health disorders, and incarcerated individuals) having estimates several fold higher (Shaffer et al. 1999). Pathological gambling (PG), representing the most severe form of problem gambling (see below), has prevalence estimates around 0.5–1% (Petry et al. 2005). Given the increased availability of legalized gambling and its popularity over the past several decades, increased attention to the health impacts of specific levels of gambling behaviours is warranted (Shaffer & Korn 2002).

Evidence of gambling exists dating back millennia and across civilizations (Potenza & Charney 2001). Early reports of gambling include descriptions of problematic levels of

* marc.potenza@yale.edu

gambling; for example, the Mahabharata relates the tale of prince Dharamputr who gambles away his kingdom, brothers, and wife (Mahabharata 1884). Although other more recent historical accounts of problematic gambling exist (Dostoyevsky 1966) and have been considered by psychiatrists like Freud (Freud 1961), it was not until 1980 that the Diagnostic and Statistical Manual (DSM) defined criteria for a gambling disorder (American Psychiatric Association 1980). The term 'pathological gambling' was selected in favour of other terms (e.g. compulsive gambling) that were arguably more widely used at the time, perhaps in an effort to distinguish the disorder from obsessive–compulsive disorder. Along with pyromania, kleptomania, trichotillomania, and intermittent explosive disorder, PG is currently classified as an 'Impulse Control Disorder Not Elsewhere Categorized' in the DSM. Similarly, in the International Classification of Disorders, the disorder is classified under 'Habit and Impulse Disorders' along with pyromania, kleptomania, and trichotillomania. Many of the current diagnostic criteria for PG share features with those for drug dependence (DD). For example, criteria targeting tolerance, withdrawal, repeated unsuccessful attempts to cut back or quit, and interference in major areas of life functioning are contained in the criteria for both PG and DD. Similarities extend to phenomenological, epidemiological, clinical, genetic, and other biological domains (Goudriaan et al. 2004; Potenza 2006; Brewer & Potenza 2008), raising questions about whether PG might best be characterized as a 'behavioural' addiction.

8.3 PG as an addiction

The term addiction, derived from the Latin word meaning 'bound to' or 'enslaved by' (Potenza 2006), was not initially linked to substance use behaviours. Over time, the word has been used to describe excessive alcohol and drug use (Maddux & Desmond 2000) such that there was general agreement in the 1980s that addiction referred exclusively to compulsive drug taking (O'Brien et al. 2006). Only relatively recently, and in large part due to neurobiological studies (Holden 2001), has PG (and other excessive behaviours in the domains of shopping, sex, and eating) been considered more seriously by the scientific community as addictive in nature (Potenza 2006; Holden 2001).

If PG represents an addiction, it should share with DD core features. Core components of addictions have been proposed including the following: (1) continued engagement in a behaviour despite adverse consequences, (2) diminished self-control over engagement in the behaviour, (3) compulsive engagement in the behaviour, and (4) an appetitive urge or craving state prior to the engagement in the behaviour (Potenza 2006). Many of these features, as well as other such as tolerance and withdrawal, appear relevant to PG and DD (Potenza 2006). Concurrent studies of both PG and DD should help define aspects that are related to drugs. That is, drugs may influence brain structure and function in ways that are central or unrelated to the addiction process. In that PG may be conceptualized as an addiction without the drug, direct comparison of both disorders may provide insight into the core neurobiological features of addiction and guide the development and testing of effective treatments.

8.4 Neurotransmitter systems and PG

Specific neurotransmitters have been hypothesized to relate to different aspects of PG (Potenza & Hollander 2002). On the basis of studies of PG and/or other disorders, norepinephrine has been hypothesized in impulse control disorders (ICDs) to be particularly relevant to aspects of arousal and excitement, serotonin to behavioural initiation and cessation, dopamine to reward and reinforcement, and opioids to pleasure or urges. These and other systems are considered below.

8.4.1 Norepinephrine

Studies performed during the 1980s compared men with PG to those without and found higher levels of norepinephrine or it metabolites in urine, blood, or cerebrospinal fluid samples in the former (Roy et al. 1988), and noradrenergic measures correlated with measures of extraversion (Roy et al. 1989). Gambling or related behaviours have been associated with autonomic arousal, with Pachinko play and casino blackjack each associated with heart rate elevations and increases in noradrenergic measures (Shinohara et al. 1999; Meyer et al. 2000). During casino blackjack gambling, heart rate and noradrenergic measures become elevated to a greater degree in men with gambling problems as compared to those without (Meyer et al. 2004). In addition to a possible role in arousal or excitement, norepinephrine may be related to other aspects of PG. For example, noradrenergic activity influences prefrontal cortical function and posterior attention networks, and medications (e.g. the norepinephrine transport inhibitor atomoxetine and the alpha-2 adrenergic agonists clonidine and guanfacine) that operate through adrenergic mechanisms have been shown to be efficacious in the treatment of attention deficit hyperactivity disorder and other psychiatric disorders (Arnsten 2006). Adrenergic drugs have been shown to influence specific aspects of impulse control in animal and human studies (Chamberlain & Sahakian 2007). These findings suggest a several possible roles for adrenergic function in PG and its treatment, and further investigation is needed in this area to examine these possibilities.

8.4.2 Serotonin

Traditionally, serotonin function has been considered of substantial importance in mediating impulse control. People with clinically relevant levels of impaired impulse control, including those with PG (Nordin & Eklundh 1999) or impulsive aggression (Linnoila et al. 1983), have demonstrated low levels of the serotonin metabolite 5-hydroxy indoleacetic acid (5-HIAA). Individuals with PG or other disorders or behaviours characterized by impaired impulse control (e.g. impulsive aggression) display different behavioural and biochemical responses to serotonergic drugs than do healthy control subjects. Following administration of meta-chlorophenylpiperazine (m-CPP), a partial serotonin receptor agonist that binds to multiple $5HT_1$ and $5HT_2$ receptors with particularly high affinity for the $5HT_{2c}$ receptor, individuals with PG reported a 'high' (DeCaria et al. 1998; Pallanti et al. 2006). This response contrasted with that of control subjects and was similar to the 'high' ratings reported previously by antisocial, borderline, and alcoholic subjects after receiving the drug. Prolactin response to m-CPP also distinguished the PG and control groups, with greater elevation observed in the former.

Serotonergic probes have been used in conjunction with brain imaging in individuals with impaired impulse control. In individuals with impulsive aggression as compared to those without, a blunted response in the ventromedial prefrontal cortex (vmPFC) is seen in response to m-CPP (New et al. 2002) or the indirect agonist fenfluramine (Siever et al. 1999), consistent with findings in alcoholics (Hommer et al. 1997). Similar studies have not been performed to date in PG, although other investigations have implicated vmPFC function in PG (see below).

Given data suggesting an important role for serotonin function in PG and impulse dyscontrol, serotonergic drugs have been investigated in the treatment of PG (Brewer et al. 2008). Serotonin reuptake inhibitors show mixed results. In one small, placebo-controlled, double-blind, crossover trial of fluvoxamine, active and placebo arms were significantly distinguished during the second half of the trial, with active drug being superior to placebo (Hollander et al. 2000). A separate small placebo-controlled trial observed no difference between active fluvoxamine and placebo (Blanco et al. 2002). Similarly, one randomized, controlled, double-blind study of paroxetine demonstrated superiority of active drug over placebo (Kim et al. 2002), whereas a larger, multi-centre, randomized, placebo-controlled, double-blind study found no significant difference between active drug and placebo (Grant et al. 2003). These initial trials typically excluded individuals with co-occurring psychiatric disorders. A small, open-label trial of escitalopram followed by double-blind discontinuation was performed in individuals with PG and co-occurring anxiety disorders (Grant & Potenza 2006). During the open-label phase, gambling and anxiety measures improved in largely a parallel fashion. Randomization to placebo was associated with a resumption of gambling and anxiety measures, whereas randomization to active drug was associated with sustained responses. Although preliminary, these findings suggest that important individual differences exist amongst individuals with PG, and that these differences have important implications for treatment response.

8.4.3 Dopamine

Dopamine is implicated in rewarding and reinforcing behaviours and drug addiction (Nestler 2004). However, few studies have investigated directly a role for dopamine in PG. Ambiguous findings have been reported for cerebrospinal fluid measures of dopamine and its metabolites in PG (Bergh et al. 1997; Nordin & Eklundh 1999). Similarly, one early molecular genetic studies in PG implicated the TaqA1 allele of the dopamine receptor gene DRD2 similarly across PG, substance abuse, and other psychiatric disorders (Comings 1998). Early molecular genetic studies of PG often included methodological limitations such as lack of stratification by race or ethnicity and incomplete diagnostic assessments, and subsequent studies using methods controlling for race/ethnicity and obtaining DSM-IV diagnoses have not observed differences in TaqA1 allelic frequencies in PG (da Silva Lobo et al. 2007). Peer-reviewed publications involving PG subjects and investigating dopamine (or other) systems using ligand-based methodologies do not exist, and such studies represent an important area of future investigation.

PG and other ICDs have been observed in individuals with Parkinson's disease (PD), a disorder characterized by degeneration of dopamine and other systems (Potenza et al. 2007; Jellinger 1991). Individuals with PD are treated with drugs that promote dopamine function (e.g. levo-dopa or dopamine agonists like pramipexole or ropinirole) or interventions (e.g. deep-brain stimulation) that promote neurotransmission through related circuitries (Lang & Obeso 2004). As such, ICDs in PD could potentially emerge from the pathophysiology of the disorder, its treatment, or some combination thereof. Two studies investigated ICDs in several hundred individuals with PD (Voon et al. 2006; Weintraub et al. 2006). ICDs were associated with the class of dopamine agonists rather than specific agents, and individuals with ICDs were younger and had earlier ages at PD onset. Individuals with and without ICDs also differed on other factors related to impaired impulse control. In one study, those with an ICD were more likely to have experienced an ICD prior to PD onset (Weintraub et al. 2006). In another, PD subjects with and without PG were distinguished by measures of impulsivity, novelty seeking, and personal or familial alcoholism (Voon et al. 2007). The potential contribution of these and other individual difference variables warrants further consideration in investigations into the pathophysiologies and treatments of ICDs in PD. Although anecdotal and case series report improvement in ICD symptomatology with discontinuation or diminished dosing of dopamine agonists (Mamikonyan et al. 2008), these studies are preliminary in nature and subject to typical biases of uncontrolled trials. Furthermore, some patients may not tolerate higher doses of levo-dopa used to control symptoms of PD, whereas others might abuse these drugs (Giovannoni et al. 2000; Evans et al. 2005). Together, these findings indicate that more research is needed into the pathophysiologies of and treatments for ICDs in PD.

8.4.4 Opioids

Opioids have been implicated in pleasurable and rewarding processes, and opioid function can influence neurotransmission in the mesolimbic pathway that extends from the ventral tegmental area to the nucleus accumbens or ventral striatum (Spanagel et al. 1992). On the basis of these findings and similarities between PG and addictions like alcohol dependence, opioid antagonists have been evaluated in the treatment of PG and other ICDs. Placebo-controlled, double-blind, randomized trials have evaluated the efficacies and tolerabilities of naltrexone and nalmefene. High-dose naltrexone (average end of study dose = 188 mg/day; range up to 250 mg/day) was superior to placebo in the treatment of PG (Kim et al. 2001). Like in alcohol dependence, the medication appeared particularly helpful for individuals with strong gambling urges at treatment onset. However, liver function test abnormalities were observed in over 20% of subjects receiving active drug during the short trial. Nalmefene, an opioid antagonist not associated with liver function impairment, was subsequently evaluated (Grant et al. 2006). Nalmefene was superior to placebo, and liver function test abnormalities were not observed. The dose showing the most efficacy and tolerability was the 25 mg/day dose, one that is roughly equivalent to the 50 mg/day dose typically used in the treatments of alcohol or opiate dependence. A subsequent analysis of treatment outcome in PG receiving opioid antagonists identified a family history of alcoholism as most strongly associated with a positive drug response, a finding consistent with the alcoholism literature (Grant et al. 2007b). The extent to which other factors associated with treatment response to opioid antagonists in alcoholism (e.g. allelic variants of the gene encoding the mu-opioid receptor (Oslin et al. 2003)) extend to the treatment of PG warrants direct investigation.

8.4.5 Glutamate

Glutamate, the most abundant excitatory neurotransmitter, has been implicated in motivational processes and drug addiction (Chambers et al. 2003; Kalivas & Volkow 2005). On the basis of these data and preliminary findings suggesting a role for glutamatergic therapies in other ICDs (Coric et al. 2007), the glutamatergic modulating agent n-acetyl cysteine was investigated in the treatment of PG (Grant et al. 2007a). The study design involved open-label treatment followed by double-blind discontinuation. During the open-label phase, gambling symptomatology improved significantly. Following double-blind discontinuation, improvement was maintained in 83% of responders randomized to active drug as compared with 29% of those randomized to placebo. These preliminary data indicate the need for additional investigations into glutamatergic contributions to PG and glutamatergic therapies for its treatment.

8.5 Neural systems

Relatively few investigations have examined how brain activities differ in individuals with PG or other ICDs as compared to those without. One initial fMRI study investigated urge or craving states in men with PG (Potenza et al. 2003b). When viewing gambling tapes and prior to the onset of subjective motivational or emotional response, the pathological gamblers (PGers) as compared to recreational ones showed relatively less blood oxygen level dependent (BOLD) signal change in frontal cortical, basal ganglionic, and thalamic brain regions. These between-group differences were not observed during the happy or sad videotape conditions during the comparable epochs of viewing, and the findings are distinct from studies of individuals with obsessive–compulsive disorder who typically showed relatively increased activation of these regions during symptom provocation studies (Breiter & Rauch 1996). During the final period of tape viewing, the time at which the most robust gambling stimuli were presented, men with PG as compared to those without were most distinguished by showing relatively diminished BOLD signal change in vmPFC. These findings appear consistent with those from studies of impaired impulse control in other behavioural domains, notably aggression (Siever et al. 1999; New et al. 2002) and decision-making (Bechara 2003).

Although other imaging studies have implicated frontal regions in PG (Crockford et al. 2005), multiple investigations have observed differences in vmPFC function in PG. A study of cognitive control using an event-related version of the Stroop colour–word interference task found that men with PG as compared to those without were most distinguished by a relatively diminished BOLD signal change in left vmPFC following the presentation of incongruent stimuli (Potenza et al. 2003a). When performing the same fMRI Stroop paradigm, individuals with bipolar disorder were distinguished most from control subjects in a similar region of vmPFC (Blumberg et al. 2003), suggesting that some elements common to the disorders (e.g. impaired impulse control, poor emotional regulation) share neural substrates across diagnostic boundaries. Analogously, individuals with substance dependence with or without PG showed less activation of vmPFC than did control subjects in a 'gambling' task assessing decision-making (Tanabe et al. 2007).

In another fMRI study, individuals with PG as compared to those without showed less activation of vmPFC during simulated gambling in contrasts comparing winning and losing conditions, and BOLD signal change in vmPFC correlated inversely with gambling severity amongst PGers (Reuter et al. 2005). In the same study and using the same contrasts, a similar pattern of diminished activation was observed in PGers in the ventral striatum, a brain region with dopaminergic innervation and that is widely implicated in drug addiction and reward processing (Everitt & Robbins 2005). On the basis of work in primates (Schultz 2000), studies of reward processing in humans have associated activation of the ventral striatum with anticipation of working for monetary reward and activation of vmPFC with receipt of monetary rewards (Knutson et al. 2003). This circuitry appears particularly relevant to the processing of immediate rewards as the selection of larger, delayed reward involves more dorsal cortical networks (McClure et al. 2004). Blackjack gambling as compared to playing blackjack for points is associated with greater cortico-striatal activations in PGers (Hollander et al. 2005). However, this study did not include subjects without PG and thus did not investigate how PG subjects differed from those without the disorder. The finding of relatively diminished activation of ventral striatum in PGers in the simulated gambling paradigm (Reuter et al. 2005) is consistent with findings from studies of reward anticipation in individuals with addictions or seemingly at-risk for such disorders. For example, relatively diminished activation of ventral striatum during anticipation of monetary rewards has been reported in individuals with alcohol dependence (Hommer 2004; Wrase et al. 2007) or cocaine dependence (CD) (Pearlson et al. 2007) as well as in adolescents as compared to adults (Bjork et al. 2004) and those with a family history of alcoholism as compared to those without (Hommer et al. 2004). Together, these findings suggest that relatively diminished activation of ventral striatum during anticipation phases of reward processing might represent an important intermediary phenotype for substance addiction and ICDs.

8.6 Appetitive urge states in PG and CD

Appetitive urge or craving states often immediately precede engagement in problematic behaviours like gambling for PGers or drug use in drug addiction. As such, an understanding of the neural correlates of these states has important clinical implications (Kosten et al. 2006). From a scientific perspective, studies of similar processes like craving states in individuals with PG or those with DD may clarify aspects that are central to the underlying motivational processes across disorders, independent of the effects of acute or chronic drug exposure.

To investigate, we employed data from our published studies of gambling urges in PG (Potenza et al. 2003b) and drug craving in CD (Wexler et al. 2001). As our gambling study involved only male subjects, we restricted analyses to men, yielding a sample including ten PG subjects and eleven recreational gamblers (C_{PG} subjects) who viewed the gambling, sad and happy videotapes during fMRI, and nine CD subjects and six non-cocaine-using, control comparison men (C_{CD} subjects) who viewed the cocaine, sad and happy scenarios, as described previously. We investigated in the following manner the extent to which brain activations in motivational and emotional processing were similar or distinct in a 'behavioural' addiction like PG as compared to the drug addiction CD. We hypothesized that brain regions whose function was influenced by cocaine exposure, such as frontal and anterior cingulate cortex, would be differentially involved in cocaine cravings in CD and gambling urges in PG.

We used a voxel-based randomization procedure to assign statistical significance in the generation of p-maps that identify differences in the manners in which affected subjects' brain function differs from that of controls across the gambling and cocaine groups during viewing of the addiction, happy and sad videotapes (Wexler et al. 2001; Potenza et al. 2003b). For each subject group viewing each tape type, we generated a t-map comparing the period of scenario viewing as compared with the average pre- and post-tape gray screen baselines. Next, for each tape type, we generated t-maps contrasting the manners in which the affected subjects (e.g. PG) differed from their respective controls (e.g. C_{PG}), generating a PG–C_{PG} contrast. Next, we contrasted the manner in which the affected groups differed from controls across the addictions ((PG–C_{PG})–(CD–C_{CD}); Table 8.1, Fig. 8.1A. At $p < 0.005$ and using a cluster of 25 to increase stringency (Friston et al. 1994), disorder-related differences in the contrasts between affected and non-affected subject groups were observed during viewing of the addiction tapes (Table 8.1, Fig. 8.1A) but not the sad or happy scenarios (not shown). Regions of ventral and dorsal anterior cingulate and right inferior parietal lobule were identified during viewing of the addiction scenarios, with relatively decreased activity in the (PG–C_{PG}) contrast as compared with the (CD–C_{CD}) comparison. Within subject-group, contributions to these differences are tabulated (Table 8.1A). The anterior cingulate cortex, a brain region implicated in emotional processing and cognitive control in healthy (Bush 2000) and CD subjects (Goldstein et al. 2007), has been shown to activate during cocaine craving (Childress et al. 1999). Cocaine administration activates the anterior cingulate

Table 8.1a Differences in addiction-related BOLD signal changes $((PG–C_{PG})–(CD–C_{CD}))$[a]

Brain region	Talaraich co-ordinates[b] (x, y, z)	Radius, mm^2	Subject groups[c]			
			Gambling tapes		Cocaine tapes	
			PG subjects	PG controls	CD subjects	CD controls
Right inferior parietal lobule	(−49, −44, 32)	4.20	No change	Increased, 0.01	No change	Decreased, 0.05
Bilateral dorsal AC	(−1, 31, 23)	4.96	Decreased, 0.05	No change	Increased, 0.02	No change
Bilateral ventral AC	(0, 36, −1)	8.05	Decreased, 0.05	No change	Increased, 0.005	No change

Table 8.1b Similarities in addiction-related BOLD signal hanges $((PG–C_{PG})+(CD–C_{CD}))$[d]

Brain region	Talaraich co-ordinates[b] (x, y, z)	Radius, mm^2	Subject groups[c]			
			Gambling tapes		Cocaine tapes	
			PG subjects	PG controls	CD subjects	CD controls
Right posterior cingulate	(−9, −39, 41)	4.21	Decreased, 0.01	Increased, 0.01	No change	Increased, 0.02
Bilateral precuneus	(3, −59, 32)	5.45	Decreased, 0.02	Increased, 0.05	No change	Increased, 0.05
Right thalamus	(−7, −23, 14)	6.62	Decreased, 0.01	Increased, 0.05	Decreased, 0.05	No change
Left insula/ ventrolateral prefrontal cortex	(34, 19, 0)	9.62	Decreased, 0.02	Increased, 0.01	No change	Increased, 0.05
Right ventral striatum/ventral PFC	(−19, 12, −5)	4.88	Decreased, 0.05	Increased, 0.01	No change	Increased, 0.02
Left lingual gyrus	(24, −59, −5)	5.09	No change	Increased, 0.05	No change	Increased, 0.02

[a]Brain activity changes differentially distinguishing addicted from control subjects were identified during the entire period of viewing of addiction videotapes (gambling for PG and C_{PG} subjects and cocaine for CD and C_{CD} subjects). No activity changes were identified in the corresponding $((PG–C_{PG})–(CD–C_{CD}))$ comparisons for the sad and happy videotapes. Directions of changes in activity indicated are those observed in individual within-group p-maps contributing to the between-group comparison maps. Individual within-group p-maps were evaluated at successive significance thresholds of $p < 0.005, 0.01, 0.02$, and 0.05 to identify contributions. P-values are listed following the direction of change to indicate the significance level of the p-map in which the indicated within-subject-group change is observed. In cases in which activity changes span across z-levels of image acquisition (as determined by the Yale fMRI imaging software), the listed value reflects the lowest significance value of a contributing map at a given z-level.

[b]Coordinates listed identify approximate Talairach coordinates for the average center of mass for an activity change. Negative x values indicate the right side of the brain and negative y values indicate brain posterior to the anterior commissure. An activity change centered on white matter (corpus collosum) at (15, 25, 14) was observed in the contrast differentially distinguishing addicted from control subjects (B). This activity change was considered artifactual, removed from further analysis, and not listed in the table.

[c]Directions of changes in activity indicated are those observed in individual within-group p maps contributing to the between-group comparison maps. Individual within-group p-maps were evaluated at successive significance thresholds of $p < 0.005, 0.01, 0.02$, and 0.05 to identify contributions. P-values listed following the direction of change to indicate the significance level of the p-map in which the indicated within-subject-group change is observed. In cases in which activity changes span across z-levels of image acquisition (as determined by the Yale fMRI imaging software), the listed value reflects the lowest significance value of a contributing map at a given z-level.

[d]Brain activity changes similarly distinguishing addicted from control subjects were identified during the initial period of viewing of addiction videotapes (gambling for PG and C_{PG} subjects and cocaine for CD and CCd subjects). No activity changes were identified in the corresponding $((PG–C_{PG})–(CD–C_{CD}))$ comparisons for the sad and happy videotapes.

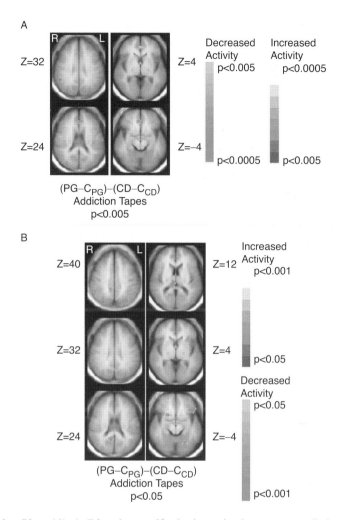

Fig. 8.1 (See also Plate 10) A Disorder-specific brain activation patterns distinguishing affected and non-affected subject groups. Shown are brain activation maps showing relatively decreased activity in the anterior cingulate (Talaraich levels $z = -4$, 4, and 24) and inferior parietal lobule ($z = 32$) for the comparison of (PG-control subjects viewing gambling scenarios) versus (CD-control subjects viewing cocaine scenarios) (($PG-C_{PG}$)$-$($CD-C_{CD}$)). Decreased activity in the PG vs. C_{PG} comparison as compared to the CD vs. C_{CD} one is indicated by blue to purple coloration indicating significance values of $p<0.005$ to 0.0005, respectively. The numbers of subjects contributing to the comparisons are: PG, 11; C_{PG}, 10; CD, 9; and C_{CD}, 6. The left side of the brain is displayed on the right. **B** Common brain activation patterns distinguishing affected and non-affected subject groups. Shown are brain regions in which both patient groups' significant differences from their respective control groups during viewing of the relevant addiction tapes. In all cases, patients showed relatively lower activity than their respective controls, with blue to purple coloration indicating significance values of $p<0.05$ to 0.001, respectively. Specific brain regions identified include left insula/inferior frontal gyrus (Talaraich $z = 4$, -4), right ventral striatum/ventral prefrontal cortex ($z = -4$), left lingual gyrus ($z = -4$), right thalamus ($z = 12$), precuneus ($z = 32$), and right posterior cingulate ($z = 40$). The numbers of subjects contributing to the comparisons are PG, 11; C_{PG}, 10; CD, 9; and C_{CD}, 6. The left side of the brain is displayed on the right.

(Febo et al. 2005), and the timing and pattern of cocaine administration influences anterior cingulate function (Harvey 2004). The difference in inferior parietal lobule activation across subject groups reflects mainly a difference in the neural responses of the control groups to the gambling and cocaine videotapes. The inferior parietal lobule has been implicated in response inhibition components of impulse regulation (Menon et al. 2001; Garavan et al. 2006). Thus, the findings indicate that viewing tapes of different content (e.g. descriptions of a socially sanctioned behaviour (gambling) as compared to an illegal activity (simulated cocaine use)) is associated with differential activation in control subjects of a brain region involved in mediating response inhibition.

We next investigated brain regions common to cocaine cravings and gambling urges, hypothesizing that we would identify brain regions that have been similarly implicated in CD and PG, such as diminished activation of the ventral striatum in reward processing in affected as compared to control subjects (Reuter et al. 2005; Pearlson et al. 2007). For each subject group viewing each tape type, we generated a t-map comparing the period of scenario viewing to the average pre- and post-tape baselines. Next, for each tape type, we created t-maps showing activation abnormalities in the patient groups by contrasting each patient group with its respective control, generating $PG-C_{PG}$ and $CD-C_{CD}$ contrasts. Computer-generated comparisons at successive significance thresholds ($p < 0.005$, $p < 0.01$, $p < 0.02$, and $p < 0.05$) were made to identify regions in which the $PG-C_{PG}$ and $CD-C_{CD}$ contrasts demonstrated similar findings. Individual group p-maps were used to identify brain regions contributing to these findings. No brain regions were identified using this procedure for the addiction, happy and sad tapes. As our prior studies demonstrated that the initial period of tape viewing, prior to the reported onset of motivational/emotional response, was associated with significant between-group differences in responses to the addiction videotapes (Wexler et al. 2001; Potenza et al. 2003b), we performed similar analyses focusing on the initial period of tape viewing as compared with the pre-tape baseline. This procedure identified multiple brain regions (Table 8.1b, Fig. 8.1B) showing similar activity changes in the contrasts between addicted and control subjects during viewing of the respective addiction tapes, and no regions were identified in comparisons involving the sad or happy tapes (not shown).

The brain regions identified as showing common activation patterns in the addicted vs. non-addicted subject groups include regions that contribute to emotional and motivational processing, reward evaluation and decision-making, response inhibition, and treatment outcome in addiction treatment. In most cases, these regions were activated in control subjects but not in addicted ones. Relatively diminished activation of ventral striatum was observed in the addicted subjects as compared to control subjects, consistent with findings on tasks involving reward processing in PG and CD subject groups (Reuter et al. 2005; Pearlson et al. 2007). Ventral components of prefrontal cortex, notably the orbitofrontal cortex, have been implicated in the processing of rewards (Schultz 2000; Knutson et al. 2003; McClure et al. 2004), and the lateral region is thought to activate when additional information is needed to guide behavioural actions or when decision-making involves the suppression of previously rewarded responses (Elliott et al. 2000). Lateral regions of ventral prefrontal cortex, such as the inferior frontal gyrus, are also considered of significant importance in response inhibition and impulse control (Chamberlain & Sahakian 2007). Other regions whose activation patterns distinguished addicted and non-addicted subjects in the present study have also been implicated in mediating impulse control. For example, in a Go/NoGo paradigm involving healthy subjects, the insula, precuneus, and posterior cingulate were activated during error processing and orbitofrontal cortex and lingual gyrus during response inhibition

(Menon et al. 2001). Insular activation also contributes to conscious urges and thus may influence decision-making processes in addiction (Craig 2002; Naqvi et al. 2007). The failure of addicted subjects to activate these regions in the early stages of response to cues that serve as triggers could contribute to poor self-control and subsequent drug use. These findings have implications for treatment outcome for both PG and drug addiction. For example, insula damage has been associated with impaired betting behaviour as evidenced by a failure to adjust bets with respect to odds of winning and thus impaired activation might be particularly relevant to PG (Clark et al., in press). Posterior cingulate activation during viewing of cocaine videotapes was associated with treatment outcome in CD subjects, with those who were able to abstain showing greater activation of this brain region (Kosten et al. 2006). Thus, although these results should be considered preliminary, given the relatively small samples of each group of subjects, the findings complement the larger literature on PG, drug addiction, impulse control, and the neural correlates of treatment outcome for drug addiction. Additional investigations involving larger and more diverse samples are needed to substantiate and extend these findings.

8.7 Conclusions and future directions

Although significant advances have been made in our understanding of PG over the past decade, substantial gaps remain in our understanding of the disorder. Most biological studies to date have involved small samples of predominantly or exclusively men, raising concerns regarding the generalizability of the findings, particularly to women. Sex differences in gambling behaviours have been reported both with respect to types of gambling problematic for women as compared to men as well as for patterns of development of gambling problems (Potenza et al. 2001). For example, the 'telescoping' phenomenon, a process referring to the foreshortened timeframe between initiation and problematic levels of behavioural engagement, was first described for alcoholism, more recently for DD, and most recently for problem and PG (Potenza et al. 2001). Given such clinically relevant differences, examinations into the underlying biology of PG should consider potential influences of sex. Similarly, different stages of gambling pathology should be considered in biological investigations, given data suggesting differential involvements of neurociruitry (e.g. ventral vs. dorsal striatum) as behaviours progress from more novel or impulsive to habitual or compulsive (Everitt & Robbins 2005; Chambers et al. 2007; Belin & Everitt 2008; Brewer & Potenza 2008). Additional considerations include the nature of impulsivity and its relationship to ICDs and substance addictions. That is, it is possible that substance use may lead to more gambling, more gambling may lead to substance use, or that common factors like impulsivity may contribute to excessive engagement in each domain. Clarifying these possibilities in animal and real-life settings represents a clinically and scientifically relevant goal (Dalley et al. 2007). Given that impulsivity is a complex, multi-faceted construct (Moeller et al. 2001), understanding how specific aspects relate to pathophysiologies and treatments for PG and drug addictions is important. Finally, PG is arguably the best studied of a group of ICDs that are currently categorized together in diagnostic manuals. Additional research is needed into other ICDs and their neurobiologies, prevention, and treatment, particularly as these disorders are associated with markers of greater psychopathology and appear currently to go frequently undiagnosed in clinical settings (Grant et al. 2005).

Acknowledgements

Bruce Wexler and Cheryl Lacadie provided assistance with the functional magnetic resonance imaging work presented. Supported in part by (1) the National Institute on Drug Abuse (R01-DA019039, R01-DA020908, P50-DA016556, P50-DA09241, P50DA16556, P50-AA12870), the National Institute of Alcohol Abuse and Alcoholism (RL1-AA017539, P50-AA015632), and the National Center for Research Resources (UL1-RR024925); (2) Women's Health Research at Yale; (3) the Office of Research on Women's Health; and (4) the US Department of Veterans Affairs VISN1 MIRECC and REAP.

Disclosures

Dr. Potenza reports that he has no conflicts of interest over the past three years to report as related to the subject of the report. Dr. Potenza has received financial support or compensation for the following: Dr. Potenza consults for and is an advisor to Boehringer Ingelheim; has consulted for and has financial interests in Somaxon; has received research support from the National Institutes of Health, Veteran's Administration, the National Center for Responsible Gaming and its affiliated Institute for Research on Gambling Disorder, Mohegan Sun Casino, and Forest Laboratories, Ortho-McNeil, and Oy-Control/Biotie pharmaceuticals; has participated in surveys, mailings, or telephone consultations related to drug addiction, ICD, or other health topics; has consulted for law offices and the federal public defender's office in issues related to ICD; has performed grant reviews for the National Institutes of Health and other agencies; has guested sections on journals has given academic lectures in grand rounds, CME events, and other clinical or scientific venues; has generated books or book chapters for publishers of mental health texts; and provides clinical care in the Connecticut Department of Mental Health and Addiction Services Problem Gambling Services Program. The contents of this chapter are solely the responsibility of the author and do not necessarily represent the official views of any of the funding agencies.

References

Arnsten, A. F. 2006 Fundamentals of attention-deficit/hyperactivity disorder: circuits and pathways. *J Clin Psychiatry* **67**(s8), 7–12.
American Psychiatric Association. 1980 *Diagnostic and Statistical Manual of Mental Disorders.* Washington, DC.
Bechara, A. 2003 Risky business: emotion, decision-making, and addiction. *J Gambling Stud* **19**, 23–51.
Belin, D. & Everitt, B. J. 2008 Cocaine seeking habits depend upon dopamine-dependent serial connectivity linking the ventral with the dorsal striatum. *Neuron* **57**, 432–41.
Bergh, C., Eklund, T., Sodersten, P. & Nordin, C. 1997 Altered dopamine function in pathological gambling. *Psychol Med* **27**(2), 473–5.
Bjork, J. M., Knutson, B., Fong, G. W., Caggiano, D. M., Bennett, S. M. & Hommer, D. W. 2004 Incentive-elicited brain activation in adolescents: similarities and differences from young adults. *J Neurosci* **24**, 1793–802.
Blanco, C., Petkova, E., Ibanez, A. & Saiz-Ruiz, J. 2002 A pilot placebo-controlled study of fluvoxamine for pathological gambling. *Ann Clin Psychiatry* **14**, 9–15.

Blumberg, H. P., Leung, H., Skudlarski, P. et al. 2003 A functional magnetic resonance imaging study of bipolar disorder: state- and trait-related dysfunction in ventral prefrontal cortices. *Arch Gen Psychiatry* **60**, 599–607.

Breiter, H. C. & Rauch, S. L. 1996 Functional MRI and the study of OCD: from symptom provocation to cognitive-behavioral probes of cortico-striatal systems and the amygdala. *Neuroimage* **4**, s127–38.

Brewer, J. A., Grant, J. E. & Potenza, M. N. 2008 The treatment of pathological gambling. *Addict Disorders Treatment* **7**, 1–14.

Brewer, J. A. & Potenza, M. N. 2008 The neurobiology and genetics of impulse control disorders: relationships to drug addictions. *Biochem Pharmacology* **75**, 63–75.

Bush, G. W., Luu, P. & Posner, M. I. 2000 Cognitive and emotional influences in anterior cingulate cortex. *Trends Cog Sci* **4**, 215–22.

Chamberlain, S. R. & Sahakian, B. J. 2007 The neuropsychiatry of impulsivity. *Curr Opin Psychiatry* **20**, 255–61.

Chambers, R. A., Bickel, W. K. & Potenza, M. N. 2007 A scale-free systems theory of motivation and addiction. *Neurosci Biobehav Rev* **31**, 1017–45.

Chambers, R. A., Taylor, J. R. & Potenza, M. N. 2003 Developmental neurocircuitry of motivation in adolescence: a critical period of addiction vulnerability. *Am J Psychiatry* **160**, 1041–52.

Childress, A. R., Mozely, P. D., McElgin, W., Fitzgerald, J., Reivich, M. & O'Brien, C. P. 1999 Limbic activation during cue-induced cocaine craving. *Am J Psychiatry* **156**, 11–18.

Clark, L., Bechara, A., Damasio, H., Aitken, M. R. F., Sahakian, B. J. & Robbins, T. W. In press. Differential effects of insular and ventromedial prefrontal cortex lesions on risky decision-making. *Brain*.

Comings, D. E. 1998 The molecular genetics of pathological gambling. *CNS Spectrums* **3**(6), 20–37.

Coric, V., Kelmendi, B., Pittenger, C., Wasylink, S. & Bloch, M. H. 2007 Beneficial effects of the antiglutamatergic agent riluzole in a patient diagnosed with trichotillomania. *J Clin Psychiatry* **68**, 170–1.

Craig, A. D. 2002 How do you feel? Interoception: the sense of the physiological condition of the body. *Nat Rev Neurosci* **3**, 655–66.

Crockford, D. N., Goodyear, B., Edwards, J., Quickfall, J., and el-Guabely, N. 2005 Cue-induced brain activity in pathological gamblers. *Biol Psychiatry* **58**, 787–95.

Dalley, J. W., Fryer, T. D., Brichard, L. et al. 2007 Nucleus accumbens D2/3 receptors predict trait impulsivity and cocaine reinforcement. *Science* **315**, 1267–70.

da Silva Lobo, D. S., Vallada, H. P., Knight, J. et al. 2007 Dopamine genes and pathological gambling in discordant sib-pairs. *J Gambling Stud* **23**, 421–33.

DeCaria, C. M., Begaz, T. & Hollander, E. 1998 Serotonergic and noradrenergic function in pathological gambling. *CNS Spectrums* **3**(6), 38–47.

Dostoyevsky, F. 1966 *The Gambler/Bobok/A Nasty Story*. Penguin Books: London, England.

Eber, G. B. & Shaffer, H. J. 2000 Trends in bio-behavioral gambling studies research: quantifying citations. *J Gambling Stud* **16**, 461–7.

Elliott, R., Dolan, R. J. & Frith, C. D. 2000 Dissociable functions in the medial and lateral orbitofrontal cortex: evidence from human neuroimaging studies. *Cereb Cortex* **10**, 308–17.

Evans, A. H., Lawrence, A. D., Potts, J., Appel, S. & Lees, A. J. 2005 Factors influencing susceptibility to compulsive dopaminergic drug use in Parkinson disease. *Neurology* **65**, 1570–4.

Everitt, B. & Robbins, T. W. 2005 Neural systems of reinforcement for drug addiction: from actions to habits to compulsion. *Nature Neuroscience* **8**(11), 1481–9.

Febo, M., Segarra, A. C., Nair, G., Schmidt, K., Duong, T. K. & Ferris, C. F. 2005 The neural consequences of repeated cocaine exposure revealed by functional mri in awake rats. *Neuropsychopharmacology* **30**, 936–43.

Freud, S. 1961 Dostoevsky and parricide. In *Complete Psychological Works of Sigmund Freud* (ed. J. Strachey). Hogarth: London, England.

Friston, K. J., Worsleym, K. J, Frackowiak, R. S. J., Mazziotta, J. C. & Evans, A. C. 1994 Assessing the significance of focal activations usg their spatial extent. *Hum Brain Mapp* **1**, 214–20.

Garavan, H., Hester, R., Murphy, K., Fassbender, C. & Kelly, C. 2006 Individual differences in the functional anatomy of inhibitory control. *Brain Res* **1105**, 130–42.

Giovannoni, G., O'Sullivan, J. D., Turner, K., Manson A. J. & Lees, A. J. L. 2000 Hedonic homeostatic dysregulation in patients with Parkinson's disease on dopamine replacement therapies. *J Neurol Neurosurg Psychiatry* **68**, 423–8.

Goldstein, R. Z., Tomasi, D., Rajaram, S. et al. 2007 Role of the anterior cingulate and medial orbito-frontal cortex in processing drug cues in cocaine addiction. *Neurosci* **144**, 1153–9.

Goudriaan, A. E., Oosterlaan, J., de Beurs, E. & van den Brink, W. 2004 Pathological gambling: a comprehensive review of biobehavioral findings. *Neurosci Biobehav Rev* **28**, 123–41.

Grant, J. E., Kim, S. W., Potenza, M. N. et al. 2003 Paroxetine treatment of pathological gambling: a multi-center randomized controlled trial. *Int Clin Psychopharmacol* **18**, 243–9.

Grant, J. E., Kim, S. W. & Odlaug, B. L. 2007a *N*-acetyl cysteine, a glutamate-modulating agent, in the treatment of pathological gambling: a pilot study. *Biol Psychiatry* **62**, 652–7.

Grant, J. E., Kim, S. W., Potenza, M. N. & Hollander, E. 2007b Predictors of response to opiate antagonists and placebo in the treatment of pathological gambling. In *American College of Neuropsychopharmacology Annual Conference*, Boca Raton, FL.

Grant, J. E., Levine, L., Kim, D. & Potenza, M. N. 2005 Impulse control disorders in adult psychiatric inpatients. *Am J Psychiatry* **162**, 2184–8.

Grant, J. E. & Potenza, M. N. 2006 Escitalopram treatment of pathological gambling with co-occurring anxiety: an open-label pilot study with double-blind discontinuation. *Int Clin Psychopharmacol* **21**, 203–209.

Grant, J. E., Potenza, M. N., Hollander, E. et al. 2006 Multicenter investigation of the opioid antago-nist nalmefene in the treatment of pathological gambling. *Am J Psychiatry* **163**, 303–12.

Harvey, J. A. 2004 Cocaine effects on the developing brain. *Neurosci Biobehav Rev* **27**, 751–64.

Holden, C. 2001 'Behavioral' addictions: Do they exist? *Science* **294**, 980–982.

Hollander, E., DeCaria, C. M., Finkell, J. N., Begaz, T., Wong, C. M., & Cartwright, C. 2000 A randomized double-blind fluvoxamine/placebo crossover trial in pathological gambling. *Biol Psychiatry* **47**, 813–17.

Hollander, E., Pallanti, S., Rossi, N. B., Sood, E., Baker, B. R. & Buchsbaum, M. S. Imaging monetary reward in pathological gamblers. 2005 *World J Biol Psychiatry* **6**, 113–20.

Hommer, D. 2004 Motivation in alcoholism. In *International Conference on Applications of Neuroimaging to Alcoholism Conference*. New Haven, CT.

Hommer, D., Andreasen, P., Rio, D. et al. 1997 Effects of m-chlorophenylpiperazine on regional brain glucose utilization: a positron emission tomographic comparison of alcoholic and control subjects. *J Neurosci* **17**, 2796–806.

Hommer, D. W., Bjork, J. M., Knutson, B., Caggiano, D., Fong, G. & Danube, C. 2004 Motivation in children of alcoholics. *Alc Clin Exper Res* **28**(5), 22A.

Jellinger, K. A. Pathology of Parkinson's disease: pathology other than the nigrostriatal pathway. *Mol Chem Neuropath* **14**, 153–97.

Kalivas, P. W. & Volkow, N. D. 2005 The neural basis of addiction: a pathology of motivation and choice. *Am J Psychiatry* **162**, 1403–13.

Kim, S. W., Grant, J. E., Adson, D. E., Shin, Y. C. & Zaninelli, R. 2002 A double-blind, placebo-controlled study of the efficacy and safety of paroxetine in the treatment of pathological gambling disorder. *J Clin Psychiatry* **63**, 501–507.

Kim, S. W., Grant, J. E., Adson, D. E. & Shin, Y. C. 2001 Double-blind naltrexone and placebo comparison study in the treatment of pathological gambling. *Biol Psychiatry* **49**, 914–21.

Knutson, B., Fong, G. W., Bennett, S. M., Adams, C. M. & Hommer, D. 2003 A region of mesial pre-frontal cortex tracks monetarily rewarding outcomes: characterization with rapid event-related fMRI. *Neuroimage* **18**, 263–72.

Kosten, T. R., Scanley, B. E., Tucker, K. A. et al. 2006 Cue-induced brain activity changes and relapse in cocaine dependent patients. *Neuropsychopharm* **31**, 644–50.

Lang, A. E. & Obeso, J. A. 2004 Challenges in Parkinson's disease: restoration of the nigrostriatal dopamine system is not enough. *Lancet Neurol* **3**, 309–16.

Linnoila, M., Virkunnen, M., Scheinen, M., Nuutila, A., Rimon, R. & Goodwin, F. 1983 Low
  cerebrospinal fluid 5 hydroxy indolacetic acid concentrations differentiates impulsive from non
  impulsive violent behavior. *Life Sci* **33**, 2609–14.
Maddux, J. F. & Desmond, D. P. 2000 Addiction or dependence? *Addiction* **95**, 661–5.
Mahabharata. Adiparva. 1884 Bharata Press and American Theological Library: Calcutta and
  Evanston.
Mamikonyan, E., Siderowf, A. D., Duda, J. E. et al. 2008 Long-term follow-up of impulse control
  disorders in Parkinson's disease. *Movement Disorders* **23**, 75–80.
McClure, S., Laibson, D. I., Loewenstein, G. & Cohen, J. D. 2004 Separate neural systems value
  immediate and delayed monetary rewards. *Science* **306**, 503–7.
Menon, V., Adleman, N. E., White, C. D., Glover, G. H. & Reiss, A. L. 2001 Error-related brain
  activation during a Go/NoGo response inhibition task. *Human Brain Mapping* **12**, 131–43.
Meyer, G., Hauffa, B. P., Schedlowski, M., Pawluk, C., Stadler, M. A. & Exton, M. S. 2000 Casino
  gambling increases heart rate and salivary cortisol in regular gamblers. *Biol Psych* **48**, 948–53.
Meyer, G., Schwertfeger, J., Exton, M. S. et al. 2004 Neuroendocrine response to casino gambling in
  problem gamblers. *Psychoneuroendocrinology* **29**, 1272–80.
Moeller, F. G., Barratt, E. S., Dougherty, D. M., Schmitz, J. M. & Swann, A. C. 2001 Psychiatric
  aspects of impulsivity. *Am J Psychiatry* **158**, 1783–93.
Naqvi, N. H., Rudrauf, D., Damasio, H. & Bechara, A. 2007 Damage to the insula disrupts addiction
  to cigarette smoking. *Science* **5811**, 531–4.
Nestler, E. J. 2004 Molecular mechanisms of drug addiction. *Neuropharmacol* **47**, 24–32.
New, A. S., Hazlett, E. A., Buchsbaum, M. S. et al. 2002 Blunted prefrontal cortical 18-fluorodeoxyglucose
  positron emission tomography response to meta-chlorophenylpiperazine in impulsive aggression.
  Arch Gen Psychiatry **59**, 621–9.
Nordin, C. & Eklundh, T. 1999 Altered CSF 5-HIAA disposition in pathologic male gamblers. *CNS
  Spectrums* **4**(12), 25–33.
O'Brien, C. P., Volkow, N. & Li, T. K. 2006 What's in a word? Addiction versus dependence in DSM-V.
  Am J Psychiatry **163**, 764–5.
Oslin, D. W., Berrettini, W., Kranzler, H. R. et al. 2003 A functional polymorphism of the mu-opioid
  receptor gene is associated with naltrexone response in alcohol-dependent patients. *Neuropsycho-
  phamacology* **28**, 1546–52.
Pallanti, S., Bernardi, S., Quercioli, L., DeCaria, C. & Hollander, E. 2006 Serotonin dysfunction in
  pathological gamblers: increased prolactin response to oral m-CPP versus placebo. *CNS Spectrums*
  11, 955–64.
Pearlson, G. D., Shashwath, M., Andre, T. et al. 2007 Abnormal fMRI activation of reward circuitry
  in current versus former cocaine abusers. In *American College of Neuropsychopharmacology Annual
  Conference*, Boca Raton, FL.
Petry, N. M., Stinson, F. S. & Grant, B. F. 2005 Co-morbidity of DSM-IV pathological gambling and
  other psychiatric disorders: results from the National Epidemiologic Survey on Alcohol and
  Related Conditions. *J Clin Psychiatry* **66**, 564–74.
Potenza, M. N. 2006 Should addictive disorders include non-substance-related conditions? *Addiction*
  101(s1), 142–51.
Potenza, M. N. & Charney, D. S. 2001 Pathological gambling: a current perspective. *Semin Clin
  Neuropsychiatry* **6**, 153–4.
Potenza, M. N. & Hollander, E. 2002 Pathological gambling and impulse control disorders. In
  Neuropsychopharmacology: The 5th Generation of Progress(ed. J. C. C. Nemeroff, D. Charney, & K.
  Davis), pp. 1725–42. Lippincott Williams and Wilkens: Baltimore, MD.
Potenza, M. N., Leung, H.-C., Blumberg, H. P. et al. 2003a. An fMRI stroop study of ventromedial
  prefrontal cortical function in pathological gamblers. *Am J Psychiatry* **160**, 1990–4.
Potenza, M. N., Steinberg, M. A., McLaughlin, S., Wu, R., Rounsaville, B. J. & O'Malley, S. S. 2001
  Gender-related differences in the charactaristics of problem gamblers using a gambling helpline.
  Am J Psychiatry **158**, 1500–5.
Potenza, M. N., Steinberg, M. A., Skudlarski, P. et al. 2003b Gambling urges in pathological gamblers:
  An fMRI study. *Arch Gen Psychiatry* **60**, 828–836.

Potenza, M. N., Voon, V. & Weintraub, D. 2007 Drug insight: impulse control disorders and dopamine therapies in Parkinson's disease. *Nat Clin Practice Neurosci* **3**, 664–72.

Reuter, J., Raedler, T., Rose, M., Hand, I., Glascher, J. & Buchel, C. 2005 Pathological gambling is linked to reduced activation of the mesolimbic reward system. *Nat Neurosci* **8**, 147–8.

Roy, A., Adinoff, B., Roehrich, L. et al. 1988 Pathological gambling. A psychobiological study. *Arch Gen Psychiatry* **45**, 369–73.

Roy, A., de Jong, J. & Linnoila, M. 1989 Extraversion in pathological gamblers: Correlates with indexes of noradrenergic function. *Arch Gen Psychiatry* **46**, 679–81.

Schultz, W., Tremblay L. & Hollerman, J. R. 2000 Reward processing in primate orbitofrontal cortex and basal ganglia. *Cerebral Cortex* **10**, 272–84.

Shaffer, H. J., Hall, M. N. & Vander Bilt, J. 1999 Estimating the prevalence of disordered gambling in the United States and Canada: a research synthesis. *Am J Public Health* **89**, 1369–76.

Shaffer, H. J., & Korn, D. A. 2002 Gambling and related mental disorders: A public health analysis. *Annu Rev Public Health* **23**, 171–212.

Shinohara, K., Yanagisawa, A., Kagota, Y. et al. 1999 Physiological changes in Pachinko players; beta-endorphin, catecholamines, immune system substances and heart rate. *Appl Human Sci* **18**, 37–42.

Siever, L. J., Buchsbaum, M. S., New, A. S. et al. 1999 d,l-fenfluaramine response in impulsive personality disorder assessed with [18F]fluorodexyglucose positron emission tomography. *Neuropsychopharmacology* **20**, 413–23.

Spanagel, R., Herz, A. & Shippenberg, T. S. 1992 Opposing tonically active endogenous opioid systems modulate the mesolimbic dopaminergic pathway. *Proc Natl Acad Sci USA* **89**, 2046–50.

Tanabe, J., Thompson, L., Claus, E., Dalwani, M., Hutchison, K. & Banich, M. T. 2007 Prefrontal cortex activity is reduced in gambling and nongambling substance users during decision-making. *Hum Brain Mapp* **28**, 1276–1286.

Voon, V., Hassan, K., Zurowski, M. et al. 2006 Prevalence of repetitive and reward-seeking behaviors in Parkinson's disease. *Neurology* **67**, 1254–57.

Voon, V., Thomsen, T., Miyasaki, J. M. et al. 2007 Factors associated with dopaminergic drug-related pathological gambling in Parkinson's disease. *Arch Neurol* **64**, 212–16.

Weintraub, D., Siderow, A., Potenza, M. N. et al. 2006 Dopamine agonist use is associated with impulse control disorders in Parkinson's Disease. *Arch Neurology* **63**, 969–73.

Wexler, B. E., Gottschalk, C. H., Fulbright, R. K. et al. 2001 Functional magnetic resonance imaging of cocaine craving. *Am J Psychiatry* **158**, 86–95.

Wrase, J., Schlagenhauf, F., Kienast, T. et al. 2007 Dysfunction of reward processing correlates with alcohol craving in detoxified alcoholics. *Neuroimage* **35**, 787–94.

9

Overlapping neuronal circuits in addiction and obesity: Evidence of systems pathology

Nora D. Volkow,* Gene-Jack Wang, Joanna S. Fowler, and Frank Telang

Drugs and food exert their reinforcing effects in part by increasing dopamine (DA) in limbic regions, which has generated interest in understanding how drug abuse/addiction relates to obesity. Here, we integrate findings from positron emission tomography imaging studies on DA's role in drug abuse/addiction and in obesity and propose a common model for these two conditions. Both in abuse/addiction and in obesity, there is an enhanced value of one type of reinforcer (drugs and food, respectively) at the expense of other reinforcers, which is a consequence of conditioned learning and resetting of reward thresholds secondary to repeated stimulation by drugs (abuse/addiction) and by large quantities of palatable food (obesity) in vulnerable individuals (i.e. genetic factors). In this model, during exposure to the reinforcer or to conditioned cues, the expected reward (processed by memory circuits) overactivates the reward and motivation circuits while inhibiting the cognitive control circuit, resulting in an inability to inhibit the drive to consume the drug or food despite attempts to do so. These neuronal circuits, which are modulated by DA, interact with one another so that disruption in one circuit can be buffered by another, which highlights the need for multi-prong approaches in the treatment of addiction and obesity.

Key Words: Dopamine; positron emission tomography; imaging; self-control; compulsion.

9.1 Introduction

Drug abuse and addiction, and certain types of obesity can be understood as resulting from habits that strengthen with repetition of the behaviour and that become increasingly harder for the individual to control despite their potentially catastrophic consequences. Consumption of food, other than eating from hunger, and some drug use are initially driven by their rewarding properties, which in both instances involves activation of mesolimbic dopamine (DA) pathways. Food and drugs of abuse activate DA pathways differently (Table 9.1). Food activates brain reward circuitry both through palatability (involves endogenous opioids and cannabinoids) and through increases in glucose and insulin concentrations (involves DA increases), whereas drugs activate this same circuitry via their pharmacological effects (via direct effects on DA cells or indirectly through neurotransmitters that modulate DA cells such as opiates, nicotine, γ-aminobutyric acid, or cannabinoids; Volkow & Wise 2005).

The repeated stimulation of DA reward pathways is believed to trigger neurobiological adaptations in other neurotransmitters and in downstream circuits that may make the behaviour increasingly compulsive and lead to the loss of control over food and drug intake. In the case of drugs of abuse, repeated supraphysiological DA stimulation from chronic use is believed to induce plastic changes in brain (i.e. glutamatergic cortico-striatal pathways), which result in enhanced emotional reactivity to drugs or their cues, poor inhibitory control over drug consumption and compulsive drug intake (Volkow & Li 2004). In parallel, dopaminergic

* nvolkow@nida.nih.gov

Table 9.1 Comparison of food and drugs as reinforcers (Modified from Volkow & Wise 2005).

	Food	Drug
Potency as a reinforcer[a]	++	Oral, ++ snorted, +++ smoked, injected ++++
Delivery	Oral	Oral, snorted, smoked, injected
Mechanisms reward	Somatosensory (palatability)	Chemical (drug)
		Chemical (glucose)
Relevance of kinetics	Not investigated	The faster the stimulation the more powerful its reinforcing effects
Regulation of intake	Peripheral and central factors	Mostly central factors
Adaptations	Physiologic	Supraphysiologic
Physiological role	Necessary for survival	Unnecessary
Learning	Habits conditioned responses	Habits conditioned responses
Role of stress	+++	+++

[a]Potency as reinforcer is estimated on the basis of the magnitude and the duration of the increases in DA induced by either food or drugs in the NAc, and is an approximate comparison since the potency will be a function of the particular foodstuff as well as the particular drug and its route of administration.

stimulation during intoxication facilitates conditioning to drugs and drug-associated stimuli (drug cues), further strengthening learned habits that then drive the behaviour to take drugs when exposed to cues or to stressors. Similarly, repeated exposure to certain foods (particularly, large quantities of energy-dense food with high-fat and sugar contents; Avena et al. 2008) in vulnerable individuals can also result in compulsive food consumption, poor food intake control, and conditioning to food stimuli. In vulnerable individuals (i.e. those with genetic or developmental predisposing factors), this can result in obesity (for food) or in addiction (for drugs).

The neurobiological regulation of feeding is much more complex than the regulation of drug abuse, since food consumption is controlled not only by reward but also by multiple peripheral, endocrinological and central factors beyond those that participate in reward (Levine et al. 2003). In this paper, we concentrate solely on the neurocircuitry linked with the rewarding properties of food, since it is likely to be a key contributor in accounting for the massive increase in obesity that has emerged over the past three decades. Our hypothesis is that adaptation in the reward circuit and also in the motivational, memory, and control circuits that occur with repeated exposure to large quantities of highly palatable food is similar to that which one observes with repeated drug exposures (Table 9.2). We also postulate that differences between individuals in the function of these circuits prior to compulsive eating or drug abuse are likely to contribute to the differences in vulnerability to food or drugs as the preferred reinforcer. These include differences in sensitivity to rewarding properties of food versus that to drugs; differences in their ability to exert inhibitory control over their intention to eat appealing food in the face of its negative consequences (gain weight) or to take an illicit drug (illegal act); and differences in the propensity to develop conditioned responses when exposed to food versus drugs.

9.2 Reward/saliency circuitry in addiction and obesity

Since DA underlies the rewarding properties of food and many drugs, we postulate that differences in the reactivity of the DA system to food or to drugs could modulate the likelihood of their consumption. To test this hypothesis, we have used positron emission

Table 9.2 Disrupted brain functions implicated in the behavioural phenotype of addiction and obesity and the brain regions believed to underlie their disruption (Modified from Volkow & O'Brien 2007).

Disrupted functions	Implicated brain region
Impaired inhibitory control	Prefrontal cortex
To drug intake in addiction	Anterior cingulate gyrus
To food intake in obesity	Lateral orbitofrontal cortex
Enhanced reward	Nucleus accumbens
To drugs in addiction	Ventral pallidum
To food in obesity	Hypothalamus
Conditioning/habits	Amygdala
To drugs and drug cues in addiction	Hippocampus
To food and food cues in obesity	Dorsal striatum
Enhanced motivation/drive	Medial orbitofrontal cortex
To consume drugs in addiction	Mesencephalic dopamine nuclei
To consume food in obesity	Dorsal striatum
Emotional reactivity	Amygdala
	Ventral cingulate gyrus

tomography (PET) and a multiple tracer approach to assess the DA system in the human brain in healthy controls as well as in subjects that are addicted to drugs and in those that are morbidly obese. Of the synaptic markers of DA neurotransmission, the availability of DA D_2 receptors in striatum is recognized to modulate the reinforcing responses to both drugs and food.

9.2.1 *Drug responses and vulnerability for drug abuse/addiction*

In healthy non-drug abusing controls, we showed that D_2 receptor availability in the striatum modulated their subjective responses to the stimulant drug methylphenidate (MP). Subjects describing the experience as pleasant had significantly lower levels of receptors compared with those describing MP as unpleasant (Volkow et al. 1999a, 2002a). This suggests that the relationship between DA levels and reinforcing responses follows an inverted U-shaped curve: too little is not optimal for reinforcement but too much is aversive. Thus, high D_2 receptor levels could protect against drug self-administration. Support for this is given by preclinical studies showing that upregulation of D_2 receptors in nucleus accumbens (NAc; region in striatum implicated in drug and food reward) dramatically reduced alcohol intake in animals previously trained to self-administer alcohol (Thanos et al. 2001), and by clinical studies showing that subjects who despite having family histories of addiction were not addicted had higher D_2 receptors in striatum than individuals without such family histories (Mintun et al. 2003; Volkow et al. 2006a).

Using PET and the D_2 receptor radioligands, we and other researchers have shown that subjects with a wide variety of drug addictions (cocaine, heroin, alcohol, and methamphetamine) have significant reductions in D_2 receptor availability in striatum that persist months after protracted detoxification (reviewed by Volkow et al. 2004). In addition, drug abusers (cocaine and alcohol) also show decreased DA release, which is likely to reflect reduced DA cell firing (Volkow et al. 1997; Martinez et al. 2005). DA release was measured using PET and [^{11}C]raclopride, which is a D_2 receptor radioligand that competes with endogenous DA for binding to D_2 receptors and thus can be used to assess the changes in DA induced by drugs. The striatal increases in DA (seen as reductions in the specific binding of [^{11}C]raclopride) induced by the intravenous administration of stimulant drugs (MP or amphetamine) in cocaine abusers and alcoholics were markedly blunted when compared with controls (more than 50% lower; Volkow et al. 1997, 2007a; Martinez et al. 2005, 2007). Since DA increases induced by MP are dependent on DA release, a function of DA cell firing, we speculated this difference probably reflected decreased DA cell activity in the cocaine abusers and alcoholics.

These studies suggest two abnormalities in addicted subjects that would result in decreased output of DA reward circuits: decreases in DA D_2 receptors, and DA release in striatum (including NAc). Each would contribute to the decreased sensitivity in addicted subjects to natural reinforcers. Indeed, drug-addicted individuals appear to suffer from an overall reduction in the sensitivity of their reward circuits to natural reinforcers. For example, a functional magnetic resonance imaging study showed reduced brain activation in response to sexual cues in cocaine-addicted individuals (Garavan et al. 2000). Similarly, a PET study found evidence suggesting that the brains of smokers react in a different way to monetary and non-monetary rewards when compared with non-smokers (Martin-Solch et al. 2001). Since drugs are much more potent at stimulating DA-regulated reward circuits than natural reinforcers, they would still be able to activate these downregulated reward circuits. Decreased sensitivity of reward circuits would result in a decreased interest for environmental stimuli, possibly predisposing subjects to seek drug stimulation as a means to temporarily activate these reward circuits.

9.2.2 Eating behavioural patterns and vulnerability for obesity

In healthy normal weight subjects, D_2 receptor availability in the striatum modulated eating behavioural patterns (Volkow et al. 2003a). Specifically, the tendency to eat when exposed to negative emotions was negatively correlated with D_2 receptor availability (the lower the D_2 receptors, the higher the likelihood that the subject would eat if emotionally stressed).

In morbidly obese subjects (body mass index (BMI) > 40), we showed lower than normal D_2 receptor availability and these reductions were proportional to their BMI (Wang et al. 2001). That is, subjects with the lower D_2 receptors had higher BMI. Similar results of decreased D_2 receptors in obese subjects were recently replicated (Haltia et al. 2007). These findings led us to postulate that low D_2 receptor availability could put an individual at risk for overeating. In fact, this is consistent with findings showing that blocking D_2 receptors (antipsychotic medications) increases food intake and raises the risk for obesity (Allison et al. 1999). However, the mechanisms by which low D_2 receptor availability would increase the risk of overeating (or how they increase the risk for drug abuse) are poorly understood.

9.3 Inhibitory control/emotional reactivity circuit in addiction and obesity

9.3.1 Drug abuse and addiction

Drug availability markedly increases the likelihood of experimentation and abuse (Volkow & Wise 2005). Thus, the ability to inhibit prepotent responses that are likely to occur in an environment with easy access to drugs is likely to contribute to the ability of the individual to restrain from taking drugs. Similarly, adverse environmental stressors (i.e. social stressors) also facilitate drug experimentation and abuse. Since not all subjects react the same to stress, differences in emotional reactivity have also been implicated as a factor that modulates the vulnerability for drug abuse (Piazza et al. 1991).

In studies on drug abusers and those on subjects at risk for addiction, we have assessed the relationships between the availability of D_2 receptors and regional brain glucose metabolism (marker of brain function) to evaluate the brain regions that have reduced activity when D_2 receptors are decreased. We have shown that the reductions in striatal D_2 receptors in the detoxified drug-addicted subjects were associated with decreased metabolic activity in orbitofrontal cortex (OFC), anterior cingulate gyrus (CG) and dorsolateral prefrontal cortex (DLPFC; Fig. 9.1; Volkow et al. 1993, 2001, 2007a). Since OFC, CG and DLPFC are involved with inhibitory control (Goldstein & Volkow 2002) and with emotional processing (Phan et al. 2002), we had postulated that their improper regulation by DA in addicted subjects could underlie their loss of control over drug intake and their poor emotional self-regulation. Indeed, in alcoholics, reductions in D_2 receptor availability in ventral striatum are associated with craving severity and greater cue-induced activation of the medial pre-frontal cortex and CG (Heinz et al. 2004). In addition, because damage to the OFC results in perseverative behaviours (Rolls 2000) and in humans impairments in OFC and CG are associated with obsessive compulsive behaviours (Insel 1992), we also postulated that DA impairment of these regions could underlie the compulsive drug intake that characterizes addiction (Volkow et al. 2005).

However, the association could also be interpreted to indicate that impaired activity in prefrontal regions could put individuals at risk for drug abuse and then the repeated drug use could result in the down-regulation of D_2 receptors. Indeed, support for the latter pos-sibility is provided by our studies, in subjects who despite having a high risk for alcoholism

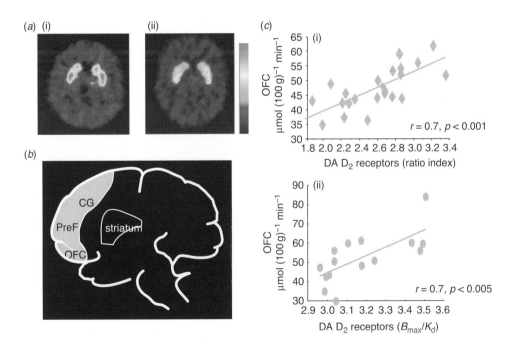

Fig. 9.1 (See also Plate 2) (*a*) Images of DA D_2 receptors (measured with [^{11}C]raclopride in striatum) in (i) a control and (ii) a cocaine abuser. (*b*) Diagram showing where glucose metabolism was associ-ated with DA D_2 receptors in cocaine abusers, which included the orbitofrontal cortex (OFC), the cingulate gyrus (CG) and the dorsolateral prefrontal cortex (PreF). (*c*) Regression slopes between D_2 receptor availability and brain glucose metabolism in OFC in a group of detoxified (i) cocaine and (ii) methamphetamine abusers. Modified from Volkow et al. (2007b).

(owing to a dense family history of alcoholism) were not alcoholics: in these, we showed higher D_2 receptors in striatum than in individuals without such family histories (Volkow et al. 2006a). In these subjects, the higher the D_2 receptors, the higher the metabolism in OFC, CG and DLPFC. In addition, OFC metabolism was also positively correlated with personality measures of positive emotionality. Thus, we postulate that high levels of D_2 receptors could protect against addiction by modulating prefrontal regions involved in inhibitory control and emotional regulation.

9.3.2 Food intake and obesity

Since food availability and variety increase the likelihood of eating (Wardle 2007), the easy access to appealing food requires the frequent need to inhibit the desire to eat it (Berthoud 2007). The extent to which individuals differ in their ability to inhibit these responses and control how much they eat is likely to modulate their risk for overeating in our current food-rich environments (Berthoud 2007).

   As described above, we had previously documented a reduction in D_2 receptors in morbidly obese subjects. This led us to postulate that low D_2 receptors could put an individual at risk for overeating. The mechanisms by which low D_2 receptors could increase the risk of over-eating is unclear but we postulated that, just as for the case with drug abuse/addiction, this could be mediated by D_2 receptor-mediated regulation of prefrontal regions.

   To assess whether the reductions in D_2 receptors in morbidly obese subjects were associated with activity in prefrontal regions (CG, DLPFC, and OFC), we assessed the relationship between D_2 receptor availability in striatum and brain glucose metabolism. Both SPM analysis (to assess correlations on a pixel-by-pixel basis with no pre-selection of regions) as well as independently drawn regions of interest revealed that D_2 receptor availability was associated with metabolism in dorsolateral prefrontal cortex (Brodmann areas (BA) 9 and 10), medial OFC (BA 11), and CG (BA 32 and 25; Fig. 9.2). The association with prefrontal metabolism suggests that decreases in D_2 receptors in obese subjects contribute to overeating in part through deregulation of prefrontal regions implicated in inhibitory control and emotional regulation.

9.4 Motivation/drive in drug abuse/addiction and obesity

9.4.1 Drug abuse and addiction

In contrast to the decreases in metabolic activity in prefrontal regions in detoxified cocaine abusers, these regions are hypermetabolic in active cocaine abusers (Volkow et al. 1991). Thus, we postulate that during cocaine intoxication or as the intoxication subsides, the drug-induced DA increases in striatum activate OFC and CG, which result in craving and compulsive drug intake. Indeed, we have shown that intravenous MP increased metabolism in OFC only in the cocaine abusers in whom it induced intense craving (Volkow et al. 1999b). Activation of the OFC and the CG in drug abusers has also been reported to occur during craving elicited by viewing a cocaine-cue video (Grant et al. 1996) and by recalling previous drug experiences (Wang et al. 1999).

9.4.2 Obesity

Imaging studies in obese subjects have documented increased activation of prefrontal regions upon exposure to a meal, which is greater in obese than lean subjects (Gautier et al. 2000).

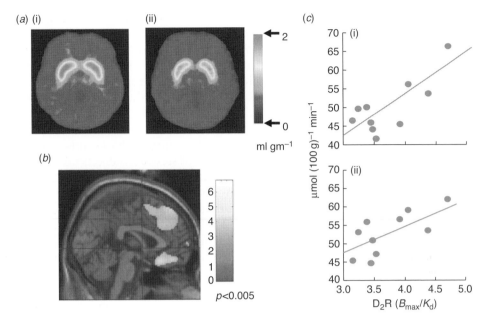

Fig. 9.2 (See also Plate 3) (*a*) Averaged images for DA D$_2$ receptors (measured with [^{11}C]raclopride) in a group of (i) controls (*n* = 10) and (ii) morbidly obese subjects (*n* = 10). *(b)* Results from SPM identifying the areas in the brain where D$_2$ receptors availability was associated with brain glucose metabolism; these included the OFC, the CG and the DLPFC (region not shown in sagittal plane). (c) Regression slopes between D$_2$ receptor availability (measured in striatum) and brain glucose metabolism in (i) CG and (ii) OFC in obese subjects. Modified from Wang et al. (2001) and Volkow et al. (2008).

When food-related stimuli are given to obese subjects (as when drug-related stimuli are given to addicts; Volkow & Fowler 2000), medial prefrontal cortex is activated and cravings are reported (Gautier et al. 2000; Wang et al. 2004; Miller et al. 2007). Several areas of the prefrontal cortex (including OFC and CG) have been implicated in motivation to feed (Rolls 2004). These prefrontal regions could reflect a neurobiological substrate common to the drive to eat or the drive to take drugs. Abnormalities of these regions could enhance either drug- or food-oriented behaviour, depending on the sensitivity to the reward and/or established habits of the subject.

9.5 Memory, conditioning, and habits to drugs and food

9.5.1 Drug abuse and addiction

Circuits underlying memory and learning, including conditioned incentive learning, habit learning, and declarative memory (reviewed by Vanderschuren & Everitt 2005), have been proposed to be involved in drug addiction. The effects of drugs on memory systems suggest ways that neutral stimuli can acquire reinforcing properties and motivational salience, i.e. through conditioned incentive learning. In research on relapse, it is important to understand why drug-addicted subjects experience an intense desire for the drug when exposed to places where they have taken the drug, to people with whom prior drug use occurred and to paraphernalia used to administer the drug. This is clinically relevant since exposure to conditioned cues (stimuli associated with the drug) is a key contributor to relapse. Since DA is involved with the prediction of reward (reviewed by Schultz 2002), we hypothesized that DA might underlie conditioned responses that trigger craving. Studies in laboratory animals support this hypothesis: when neutral stimuli are paired with a drug they will, with repeated associations, acquire the ability to increase DA in NAc and dorsal striatum (becoming conditioned cues). Furthermore, these neurochemical responses are associated with drug-seeking behaviour (reviewed by Vanderschuren & Everitt 2005).

In humans, PET studies with [^{11}C]raclopride recently confirmed this hypothesis by showing that in cocaine abusers drug cues (cocaine-cue video of scenes of subjects taking cocaine) significantly increased DA in dorsal striatum and these increases were associated with cocaine craving (Fig. 9.3; Volkow et al. 2006b; Wong et al. 2006). Because the dorsal striatum is implicated in habit learning, this association is likely to reflect the strengthening of habits as chronicity of addiction progresses. This suggests that a basic neurobiological disruption in addiction might be DA-triggered conditioned responses that result in habits leading to compulsive drug consumption. It is likely that these conditioned responses involve

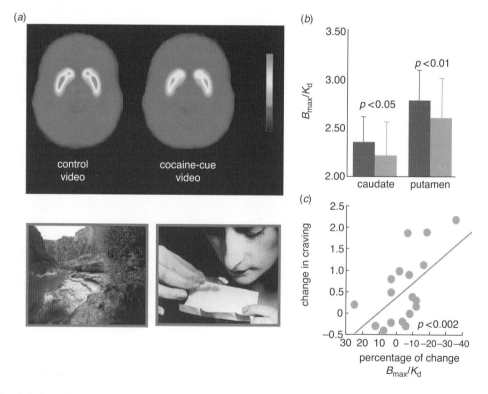

Fig. 9.3 (See also Plate 4) (*a*) Averaged images of DA D$_2$ receptors (measured with [^{11}C]raclopride) in a group of cocaine-addicted subjects (*n* = 16) tested while viewing a neutral video and while viewing a cocaine-cue video. (*b*) Histogram showing the measures of DA D$_2$ receptor availability (*B*$_{max}$/*K*$_d$) in caudate and putamen when viewing the neutral (blue bars) and cocaine-cue (red bars) videos. (*c*) Regression slopes between DA changes (assessed as changes in B$_{max}$/K$_d$) induced by the cocaine video and the self-reports of craving. Modified from Volkow et al. (2006b).

adaptations in cortico-striatal glutamatergic pathways that regulate DA release (reviewed Kalivas et al. 2005). Thus, while drugs (as well as food) may initially lead to DA release in ventral striatum (signalling reward), with repeated administration and as habits develop there appears to be a shift in the DA increases occurring into the dorsal striatum.

9.5.2 Food and obesity

DA regulates food consumption not only through modulation of its rewarding properties (Martel & Fantino 1996) but also by facilitating conditioning to food stimuli that then drive the motivation to consume the food (Kiyatkin & Gratton 1994; Mark et al. 1994). One of the first descriptions of a conditioned response was by Pavlov who showed that when dogs were exposed to repeated pairing of a tone with a piece of meat the tone by itself would elicit salivation in these animals. Since then, voltammetry studies have shown that the presentation of a neutral stimulus that has been conditioned to food results in increases in striatal DA and that the DA increases are linked to the motoric behaviour required to procure the food (lever pressing; Roitman et al. 2004).

   We have used PET to evaluate these conditioned responses in healthy controls. We hypothesize that food cues would increase extracellular DA in striatum and that these increases would predict the desire for food. Food-deprived subjects were studied while stimulated with a neutral or food-related stimulus (conditioned cues). To amplify the DA changes, we pretreated the subjects with MP (20 mg orally), a stimulant drug that blocks DA transporters (the main mechanism for the removal of extracellular DA; Giros et al. 1996). Food stimulation significantly increased DA in striatum and these increases correlated with the increases in self-reports of hunger and desire for food (Volkow et al. 2002b; Fig. 9.4). Similar findings were reported when food cues were presented to healthy controls without pretreatment with MP. These findings corroborate the involvement of striatal DA signalling in conditioned responses to food and the participation of this pathway in food motivation in humans. Since these responses were obtained when subjects did not consume the food, this identifies these responses as distinct from the role of DA in regulating reward through NAc.

   We are currently evaluating these conditioned responses in obese subjects in whom we hypothesize an accentuated increase in DA when exposed to cues compared with those of normal weight individuals.

9.6 A systems model of abuse/addiction and of obesity

As summarized previously, several common brain circuits have been identified by imaging studies as being relevant in the neurobiology of drug abuse/addiction and obesity. Here, we highlight four of these circuits: (i) reward/saliency, (ii) motivation/drive, (iii) learning/conditioning, and (iv) inhibitory control/emotional regulation/executive function. Note that the two other circuits (emotion/mood regulation and interoception) also participate in modulating the propensity to eat or take drugs but for simplicity are not incorporated into the model. We propose that a consequence of the disruption of these four circuits is an enhanced value of one type of reinforcer (drugs for the drug abuser and high-density food for the obese individual) at the expense of other reinforcers, which is a consequence of conditioned learning and resetting of reward thresholds secondary to repeated stimulation by drugs (drug abuser/addict) and by large quantities of high-density food (obese individual) in vulnerable individuals.

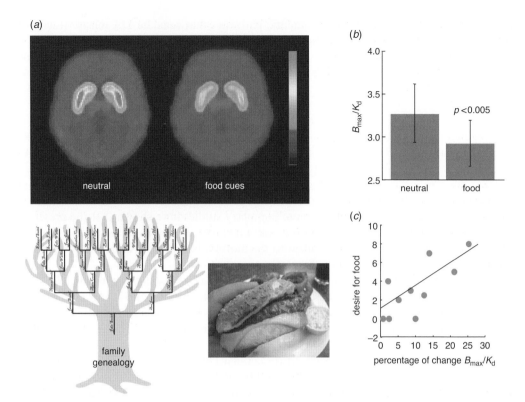

Fig. 9.4 (See also Plate 5) (*a*) Averaged images of DA D$_2$ receptors (measured with [^{11}C]raclopride) in a group of controls (nZ 10) tested while reporting on their family genealogy (neutral stimuli) or while being exposed to food. (*b*) Histogram showing the measures of DA D$_2$ receptor availability (B$_{max}$/K$_d$) in striatum (average caudate and putamen) when viewing the neutral and cocaine-cue videos. (*c*) Regression slopes between DA changes (assessed as changes in B$_{max}$/K$_d$) induced by the food stimuli and the self-reports of desire for the food. [a]To enhance the DA signal, subjects were pretreated with oral MP to block DA transporters and so amplify the DA signal. Modified from Volkow et al. (2002b).

A consequence of the impairment in the reward/saliency circuit (processes mediated in part through NAc, ventral pallidum, medial OFC, and hypothalamus), which modulates our response to both positive and negative reinforcers, is a decreased value to stimuli that otherwise would motivate behaviours likely to result in beneficial outcomes while avoiding behaviours that could result in punishment. For the case of drug abuse/addiction, one can predict that as a result of dysfunction in this neurocircuit the person would be less likely to be motivated to abstain from drug use because alternative reinforcers (natural stimuli) are much less exciting and negative consequences (e.g. incarceration, divorce) are less salient. For the case of obesity, one can predict that as a result of dysfunction in this neurocircuit the person would be less likely to be motivated to abstain from eating because alternative reinforcers (physical activity and social interactions) are less exciting and negative consequences (e.g. gaining weight, diabetes) are less salient.

A consequence of disruption of the inhibitory control/emotional regulation circuit is the impairment of the individual to exert inhibitory control and emotional regulation (processes mediated in part through the DLPFC, CG, and lateral OFC), which are critical components of the substrates necessary to inhibit prepotent responses such as the intense desire to take the drug in an addicted subject or to eat high-density food in an obese individual. As a result, the person is less likely to succeed in inhibiting the intentional actions and to regulate the emotional reactions associated with the strong desires (either to take the drug or to eat the food).

The consequences of the involvement of memory/conditioning/habits circuit (mediated in part through hippocampus, amygdala, and dorsal striatum) are that repeated use of drugs (drug abuser/addict) or repeated consumption of large quantities of high-density food (obese individual) results in the formation of new linked memories (processes mediated in part through hippocampus and amygdala), which condition the individual to expect pleasurable responses, not only when exposed to the drug (drug abuser/addict) or to the food (obese individual) but also from exposure to stimuli conditioned to the drug (i.e. smell of cigarettes) or conditioned to the food (i.e. watching TV). These stimuli trigger automatic responses that frequently drive relapse in the drug abuser/addict and food bingeing, even in those who are motivated to stop taking drugs or to lose weight.

The motivation/drive and action circuit (mediated in part through OFC, dorsal striatum, and supplementary motor cortices) is involved both in executing the act and in inhibiting it and its actions are dependent on the information from the reward/saliency, memory/conditioning, and inhibitory control/emotional reactivity circuits. When the value of a reward is enhanced owing to its previous conditioning, it has greater incentive motivation and if this occurs in parallel to a disruption of the inhibitory control circuit this could trigger the behaviour in a reflexive fashion (no cognitive control; Fig. 9.5). This could explain why drug-addicted subjects report taking drugs even when they were not aware of doing so and why obese individuals have such a difficult time in controlling their food intake and why some individuals claim that they take the drug or the food compulsively even when it is not perceived *per se* as pleasurable.

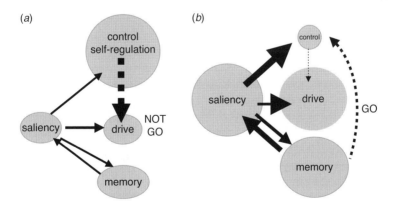

Fig. 9.5 Model of brain circuits involved with addiction and obesity: reward/saliency motivation/ drive, memory/conditioning and inhibitory control/emotional regulations. Disrupted activity in brain regions involved with inhibitory control/emotional regulation when coupled with enhanced activation of reward/saliency and memory/conditioning leads to enhanced activation of the motivational/drive circuit and the resultant compulsive behaviour (drug taking or food ingestion) when the individual is exposed to the reinforcer (drug or food), conditioned cues or a stressor. Note that circuits that regulate mood as well as internal awareness (interoception) are also likely to modulate the ability to exert control over incentive drives. (*a*) Healthy brain, (*b*) dysregulated brain. Modified from Volkow et al. (2003b).

In this model, during exposure to the reinforcer or to the cues conditioned to the reinforcer, the expected reward (processed by memory circuit) results in overactivation of the reward and motivation circuits while decreasing the activity in the cognitive control circuit. This contributes to an inability to inhibit the drive to seek and consume the drug (drug abuser/addict) or the food (obese person) despite the attempt to do so (Fig. 9.5). Because these neuronal circuits, which are modulated by DA, interact with one another, disruption on one circuit can be buffered by the activity of another, which would explain why an individual may be better able to exert control over their behaviour to take drugs or food on some occasions but not on others.

9.7 Clinical significance

This model has therapeutic implications for it suggests a multi-prong approach that targets strategies to: decrease the rewarding properties of the problem reinforcer (drug or food); enhance the rewarding properties of alternative reinforcers (i.e. social interactions, physical activity); interfere with conditioned-learned associations (i.e. promoting new habits to substitute for old ones); and strengthen inhibitory control (i.e. biofeedback), in the treatment of drug abuse/addiction and obesity Volkow et al. (2003b).

References

Allison, D. B., Mentore, J. L., Heo, M., Chandler, L. P., Cappelleri, J. C., Infante, M. C. & Weiden, P. J. 1999 Antipsychotic-induced weight gain: a comprehensive research synthesis. *Am. J. Psychiatry* **156**, 1686–96.

Avena, N. M., Rada, P. & Hoebel, B. G. 2008 Evidence for sugar addiction: behavioral and neurochemical effects of intermittent, excessive sugar intake. *Neurosci. Biobehav. Rev.* **32**, 20–39. (doi:10.1016/j.neubiorev.2007.04.019)

Berthoud, H. R. 2007 Interactions between the 'cognitive' and 'metabolic' brain in the control of food intake. *Physiol. Behav.* **91**, 486–98. (doi:10.1016/j.physbeh.2006.12. 016)

Garavan, H. et al. 2000 Cue-induced cocaine craving: neuroanatomical specificity for drug users and drug stimuli. *Am. J. Psychiatry* **157**, 1789–98. (doi:10.1176/appi.ajp.157.11.1789)

Gautier, J. F., Chen, K., Salbe, A. D., Bandy, D., Pratley, R. E., Heiman, M., Ravussin, E., Reiman, E. M. & Tataranni, P. A. 2000 Differential brain responses to satiation in obese and lean men. *Diabetes* **49**, 838–46. (doi:10.2337/diabetes.49.5.838)

Giros, B., Jaber, M., Jones, S. R., Wightman, R. M. & Caron, M. G. 1996 Hyperlocomotion and indifference to cocaine and amphetamine in mice lacking the dopamine transporter. *Nature* **379**, 606–12. (doi:10.1038/379606a0)

Goldstein, R. Z. & Volkow, N. D. 2002 Drug addiction and its underlying neurobiological basis: neuroimaging evidence for the involvement of the frontal cortex. *Am. J. Psychiatry* **159**, 1642–52. (doi:10.1176/appi.ajp.159.10.1642)

Grant, S., London, E. D., Newlin, D. B., Villemagne, V. L., Liu, X., Contoreggi, C., Phillips, R. L., Kimes, A. S. & Margolin, A. 1996 Activation of memory circuits during cue-elicited cocaine craving. *Proc. NatlAcad. Sci. USA* **93**, 12040–5. (doi:10.1073/pnas.93.21.12040)

Haltia, L. T., Rinne, J. O., Merisaari, H., Maguire, R. P., Savontaus, E., Helin, S., Någren, K. & Kaasinen, V. 2007 Effects of intravenous glucose on dopaminergic function in the human brain *in vivo. Synapse* **61**, 748–56. (doi:10. 1002/syn.20418)

Heinz, A. et al. 2004 Correlation between dopamine D(2) receptors in the ventral striatum and central processing of alcohol cues and craving. *Am. J. Psychiatry* **161**, 1783–9. (doi:10.1176/appi.ajp.161.10.1783)

Insel, T. R. 1992 Towards a neuroanatomy of obsessive-compulsive disorder. *Arch. Gen. Psychiatry* **49**, 739–44.

Kalivas, P. W., Volkow, N. D. & Seamans, J. 2005 Unmanageable motivation in addiction: a pathology in prefrontal-accumbens glutamate transmission. *Neuron* **45**, 647–50. (doi:10.1016/j.neuron. 2005.02.005)

Kiyatkin, E. A. & Gratton, A. 1994 Electrochemical monitoring of extracellular dopamine in nucleus accumbens of rats lever-pressing for food. *Brain Res.* **652**, 225–34. (doi:10.1016/0006–8993 (94)90231–3)

Levine, A. S., Kotz, C. M. & Gosnell, B. A. 2003 Sugars: hedonic aspects, neuroregulation, and energy balance. *Am. J. Clin. Nutr.* **78**, 834S–42S.

Mark, G. P., Smith, S. E., Rada, P. V. & Hoebel, B. G. 1994 An appetitively conditioned taste elicits a preferential increase in mesolimbic dopamine release. *Pharmacol. Biochem. Behav.* **48**, 651–60. (doi:10.1016/0091–3057 (94)90327–1)

Martel, P. & Fantino, M. 1996 Mesolimbic dopaminergic system activity as a function of food reward: a micro-dialysis study. *Pharmacol. Biochem. Behav.* **53**, 221–6. (doi:10.1016/0091–3057(95) 00187–5)

Martin-Solch, C., Magyar, S., Kunig, G., Missimer, J., Schultz, W. & Leenders, K. L. 2001 Changes in brain activation associated with reward processing in smokers and nonsmokers. A positron emission tomography study. *Exp. Brain Res.* **139**, 278–86. (doi:10.1007/s00221 0100751)

Martinez, D. et al. 2005 Alcohol dependence is associated with blunted dopamine transmission in the ventral striatum. *Biol. Psychiatry* **58**, 779–86. (doi:10.1016/j.biopsych.2005.04.044)

Martinez, D. et al. 2007 Amphetamine-induced dopamine release: markedly blunted in cocaine dependence and predictive of the choice to self-administer cocaine. *Am. J. Psychiatry* **164**, 622–9. (doi:10.1176/appi.ajp.164.4. 622)

Miller, J. L., James, G. A., Goldstone, A. P., Couch, J. A., He, G., Driscoll, D. J. & Liu, Y. 2007 Enhanced activation of reward mediating prefrontal regions in response to food stimuli in Prader-Willi syndrome. *J. Neurol. Neurosurg. Psychiatry* **78**, 615–19. (doi:10.1136/jnnp.2006.099044)

Mintun, M. A., Bierut, L. J. & Dence, C. 2003 A family study of cocaine dependences using PET measures of striatal [^{11}C]raclopride binding: preliminary evidence that non-dependent siblings may be unique group with elevated [^{11}C]raclopride binding. In paper presented at: *American College of Neuropsychopharmacology 42nd Annual Meeting, San Juan, Puerto Rico.*

Phan, K. L., Wager, T., Taylor, S. F. & Liberzon, I. 2002 Functional neuroanatomy of emotion: a meta-analysis of emotion activation studies in PET and fMRI. *Neuroimage* **16**, 331–48. (doi:10.1006/nimg.2002.1087)

Piazza, P. V., Maccari, S., Deminiere, J. M., Le Moal, M., Mormede, P. & Simon, H. 1991 Corticosterone levels determine individual vulnerability to amphetamine self-administration. *Proc. Natl Acad. Sci. USA* **88**, 2088–92. (doi: 10.1073/pnas.88.6.2088)

Roitman, M. F., Stuber, G. D., Phillips, P. E., Wightman, R. M. & Carelli, R. M. 2004 Dopamine operates as a subsecond modulator of food seeking. *J. Neurosci.* **24**, 1265–71. (doi:10.1523/JNEUROSCI.3823–03.2004)

Rolls, E. T. 2000 The orbitofrontal cortex and reward. *Cereb. Cortex* **10**, 284–94. (doi:10.1093/cercor/10.3.284)

Rolls, E. T. 2004 The functions of the orbitofrontal cortex. *Brain Cogn.* **55**, 11–29. (doi:10.1016/S0278–2626(03) 00277–X)

Schultz, W. 2002 Getting formal with dopamine and reward. *Neuron* **36**, 241–63. (doi:10.1016/S0896–6273(02) 00967–4)

Thanos, P. K., Volkow, N. D., Freimuth, P., Umegaki, H., Ikari, H., Roth, G., Ingram, D. K. & Hitzemann, R. 2001 Overexpression of dopamine D$_2$ receptors reduces alcohol self-administration. *J. Neurochem.* **78**, 1094–103. (doi:10.1046/j.1471–4159.2001.00492.x)

Vanderschuren, L. J. M. J. & Everitt, B. J. 2005 Behavioral and neural mechanisms of compulsive drug seeking. *Eur. J. Pharmacol.* **526**, 77–88. (doi:10.1016/j.ejphar. 2005.09.037)

Volkow, N. D. & Fowler, J. S. 2000 Addiction, a disease of compulsion and drive: involvement of the orbitofrontal cortex. *Cereb. Cortex* **10**, 318–25. (doi:10.1093/cercor/10. 3.318)

Volkow, N. D. & Li, T. K. 2004 Science and society: drug addiction: the neurobiology of behaviour gone awry. *Nat. Rev. Neurosci.* **5**, 963–70. (doi:10.1038/nrn1539)

Volkow, N. D. & O'Brien, C. P. 2007 Issues forDSM-V: should obesity be included as a brain disorder? *Am. J. Psychiatry* **164**, 708–10. (doi:10.1176/appi.ajp.164.5.708)

Volkow, N. D. & Wise, R. A. 2005 How can drug addiction help us understand obesity? *Nat. Neurosci.* 8, 555–60. (doi:10.1038/nn1452)

Volkow, N. D., Fowler, J. S., Wolf, A. P., Hitzemann, R., Dewey, S., Bendriem, B., Alpert, R. & Hoff, A. 1991 Changes in brain glucose metabolism in cocaine dependence and withdrawal. *Am. J. Psychiatry* **148**, 621–6.

Volkow, N. D., Fowler, J. S., Wang, G.-J., Hitzemann, R., Logan, J., Schlyer, D. J., Dewey, S. L. & Wolf, A. P. 1993 Decreased dopamine D$_2$ receptor availability is associated with reduced frontal metabolism in cocaine abusers. *Synapse* **14**, 169–77. (doi:10.1002/syn.890140210)

Volkow, N. D., Wang, G.-J., Fowler, J. S., Logan, J., Gatley, S. J., Hitzemann, R., Chen, A. D., Dewey, S. L. & Pappas, N. 1997 Decreased striatal dopaminergic responsivity in detoxified cocaine abusers. *Nature* **386**, 830–3. (doi: 10. 1038/386830a0)

Volkow, N. D., Wang, G.-J., Fowler, J. S., Logan, J., Gatley, S. J., Gifford, A., Hitzemann, R., Ding, Y.-S. & Pappas, N. 1999a Prediction of reinforcing responses to psychostimulants in humans by brain dopamine D$_2$ receptor levels. *Am. J. Psychiatry* **156**, 1440–3.

Volkow, N. D., Wang, G.-J., Fowler, J. S., Hitzemann, R., Angrist, B., Gatley, S. J., Logan, J., Ding, Y.-S. & Pappas, N. 1999b Association of methylphenidate-induced craving with changes in right striato-orbitofrontal metabolism in cocaine abusers: implications in addiction. *Am. J. Psychiatry* **156**, 19–26.

Volkow, N. D. et al. 2001 Low levels of brain dopamine D(2) receptors in methamphetamine abusers: association with metabolism in the orbitofrontal cortex. *Am. J. Psychiatry* **158**, 2015–21. (doi:10.1176/appi.ajp.158.12.2015)

Volkow, N. D. et al. 2002a Brain DA D$_2$ receptors predict reinforcing effects of stimulants in humans: replication study. *Synapse* **46**, 79–82. (doi:10.1002/syn.10137)

Volkow, N. D. et al. 2002b "Nonhedonic" food motivation in humans involves dopamine in the dorsal striatum and methylphenidate amplifies this effect. *Synapse* **44**, 175–80. (doi:10.1002/syn.10075)

Volkow, N. D. et al. 2003a Brain dopamine is associated with eating behaviors in humans. *Int. J. Eat. Disord.* **33**, 136–42. (doi:10.1002/eat.10118)

Volkow, N. D., Fowler, J. S. & Wang, G.-J. 2003b The addicted human brain: insights from imaging studies. *J. Clin. Invest.* **111**, 1444–51.

Volkow, N. D., Fowler, J. S., Wang, G.-J. & Swanson, J. M. 2004 Dopamine in drug abuse and addiction: results from imaging studies and treatment implications. *Mol. Psychiatry* **9**, 557–69. (doi:10.1038/sj.mp.4001507)

Volkow, N. D., Wang, G.-J., Ma, Y., Fowler, J. S., Wong, C., Ding, Y.-S., Hitzemann, R., Swanson, J. M. & Kalivas, P. 2005 Activation of orbital and medial prefrontal cortex by methylphenidate in cocaine-addicted subjects but not in controls: relevance to addiction. *J. Neurosci.* **25**, 3932–9. (doi:10.1523/JNEUROSCI.0433–05.2005)

Volkow, N. D. et al. 2006a High levels of dopamine D$_2$ receptors in unaffected members of alcoholic families: possible protective factors. *Arch. Gen. Psychiatry* **63**, 999–1008. (doi:10.1001/archpsyc.63.9.999)

Volkow, N. D., Wang, G.-J., Telang, F., Fowler, J. S., Logan, J., Childress, A. R., Jayne, M., Ma, Y. & Wong, C. 2006b Cocaine cues and dopamine in dorsal striatum: mechanism of craving in cocaine addiction. *J. Neurosci.* **26**, 6583–8. (doi:10.1523/JNEUROSCI.1544–06.2006)

Volkow, N. D., Wang, G.-J., Telang, F., Fowler, J. S., Logan, J., Jayne, M., Ma, Y., Pradhan, K. & Wong, C. 2007a Profound decreases in dopamine release in striatum in detoxified alcoholics: possible orbitofrontal involvement. *J. Neurosci.* **27**, 12 700–6. (doi:10.1523/JNEUR–OSCI.3371–07.2007)

Volkow, N. D., Fowler, J. S., Wang, G.-J., Swanson, J. M. & Telang, F. 2007b Dopamine in drug abuse and addiction: results of imaging studies and treatment implications. *Arch. Neurol.* **64**, 1575–9. (doi:10.1001/archneur.64. 11.1575)

Volkow, N. D., Wang, G.-J., Telang, F., Fowler, J. S., Thanos, P. K., Logan, J., Alexoff, D., Ding, Y.-S. & Wong, C. 2008. Low dopamine striatal D2 receptors are associated with prefrontal metabolism in obese subjects: possible contributing factors. *Neuroimage* **42**, 1337–43. (doi:10.1016/j.neuroimage. 2008.06.002)

Wang, G.-J., Volkow, N. D., Fowler, J. S., Cervany, P., Hitzemann, R. J., Pappas, N., Wong, C. T. & Felder, C. 1999 Regional brain metabolic activation during craving elicited by recall of previous drug experiences. *Life Sci.* **64**, 775–84. (doi:10.1016/S0024–3205(98)00619–5)

Wang, G.-J., Volkow, N. D., Logan, J., Pappas, N. R., Wong, C. T., Zhu, W., Netusil, N. & Fowler, J. S. 2001 Brain dopamine and obesity. *Lancet* **357**, 354–7. (doi:10. 1016/S0140–6736(00)03643–6)

Wang, G.-J. et al. 2004 Exposure to appetitive food stimuli markedly activates the human brain. *Neuroimage* **21**, 1790–7. (doi:10.1016/j.neuroimage.2003.11.026)

Wardle, J. 2007 Eating behaviour and obesity. *Obesity Rev.* **8**, 73–5. (doi:10.1111/j.1467–789X. 2007.00322.x)

Wong, D. F. et al. 2006 Increased occupancy of dopamine receptors in human striatum during cue-elicited cocaine craving. *Neuropsychopharmacology* **31**, 2716–27. (doi:10.1038/sj.npp.1301194)

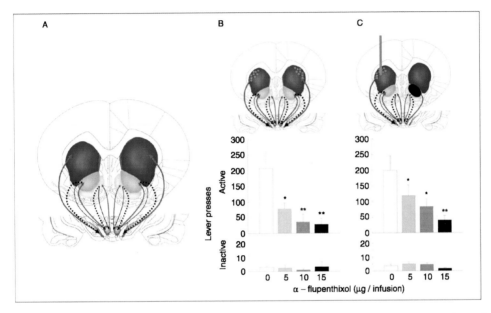

Plate 1 (See also Fig. 3.1) Within striatum, serial processing underlies the establishment of cocaine seeking habits. **A** Schematic representation of the intrastriatal dopamine-dependent spiralling circuitry functionally connecting the ventral with the dorsal striatum in the rat (modified from Belin & Everitt 2008). The spiralling loop organization is depicted as the alternation of pink and black arrows from the ventral to the more dorsal parts of the circuit, i.e. from the Acb Shell (yellow) to the AcbC (light blue) via the ventral tegmental area (pink) and from the AcbC via the substantia nigra to the dorsal striatum (dark blue). **B** Cocaine-seeking is dose-dependently impaired by bilateral infusions of the DA receptor antagonist α-flupenthixol (depicted as green dots in the diagram) into the DL striatum. α-flupenthixol infusions into the DL striatum dose-dependently decreased responding on the active lever under a second-order schedule of cocaine reinforcement, but had no effect on responding on the inactive lever (Belin & Everitt, 2008). **C** Disconnecting the AcbC from the dopaminergic innervation of the dorsal striatum impairs habitual cocaine-seeking. In unilateral AcbC-lesioned rats, the AcbC relay of the loop is lost on one side of the brain. However, on the non-lesioned side, the spiralling circuitry is intact and functional. When α-flupenthixol (green dots in the diagram) is infused in the DL striatum contralateral to the lesion it blocks the DAergic innervation from the midbrain, impairing the output structure of the spiralling circuitry on the non-lesioned side of the brain. Therefore, this asymmetric manipulation disconnects the core of the nucleus accumbens from the DL striatum and greatly diminishes cocaine seeking (Belin & Everitt 2008).

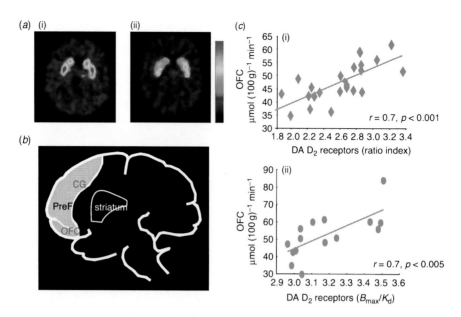

Plate 2 (See also Fig. 9.1) (*a*) Images of DA D$_2$ receptors (measured with [^{11}C]raclopride in striatum) in (i) a control and (ii) a cocaine abuser. (*b*) Diagram showing where glucose metabolism was associated with DA D$_2$ receptors in cocaine abusers, which included the orbitofrontal cortex (OFC), the cingulate gyrus (CG) and the dorsolateral prefrontal cortex (PreF). (*c*) Regression slopes between D$_2$ receptor availability and brain glucose metabolism in OFC in a group of detoxified (i) cocaine and (ii) methamphetamine abusers. Modified from Volkow et al. (2007b).

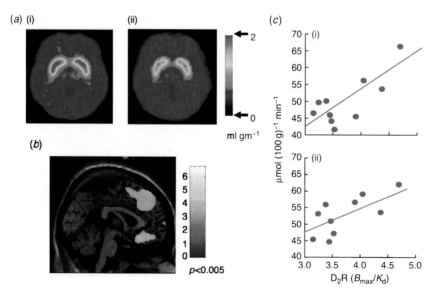

Plate 3 (See also Fig. 9.2) (*a*) Averaged images for DA D$_2$ receptors (measured with [^{11}C]raclopride) in a group of (i) controls (*n* = 10) and (ii) morbidly obese subjects (*n* = 10). (*b*) Results from SPM identifying the areas in the brain where D$_2$ receptors availability was associated with brain glucose metabolism; these included the OFC, the CG and the DLPFC (region not shown in sagittal plane). (*c*) Regression slopes between D$_2$ receptor availability (measured in striatum) and brain glucose metabolism in (i) CG and (ii) OFC in obese subjects. Modified from Wang et al. (2001) and Volkow et al. (in press).

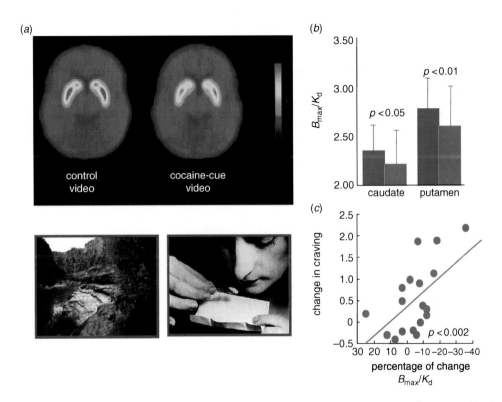

Plate 4 (See also Fig. 9.3) (*a*) Averaged images of DA D_2 receptors (measured with [¹¹C]raclopride) in a group of cocaine-addicted subjects (*n*= 16) tested while viewing a neutral video and while viewing a cocaine-cue video. (*b*) Histogram showing the measures of DA D_2 receptor availability ($\boldsymbol{B}_{max}/K_d$) in caudate and putamen when viewing the neutral (blue bars) and cocaine-cue (red bars) videos. (*c*) Regression slopes between DA changes (assessed as changes in B_{max}/K_d) induced by the cocaine video and the self-reports of craving. Modified from Volkow et al. (2006b).

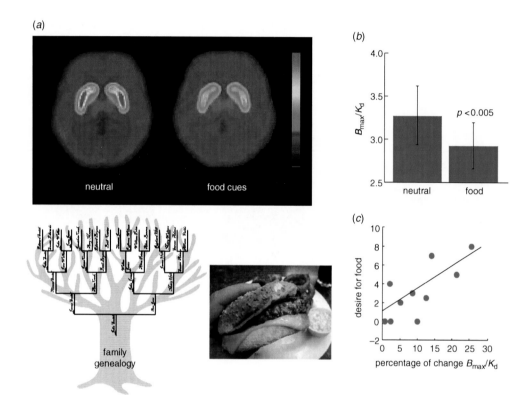

Plate 5 (See also Fig. 9.4) (*a*) Averaged images of DA D$_2$ receptors (measured with [^{11}C]raclopride) in a group of controls (nZ 10) tested while reporting on their family genealogy (neutral stimuli) or while being exposed to food. (*b*) Histogram showing the measures of DA D$_2$ receptor availability (B$_{max}$/K$_d$) in striatum (average caudate and putamen) when viewing the neutral and cocaine-cue videos. (*c*) Regression slopes between DA changes (assessed as changes in B$_{max}$/K$_d$) induced by the food stimuli and the self-reports of desire for the food. [a]To enhance the DA signal, subjects were pretreated with oral MP to block DA transporters and so amplify the DA signal. Modified from Volkow et al. (2002b).

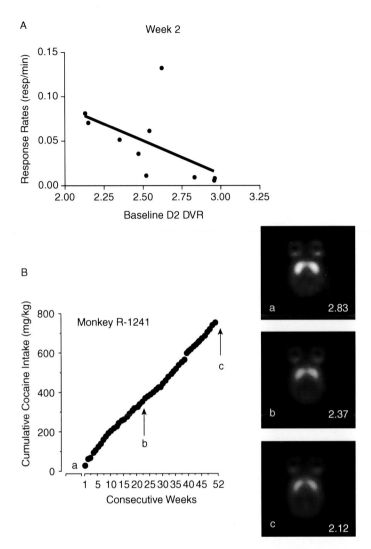

Plate 6 (See also Fig. 12.1) Correlation between baseline D2 receptor availability and rates of cocaine self-administration in male rhesus monkeys. (**B**) Representative data from one monkey (R-1241) showing cumulative cocaine intake and associated changes in D2 receptor availability. From Nader et al. (2006).

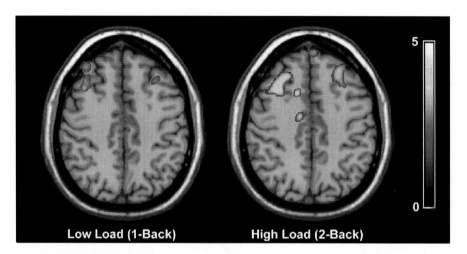

Plate 7 (See also Fig. 15.2) BOLD signal in the superior frontal gyrus is greater in non-drug using controls than cocaine users during performance of a standard verbal working memory task. This difference is amplified in conditions of higher cognitive demand (high load, right image). The color bar indicates *z* scores from the group-level analysis (Hanlon et al., unpublished observations).

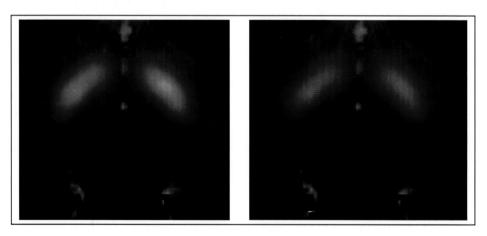

Plate 8 (See also Fig. 3.2) Reduced [18F]fallypride binding in the ventral striatum of highly impulsive (right panel) compared to non-impulsive (left panel) rats (Dalley et al., 2007).

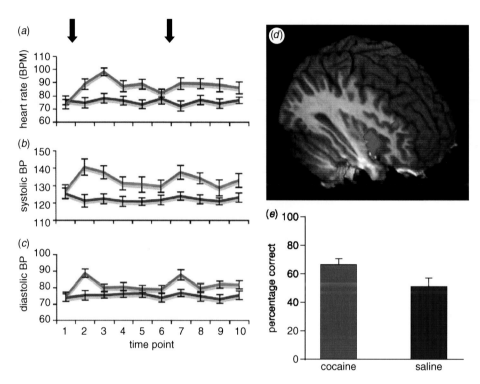

Plate 9 (See also Fig. 16.2) Physiological, behavioural, and functional brain effects of cocaine in performing an inhibitory control Go/No-Go task. Cocaine administration increased (*a*) HR, (*b*) systolic BP, and (*c*) diastolic BP and (*e*) improved the user's ability to inhibit a prepotent behaviour (all error bars are standard errors of the mean). Improved inhibitory control (successful inhibitions) was associated with increased activity in (*d*) right insula/inferior frontal gyrus (coronal section, yZ14) and right dorsolateral prefrontal cortex. Drug infusions occurred between time points 1 and 2 as well as between time points 6 and 7. The four runs of the Go/No-Go task commenced following time points 3, 5, 8, and 10. The event-related finger-tapping control task was performed following time points 4 and 9. Red, cocaine; blue, saline.

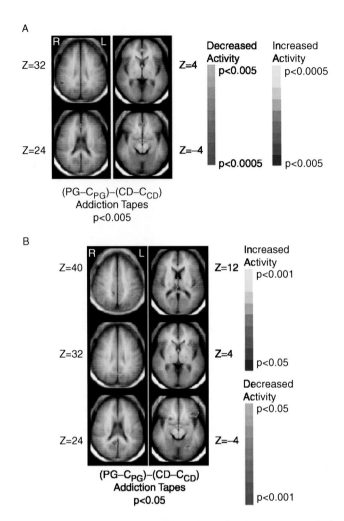

Plate 10 (See also Fig. 8.1) **A** Disorder-specific brain activation patterns distinguishing affected and non-affected subject groups. Shown are brain activation maps showing relatively decreased activity in the anterior cingulate (Talaraich levels $z = -4$, 4, and 24) and inferior parietal lobule ($z = 32$) for the comparison of (PG-control subjects viewing gambling scenarios) versus (CD-control subjects viewing cocaine scenarios) (($PG-C_{PG}$)-($CD-C_{CD}$)). Decreased activity in the PG vs. C_{PG} comparison as compared to the CD vs. C_{CD} one is indicated by blue to purple coloration indicating significance values of $p<0.005$ to 0.0005, respectively. The numbers of subjects contributing to the comparisons are: PG, 11; C_{PG}, 10; CD, 9; and C_{CD}, 6. The left side of the brain is displayed on the right. **B** Common brain activation patterns distinguishing affected and non-affected subject groups. Shown are brain regions in which both patient groups' significant differences from their respective control groups during viewing of the relevant addiction tapes. In all cases, patients showed relatively lower activity than their respective controls, with blue to purple coloration indicating significance values of $p<0.05$ to 0.001, respectively. Specific brain regions identified include left insula/inferior frontal gyrus (Talaraich $z = 4$, -4), right ventral striatum/ventral prefrontal cortex ($z = -4$), left lingual gyrus ($z = -4$), right thalamus ($z = 12$), precuneus ($z = 32$), and right posterior cingulate ($z = 40$). The numbers of subjects contributing to the comparisons are PG, 11; C_{PG}, 10; CD, 9; and C_{CD}, 6. The left side of the brain is displayed on the right.

Part 3

Vulnerability to Drug Abuse

10

Neurogenetic studies of alcohol addiction

John C. Crabbe*

Neurogenetic studies of alcohol dependence have relied substantially on genetic animal models, particularly rodents. Studies of inbred strains, selectively bred lines, and mutants bearing genes whose function has been targeted for over or under expression are reviewed. Studies focused on gene expression changes are the most recent contributors to this literature, and some genetic effects may work through epigenetic mechanisms. In a few instances, interesting parallels have been revealed between genetic risk in humans and studies in non-human animal models. Future approaches are likely to be increasingly complex.

Key Words: Alcohol; genetic animal models; candidate genes.

10.1 Introduction

There is clear evidence of genetic contributions to alcohol dependence in humans, but studies must cope with diagnostic and aetiologic heterogeneity, as well as comorbidities with other psychiatric disorders and the role of other genetically influenced risk factors such as personality traits (e.g. impulsivity). Genes of influence are manifold, and their individual effects on risk are small. Environmental factors such as major life stressors, work, and peer influences are equally important. Although it is more difficult to document, most believe that risk-promoting genes are likely to be of importance only under certain (and possibly specific) risk-promoting environmental conditions: that is, there are important gene–environment interactions. Given the genetic heterogeneity of human populations, their long generation time and their unwillingness to cooperate with useful experimental mating schemes, it is a wonder that we have been able to find clear examples of genetic risk. The best such example is the increased frequency of the aldehyde dehydrogenase isoform leading to accumulation of acetaldehyde upon drinking alcohol. Among hundreds of individuals genotyped from the East Asian gene pools where this isoform is predominant, only a single homozygous individual for the slow aldehyde dehydrogenase variant has been reported to earn a diagnosis of alcoholism (Enoch & Goldman 2001).

Research on genetic risk has concentrated on laboratory animals, particularly rodents. Most symptoms important for a diagnosis of alcoholism or an alcohol use disorder as currently defined are behavioural. These include failure to control quantity or frequency of drinking, and continuing to drink in the face of consequential medical, legal, or social/familial problems. It is clearly difficult to envision completely believable rodent models for such behaviours as getting into trouble at work, a limit to the usefulness of such models (Lovinger & Crabbe 2005). Nonetheless, the tractability of rodent neurobiology, and especially the flowering of mouse genetics and genomics, has made studies of these species attractive. While I will mention other species and attempt to draw parallels with human genetic data where possible, the focus of this review will be on rodent genetic studies.

* crabbe@ohsu.edu

Results from four methods for approaching the neurogenetics of alcoholism will be assessed—inbred strain studies, work with selectively bred lines, candidate gene targeting approaches and gene expression profiling.

I do not believe that there is a rodent model that resembles human alcoholism in all important aspects. The inherent fallacies in attempting such simulacra were eloquently outlined many years ago (McClearn 1979). Rather, I advocate concentrating on specific aspects of the disorder that can be convincingly modelled in rats and mice. These include aspects of the pharmacology of ethyl alcohol (neural sensitivity to the drug, the development of tolerance to its effects with repeated administration, and withdrawal symptoms shared across mammalian species, e.g. seizures or convulsions, autonomic dysregulation). Extensive studies of the neuroadaptations accompanying tolerance development have shown genetic influences to be strong (Kalant et al. 1971; Kalant 1998). Recent studies using the powerful genetic manipulations available in invertebrate species have extended the range of genetic influences thought to be responsible (Scholz et al. 2000; Cowmeadow et al. 2005).

Despite the use of reductionist approaches, the complex behavioural disorder, alcoholism, demands an attempt to model some of the key behavioural features. Foremost among these is self-administration of the drug. Genetic animal model research in alcoholism has focused extensively on voluntary oral ethanol self-administration, using the two-bottle preference test. Mice or rats are offered a bottle containing (typically) 10% ethanol and one containing tap water, usually ad libitum. The amount of alcohol drunk is taken to indicate the reinforcing effect of the drug. The majority of published studies on the genetics of alcohol in rodents have targeted this phenotype and its variants. This offers the theoretical advantage of allowing comparisons of results across methodological approaches. For example, if gene X is knocked out and found to reduce alcohol consumption, is it also found to be up- or down-regulated on a microarray analysis of brain tissue DNA after chronic drinking? I will attempt to identify such consonances in the literature.

10.2 Inbred strains

In a seminal study, inbred C57BL/6 mice were compared with four other inbred strains for two-bottle preference for ethanol (McClearn & Rodgers 1959). They drank more than the other strains, one of which (DBA/2) nearly completely refused to drink ethanol. These strains have been repeatedly characterized over the years, and C57BL/6 and DBA/2 have nearly the highest and lowest preference levels, respectively, of the more than 40 inbred strains subsequently tested in almost all studies. The pattern of strain differences has been replicated many times over the past 45 years, with highly reliable results (Wahlsten et al. 2006).

An inbred strain results when brothers and sisters are mated, generation after generation. In each generation, half the allelic genetic variability is lost, until after 20 generations, all same-sex animals have two copies of the same allele for any gene—they are obligatory homozygotes throughout their genome (Falconer & Mackay 1996). However, each inbred strain is genetically unique, and different from all others. The degree of difference depends upon the pedigree history of the strain's derivation, and there are seven major lineages for the more than 100 standard inbred strains that are commercially available (Petkov et al. 2004). If a panel of inbred strains is tested under controlled environmental conditions, the differences in a behaviour (or a neurochemical phenotype, for example) are taken to be of allelic genetic origin. To the extent that they exceed the average individual differences within a strain, they serve as an estimate of the aggregate effect of genetics on the phenotype.

Within an inbred strain, however, there are always individual differences. Most C57BL/6J mice show increasing alcohol drinking over a period of two to three weeks, for example, which was noted in the earliest paper (McClearn & Rodgers 1959). The source of these differences cannot be allelic, and must derive from environmental factors (e.g. social dominance in group-housed animals, food, how well they slept the night before testing). Alternatively, they may be epigenetically based, whether or not they are transmitted to their offspring (Francis et al. 1999, 2003).

What have we learned from inbred strain studies of alcohol-related phenotypes since 1959? When the inbred strain literature on behavioural responses (Phillips & Crabbe 1991) and neurochemical strain differences (Allan & Harris 1991) were first comprehensively reviewed in 1991, only a handful of studies were published and these were nearly all limited to comparisons of the C57BL/6J and DBA/2J strains, previously identified as outliers for alcohol drinking and for the severity of alcohol withdrawal (Kakihana 1979). However, the development of recombinant inbred (RI) strains (Bailey 1971) extended the use of inbred strains to a new purpose. RI strains are derived from re-inbreeding after intercrossing two inbred strains to obtain an F2 generation. The F2 population shows a mosaic pattern of DNA segments on each chromosome due to crossovers during meiosis. After inbreeding to form a new RI strain is complete, the order of genetic segments randomly reshuffled in the genome of the F2 animals is preserved in future generations with the same fidelity as in standard inbreds (Silver 1995). With the advent of high-throughput genomics enabled by the Human Genome Project, genomic markers were rapidly developed. These started with restriction fragment length polymorphisms, soon thereafter succeeded by microsatellite repeat markers, and most recently by single nucleotide polymorphisms, or SNPs. The stability of inbred strains thus allowed genome scientists to build a mouse genome map in parallel with the human genome map.

The mouse map was completed in 2002, but long before that, the genetic marker map was sufficiently dense to allow mapping the location of genes whose alleles were correlated with high or low values on any measured phenotype. Thus, it was possible to study the 26 B × D RI strains then in existence, each derived from crossing (high-drinking strain) C57BL/6J mice with (low-drinking strain) DBA/2J mice. These B×D RI strains differed markedly in their preference for ethanol, and because each possessed a stable mixture of marker alleles that were inherited from either C57BL/6J or DBA/2J progenitors, the location of segments of DNA associated with high and low drinking could be 'read' directly from the patterns of RI strain phenotypic differences (Phillips et al. 1998). These locations are initially deemed 'loci', called 'quantitative trait loci' (QTL) for two reasons: first, because the trait, drinking, is influenced by many genes, its inheritance pattern is not all or none (Mendelian), but rather graded or quantitative; and second, because any QTL comprises a substantial stretch of chromosomal DNA and includes multiple genes. The stability of inbred strains across generations and laboratories has allowed several groups to combine similar analyses, and several QTL affecting preference drinking have been firmly supported in multiple studies (Rodriguez et al. 1994; Melo et al. 1996; Phillips et al. 1998; Tarantino et al. 1998). However, none of these QTL for drinking has as yet been resolved to the level of a single quantitative trait gene (QTG). This is for several reasons, including (but not limited to) the difficulty of manipulating all the candidate genes in the QTL interval to rule in or out their role; the possibility that multiple genes may reside in a single QTL interval; and the small effect size for any QTL.

QTL mapping has led to at least one QTG. Acute withdrawal from ethanol and pentobarbital has been studied in standard inbreds and the B×D RI strains, and provisional QTL identified (Buck et al. 1997). Subsequent studies winnowed one QTL on chromosome 4 to a few genes (Fehr et al. 2002). Finally, comparisons of purpose-bred mice and standard inbred strains ruled out all but a single gene, *Mpdz*, as the source of the effects on withdrawal severity (Shirley et al. 2004). This gene encodes a scaffolding protein that participates in neurotransmitter–receptor interactions, and current studies are exploring possible specific partners affected by the *Mpdz* polymorphism. There are many new methods for mapping QTL and isolating the specific genes of importance. Inbred strains can be surveyed directly for associations between markers and phenotypes (Grupe et al. 2001; Liao et al. 2004), although the statistical mapping power of such analyses has been questioned due to the close pedigree relationships among standard inbred strains, leading to large haplotype similarities. Mapping studies are more difficult, but more powerful, in outbred stocks (Mott et al. 2000; Flint et al. 2005; Valdar et al. 2006).

Another feature of inbred strains that is very useful is their cumulative power. A recent effort has sought to enter phenotypic information for many of the widely used strains into a database. The Mouse Phenome Database (MPD) http://phenome.jax.org/pub-cgi/phe-nome/mpdcgi?rtn = docs/home contains nearly 1200 phenotypes as of this writing (May 2008) which have been collected on at least eight inbred strains (average of 18 strains/phenotype), and targets 36 strains as high priority. The phenotypes range from behavioural to neurochemical, anatomical, and physiological and are derived from 68 projects; some data are available for 598 strains. Owing to the inherent replicability of inbred strain data (Wahlsten et al. 2006), strain mean data can be correlated across phenotypes, and a significant correlation across strain means suggests that some genes affect both phenotypes. The increasing availability of SNP data in the MPD and elsewhere further strengthens the usefulness of this resource.

For example, several studies have explored the negative genetic relationship suggested by McClearn's group between high drinking (McClearn & Rodgers 1959) and low withdrawal (Kakihana 1979). A meta-analysis of strain differences on these two phenotypes found them to be significantly negatively genetically correlated. This correlation was obtained despite differences in the specific preference phenotypes examined (short versus long exposure ethanol preference tests), and acute versus chronic ethanol withdrawal (Metten et al. 1998). A later study surveyed strains for their sensitivity to ethanol's effectiveness in conditioning a taste aversion (CTA) to a paired, novel flavour. Ethanol's efficacy in the CTA paradigm was correlated with high withdrawal and low preference drinking (Broadbent et al. 2002). A recent meta-analysis of dozens of published studies with genetically defined rats and mice has included assessment of panels of inbred mouse strains (Green & Grahame 2008). This analysis confirmed the high preference–low withdrawal–low CTA triad of association, which was also seen in lines selectively bred for drinking (see §10.3). The authors argue that genetically high drinkers appear to be more sensitive to some aversive properties of ethanol, which limit preference drinking. Interestingly, although there was a strong and consistent association between home cage drinking and intravenous self-administration across genotypes, there was a weaker association between these consummatory responses and the efficacy of ethanol to condition a place preference. The place preference data are complicated by a species difference: while mice prefer ethanol-associated locations, rats generally learn to avoid them, for reasons as yet not understood (Green & Grahame 2008). An older study of several inbred mouse strains documented differences in their ability to withhold a rewarded nose poke response for a few seconds. There was a strong correlation between this behavioural analogue of impulsivity and the preference of the strains for alcohol (Logue et al. 1998). A study of impulsive action in multiple mouse strains is finding their response inhibition to a no-go signal in a go/no-go task to be well correlated with the pre-signal impulsive nose-poke data (S. H. Mitchell et al. 2008, personal communication).

Inbred strains will continue to provide useful data in the search for genetic influences on alcohol responses. Their use is insured by their usefulness as stable backgrounds for placement of spontaneous mutants, or those engineered (e.g. as knockouts, see §10.4) or induced, e.g. by ethylnitrosourea (ENU) mutagenesis (see Hamre et al. 2007). They are also increasingly used in gene expression profiling studies (e.g. Letwin et al. 2006; see §10.5).

10.3 Selective breeding

The technique of selective breeding is the oldest in behavioural genetics, and was refined through many years of usage in agricultural settings. When extremely high-scoring individuals are selected from a population and mated together, the effect is to increase the frequency of alleles in their offspring that support high scores. Over many generations, the population under directional selection shows a gradual increase in their scores. The rate of response to selection is proportional to the degree of genetic influence, or heritability. Selected lines are extremely useful for studying the biological mechanisms underlying the selected response, and any trait not directly selected which changes over generations in parallel to the selected response increases is demonstrably influenced by the selected alleles. This is called a correlated response to selection.

Starting in the 1940s, Mardones successfully bred rats for high ethanol preference, proving that the trait was heritable (Mardones & Segovia-Riquelme 1983). The basic experimental design has been used many times since to create other high-preferring rat and mouse lines. High-preferring mice or rats may reach high blood alcohol levels (BALs), but usually only after many months of drinking. More typically, they stop drinking at BALs of approximately 60mg%. In other words, rodents appear to have some internal controls limiting intake which are not shared by susceptible humans. Neurobiological and genetic findings from these selected lines are discussed in a series of recent reviews (Murphy et al. 2002; Bell et al. 2006; Colombo et al. 2006; Quintanilla et al. 2006; Sommer et al. 2006). UChB (versus UChA), P (versus NP), AA (versus ANA), HAD (versus LAD), sP (versus sNP), and msP (versus msNP) rats (and HAP versus LAP mice) were all bred for the same trait using a nearly identical protocol; one could reasonably expect that strong genetic correlates of high alcohol preference should have emerged from these multiple replications.

Much of the early work with the selectively bred rat lines was focused on assessments of neurotransmitter levels, their activity, their interactions with brain receptors and the neuroanatomical differences in these brain systems, in comparisons with naive animals. There is substantial agreement across models that low limbic system levels of serotonin and other serotonergic differences characterize high drinkers (Murphy et al. 2002). Interestingly, dopaminergic differences have not been reported as consistently (Sommer et al. 2006). Differences in endocannabinoid, opioid, GABA, glutamate, and other systems remain to be established clearly in multiple models. Somewhat more clarity has evolved from behavioural comparisons of the multiple pairs of selected lines. High drinkers are more sensitive to low-dose alcohol and less sensitive to higher dose, sedative effects in some studies, but these results have not been generalized consistently across studies. There is good agreement that high drinkers tend to develop tolerance more readily than non-drinkers, and that it persists longer.

As noted in analyses of inbred strain panels, the relationship between ethanol-induced CTA and drinking is shared across selections (Phillips et al. 2005; Green & Grahame 2008). Finally, mice were bred from the F2 cross of C57BL/6J×DBA/2J in a short-term selection for high- or low-preference drinking. Mice from the high drinking line were found to be more impulsive in a go/no-go response inhibition task than the low drinkers, but the lines did not differ in a task of impulsive choice, delay discounting (Wilhelm et al. 2007).

Rats have also been bred for their intake of ethanol in a limited access paradigm. HARF rats drink substantial amounts of ethanol in a 20 min access period, versus the low-drinking LARF line (Lê et al. 2001). However, these animals have been rarely studied (Shram et al. 2004; Turek et al. 2005). To overcome some limitations of the older selected lines, we have developed a new model for binge drinking. C57BL/6J mice had been shown to self-administer substantial ethanol in a limited access paradigm during the circadian dark (Sharpe et al. 2005). Mice drink and eat mostly during their circadian dark period. In our paradigm, C7BL/6J mice drinking in the dark (DID) readily self-administered approximately 7–8 g ethanol kg^{-1} body weight in 4 hours and became intoxicated (Rhodes et al. 2005). We later showed that inbred strains differed in DID and the response was both reliable and heritable (Rhodes et al. 2007). We are currently selectively breeding mice for this trait: after nine selected generations, average BAL has doubled (because average intake has increased 150%) and the high DID (HDID-1) mice also become intoxicated (Crabbe et al. 2009). These mice should be useful for mechanistic studies of the biological and genetic contributions to excessive drinking. They have not been tested for many other traits. However, the DID phenotype is proving to be a useful way to explore mechanisms underlying binge-like drinking. DID was shown to be reduced by intraperitoneal naltrexone doses that did not affect water or sugar–water intake (Kamdar et al. 2007). Another group has shown that the $GABA_B$ agonist baclofen reduced ethanol DID without affecting water drinking, while two $GABA_A$ agonists, THIP, and muscimol, reduced drinking non-specifically (Moore et al. 2007). A CRF_1 receptor antagonist also reduced ethanol DID without affecting sucrose drinking (Sparta et al. 2008). Finally, infusion of urocortin 1 into lateral septum selectively reduced ethanol DID, while CRF reduced intake of both ethanol and water (Ryabinin et al. 2008).

Many other lines have been selectively bred for differential responses to alcohol. These include the long-sleep (LS) and short-sleep (SS) mice, which were selected for differences in the duration of the loss of the righting reflex after high-dose ethanol. These mice have been the subject of hundreds of papers, and have been used effectively to map QTL underlying this response (Bennett et al. 2006). A large panel of RI strains has been developed from an LS×SS cross, and these RI strains have also been used to map QTL for ethanol-induced locomotor activation and acute functional tolerance development (Downing et al. 2006; Bennett et al. 2007). The locomotor activating response to ethanol is taken as an analogue of ethanol's euphoric effects in humans. Mice selected for high ethanol-induced activity (FAST) have been compared with low responders (SLOW) in many studies. These findings have been reviewed elsewhere (Palmer & Phillips 2002; Cunningham & Phillips 2003). Selection for differences in the severity of withdrawal after chronic ethanol treatment has been the subject of multiple selective breeding efforts. The Withdrawal Seizure-Prone and -Resistant selected lines remain under active investigation in several laboratories. Early work with these lines has been comprehensively reviewed (Metten & Crabbe 1996) and much of the recent work has focused on the role of neurosteroid systems in withdrawal (Finn et al. 2004; Beckley et al. 2008).

The use of selective breeding has seen a good deal of use in recent years since Belknap noted its efficacy in the aid of gene mapping efforts (Belknap et al. 1997). Especially when starting with a simple cross of two inbred strains, where there are only two possible alleles at each gene, intense directional selection based on phenotype usually produces very rapid changes in both the phenotype and the underlying important gene frequencies. The parallel changes in phenotype and genotype have provided strong support for several QTL analyses (Buck et al. 1997). More recently, interest has turned towards using genome-wide expression analyses to identify genes of interest. Here, too, short-term selective breeding has rapidly uncovered genes important for the phenotype (Mulligan et al. 2006). An interesting use of selected lines has recently employed the oldest selected rat line, high-drinking UChB rats. Individuals from East Asian gene pools possessing alleles coding for relatively inactive ALDH 2*2 activity experience aversive side effects when they drink alcohol because they generate high levels of blood acetaldehyde. These subjects are highly protected from developing alcohol dependence. The Chilean group developed an *anti-Aldh2* antisense gene, injected it into UChB rats and saw pronounced suppression of ethanol intake (Ocaranza et al. 2008).

10.4 Candidate genes

The first study reporting the effects of a targeted gene deletion found that serotonin 1B receptor null mutants drank more ethanol, were less sedated by an acute dose of ethanol and developed tolerance to a lesser extent than wild-types (Crabbe et al. 1996). This finding has proven to depend upon genotype at other loci, an example of epistasis or gene–gene interaction (Phillips & Belknap 2002). A review 10 years hence found that 141 published reports assessed 93 targeted genes (Crabbe et al. 2006). Seventy-six mutants were tested for two-bottle preference. One quarter drank more than wild-types, one-third less and 40% about the same. The genes showing a major effect were not clustered in any pattern that offered clues to the underlying neurobiology.

Since the initial review, 34 additional papers have appeared, adding information about alcohol responses for several previously targeted genes, but also introducing 14 new genes to the mix. Two studies used ENU mutagenesis to generate novel mutants, some of which were found to differ in alcohol responses (Pawlak et al. 2005; Hamre et al. 2007). In one study, cerebellar tissue from ethanol-treated mice with or without a protein kinase C (PKC) gamma null mutation was compared in a gene expression profiling analysis. Several genes of potential relevance to the failure of PKC gamma mutants to develop ethanol tolerance were identified (Bowers et al. 2006). With no disrespect intended to the authors of the new studies, the increase in knowledge since 2006 has not revealed any new striking findings (not reviewed here). Gene targeting will remain a very useful tool for confirming the importance of a gene for which there are parallel lines of evidence for its importance. However, it is unlikely to be a sufficient tool for proving gene involvement on an alcohol response.

A clear example of how a strong case can be built for the involvement of a specific gene product in alcohol responses is offered by studies of mice engineered to lack the PKC epsilon isoform. Several previous studies had consistently established that PKC epsilon null mutants drank less ethanol than wild-types, and this effect was postulated to reflect the insensitivity of these mutants to ethanol's enhancement of $GABA_A$ receptor function in neurochemical and electrophysiological assays (Crabbe et al. 2006). The null mutants were also shown to self-administer less ethanol in an oral operant paradigm (Olive et al. 2000). Mice had been shown to develop either a conditioned place preference (CPP) or aversion (CPA) for a location paired with an ethanol injection, depending on whether the injection is before or after each daily training session, respectively (Cunningham et al. 1998). In dose-response studies, PKC epsilon mutants were found to be more sensitive to ethanol-induced CPA and less sensitive to CPP than wild-types (Newton & Messing 2007). In studies attempting to regu-late ethanol preference drinking through administration of diazepam, zolpidem or L-655,708, PKC epsilon mutants, unlike wild-type controls, were insensitive to all three $GABA_A$ recep-tor modulators. The authors concluded that PKC epsilon is necessary for ethanol's modula-tory effects on $GABA_A$ receptors (Besheer et al. 2006). Because no drug was available that selectively inhibited PKC epsilon activity over other PKC isoforms, the authors used a chemical strategy to generate an ATP analogue-sensitive PKC epsilon mutant to selectively inhibit catalytic activity of PKC epsilon (Qi et al. 2007). Using this mutant, they showed that PKC epsilon affects $GABA_A$ receptors by phosphorylating the $\gamma2$ subunit, thereby affecting receptors with the $\alpha1\beta2\gamma2$ subunit composition, an abundant variant in brain. This may explain the low ethanol withdrawal severity of PKC epsilon mutants (Olive et al. 2001) and the increased withdrawal in $\gamma2$ hemizygotes (Hood et al. 2006).

10.5 Gene expression analyses

The area of genetic analysis changing most rapidly in alcohol studies is exploration of the role of gene expression. Studies of gene expression changes, particularly following chronic ethanol administration, have been pursued for many years. The limiting nature of gene-by-gene expression assessment technology (e.g. Northern analysis of mRNA, RNAse protec-tion analyses) kept progress to a slow pace. However, many useful findings were carefully documented (for a review, see Reilly et al. 2001). Early studies used banked tissue from human brain to compare alcoholics and controls (Lewohl et al. 2000) or cultured cells to which alcohol was applied (Thibault et al. 2000). With the advent of gene chip technologies, it became possible to survey nearly the entire genome for expression differences, and some similarities emerged between microarray analyses and earlier studies (Lewohl et al. 2000; Liu et al. 2006). Microarrays also facilitated the spread of global expression analyses to their use in genetically defined rodent lines, such as the LS and SS mice (Xu et al. 2001) and the PKC gamma mutants just discussed (Bowers et al. 2006).

Gene expression profiling analyses typically discover numerous genes differentially expressed between control and treatment tissues, or between genotypes with high and low sensitivity to alcohol. Increasingly, the resulting lists of genes are being replaced with more sophisticated bioinformatics analyses of the output that seek gene clusters, gene families and/or similarity across multiple studies. For example, data banks containing the whole brain gene expression outputs from three pairs of lines selectively bred for high- or low-preference drinking were explored in conjunction with data from six inbred or isogenic strains of mice. A meta-analysis found nearly 4000 genes consistently differentially expressed in high versus low drinkers (Mulligan et al. 2006). Functional groups were proposed based on analysis of the proteins coded by those genes (the transcriptome). Using congenic strains, which differed from the background strain only in one small piece of DNA from chromo-some 9 that contained a QTL for preference drinking first reported in an analysis of B×D RI strains (Phillips et al. 1994), more microarray analyses were performed. Comparison of the datasets reduced the number of candidate genes within the QTL to 16 plus 4 expressed sequence tags (ESTs). These candidates included *Scn4b*, encoding a sodium channel.

Several other expression-based analyses have recently appeared. AA and ANA rats show many differentially expressed genes whose patterns of function have been discussed

(Sommer et al. 2006). Candidate genes for preference drinking were explored in NP rats with a congenic interval containing a QTL for high preference from the P line. Several genes in several brain regions were differentially expressed (Carr et al. 2007). QTL effects can also be based on differences in gene expression rather than sequence. Several studies are actively pursuing these loci, deemed 'expression QTL' or 'eQTL'. eQTL are often likely to be caused by transcription factors in the interval, and those transcription factors can either act on an adjacent or nearby gene (deemed 'cis-acting') or on genes on other chromosomes (deemed 'trans-acting'). Most such studies are integrating the results from sequence-based and eQTL results to obtain a more complete picture of genetic influences (Hitzemann et al. 2004; Chesler et al. 2005; Letwin et al. 2006; Peirce et al. 2006; Tabakoff et al. 2008). One recent study has combined results from studies of alcohol and other drugs of abuse (Li et al. 2008).

10.6 Epigenetic changes

Epigenetic modification of chromatin has been proposed to translate environmental stimuli into persistent 'cellular memories'. The acetylation state can be pharmacologically modulated by histone deacetylases (HDACs) and histone acetyltransferases that catalyse reversible histone acetylation. There are several studies reporting chromatin remodelling and regulation of transcription after chronic ethanol through dynamic histone acetylation. One study has shown changes in histone deacetylation or DNA methylation in chronic alcoholics (Bonsch et al. 2004a). Chromatin remodelling was also shown in rat brain after chronic alcohol (Mahadev & Vemuri 1998; Kim & Shukla 2006). A recent study in *Drosophila* showed that a single anaesthetic dose of benzyl alcohol could induce tolerance and showed a pattern of histone H4 acetylation across the promoter region of a gene (*slo*) of known importance for the phenotype. This gene encodes the pore-forming region of BK potassium channels and an HDAC inhibitor produced parallel effects on histone acetylation, *slo* expression, and produced a tolerance-mimicking phenotype, probably through a CREB transcription site (Wang et al. 2007).

Recent work from Nestler's group has shown that chronic cocaine administration leads to increases in histone modifications at genes known to be crucial for cocaine's chronic effects. The *Bdnf* and *Cdk5* genes showed H3 hyperacetylation in their promoter regions after chronic, but not acute, cocaine. Furthermore, HDAC inhibitor treatment affected chronic cocaine responses (Kumar et al. 2005). Other work has shown that HDAC5 epigenetically controls behavioural adaptations to chronic emotional stimuli and histone acetylation plays a role in the behavioural response to cocaine (Renthal et al. 2007).

10.7 Conclusions

The pace of accumulation of information regarding genetic modulation of responses to and oriented towards alcohol continues to accelerate. I have reviewed progress derived from several methods for linking specific genes to alcohol-related behaviours. I conclude with selected examples of directions where, I think, promising leads are being developed. In each case, the developing story has used multiple methods to further the theorized link between gene and behaviour.

One area of promise is the link between endogenous opioids and alcohol dependence. Substantial data from animal models implicate common genetic contributors to endogenous opioid function and alcohol self-administration or dependence (Town et al. 2000). Numerous gene targeting studies suggest a specific role for the mu opioid receptor in ethanol preference, as its deletion reduces intake in many studies (Crabbe et al. 2006). However, there does not appear to be a straightforward homology with the human receptor. A meta-analysis of many studies seeking to test an association between the specific Asn40Asp polymorphism in the mu opioid receptor, OPRM1, and substance dependence failed to find a significant elevation in relative risk (Arias et al. 2006), even in the several studies of alcohol-dependent subjects. Nonetheless, naltrexone remains an effective therapy for some alcoholics (Heilig & Egli 2006), and a recent study reported an association between response to naltrexone therapy and the Asn40Asp polymorphism in a population of alcoholics (Anton et al. 2008). It should be noted that a smaller study of patients in several Veterans Affairs hospitals saw no similar association (Gelernter et al. 2007).

Animal studies have provided a convincing link between the stress axis and ethanol drinking. Mice lacking functional CRF-1 receptors show normal ethanol preference, but the increase in preference following stress may be attenuated (Sillaber et al. 2002). A similar effect is seen when a CRF-1 receptor antagonist is administered to normal mice (Lowery et al. 2008), and, as noted above, an antagonist also attenuates ethanol DID (Sparta et al. 2008). Also as noted above, intra-septal CRF and urocortin 1 both reduce DID (Ryabinin et al. 2008). Ethanol intake can also be potentiated following induction of physical dependence (Lopez & Becker 2005), and these increases are also blocked by CRF_1 antagonists (Chu et al. 2007; Finn et al. 2007; Richardson et al. 2008) or are absent in the knockout (Chu et al. 2007). A recent study has suggested that a polymorphism in the human CRHR1 gene is associated with heavy drinking in a sample of German 15 year olds in some measures, only if associated with more stressful life events (Blomeyer et al. 2008). It should be noted that two previous studies with adult samples have failed to find significant associations (Dahl et al. 2005; Treutlein et al. 2006).

Finally, I mention the interesting story of alpha synuclein. QTL mapping studies in crosses between P and NP rats identified a region of rat chromosome 4, among others (Bice et al. 1998; Carr et al. 1998). A subsequent gene expression profiling analysis compared tissue from multiple brain areas from inbred P and NP rats, and found many genes and ESTs to be differentially expressed (Liang et al. 2003). Although alpha synuclein had not been mapped in the rat, it was selected as a candidate gene based on its location in the homologous portion of mouse chromosome 6, and it was shown to be expressed more highly in P hippocampus than in NP. Levels of mRNA in the blood of alcohol self-administering cynomolgus monkeys were higher than in controls (Walker & Grant 2006). Subsequent studies reported increased alpha synuclein mRNA (Bonsch et al. 2004b) and protein (Bonsch et al. 2005a) levels in the blood of alcoholics versus that of controls. This group also reported increased levels of homocysteine in plasma of alcoholics, and further that these patients showed a correlated increase in levels of DNA methylation (Bonsch et al. 2004a). Increased plasma homocysteine levels were also correlated with cognitive deficits in early withdrawal (Wilhelm et al. 2006). The DNA hypermethylation is pronounced in the area of the alpha synuclein, but not the presenilin 1, promoter (Bonsch et al. 2005b). Thus, the alpha synuclein story may depend upon epigenetic modifications of the expression of other genes as yet unidentified.

This story, like all others, has its qualifications. A study of 219 multiplex families reported both a SNP and a haplotype association of alpha synuclein polymorphisms with alcohol craving, but not with alcohol dependence (Foroud et al. 2007). However, a subsequent study of two American Indian populations found scattered, weak associations with addiction-related variables, but none survived correction for multiple comparisons (Clarimon et al. 2007). In addition it must be noted that the original difference between P and NP rats was not seen in comparisons of the two pairs of HAD and LAD lines selected for the same phenotype. Nor has any association with the region of mouse chromosome 6 that harbours the gene ever emerged from the many QTL studies in the literature.

In conclusion, we continue to gain ground in our understanding of the effects of specific genes on alcoholism risk. The goal of genomically personalized therapies remains beyond our reach at the moment. The most hopeful sign is the increasing cooperative assembly and evaluation of large phenotypic and genetic datasets. It seems likely that a disease as genetically complex as alcohol dependence will require such a large-scale effort to solve its pathophysiology and aetiology. I have discussed elsewhere the parallel need for thinking carefully about the many behavioural assays employed with rodent animal model work (Crabbe & Morris 2004; Wahlsten & Crabbe 2007). We certainly are in need of continuing development of more relevant phenotypes than those currently available. In particular, the lack of parallelism between phenotypes studied in human genetic and animal model research is distressing, and there is room for much work on this front.

The author is supported by the US Department of Veterans Affairs, and by grants AA10760 and AA12714 from the National Institute on Alcohol Abuse and Alcoholism (NIAAA) of the NIH. Some of the work discussed here was supported by grant AA13519 as part of the consortium effort, the Integrative Neuroscience Initiative on Alcoholism, funded by the NIAAA.

References

Allan, A. M. & Harris, R. A. 1991 Neurochemical studies of genetic differences in alcohol action. In *The genetic basis for alcohol and drug actions* (eds J. C. Crabbe & R. A. Harris), pp. 105–52. New York, NY: Plenum Press.

Anton, R. F., Oroszi, G., O'Malley, S. et al. 2008 An evaluation of μ-opioid receptor (OPRM1) as a predictor of naltrexone response in the treatment of alcohol dependence: results from the Combined Pharmacotherapies and Behavioral Interventions for Alcohol Dependence (COMBINE) study. *Arch. Gen. Psychiatry* **65**, 135–44. (doi:10.1001/ archpsyc.65.2.135)

Arias, A., Feinn, R. & Kranzler, H. R. 2006 Association of an Asn40Asp (A118G) polymorphism in the μ-opioid receptor gene with substance dependence: a meta-analysis. *Drug Alcohol Depend.* **83**, 262–8. (doi:10. 1016/j.drugalcdep.2005.11.024)

Bailey, D. W. 1971 Recombinant-inbred strains. An aid to finding identity, linkage, and function of histocompatibility and other genes. *Transplantation* **11**, 325–7.

Beckley, E. H., Fretwell, A. M., Tanchuck, M. A., Gililland, K. R., Crabbe, J. C. & Finn, D. A. 2008 Decreased anticonvulsant efficacy of allopregnanolone during ethanol withdrawal in female Withdrawal Seizure-Prone vs. Withdrawal Seizure-Resistant mice. *Neuropharmacology* **54**, 365–74. (doi:10.1016/j.neuropharm.2007.10.006)

Belknap, J. K., Richards, S. P., O'Toole, L. A., Helms, M. L. & Phillips, T. J. 1997 Short-term selective breeding as a tool for QTL mapping: ethanol preference drinking in mice. *Behav. Genet.* **27**, 55–66. (doi:10.1023/A:1025615409383)

Bell, R. L., Rodd, Z. A., Lumeng, L., Murphy, J. M. & McBride, W. J. 2006 The alcohol-preferring P rat and animal models of excessive alcohol drinking. *Addict. Biol.* **11**, 270–88. (doi:10.1111/ j.1369-1600.2005.00029.x)

Bennett, B., Carosone-Link, P., Zahniser, N. R. & Johnson, T. E. 2006 Confirmation and fine mapping of ethanol sensitivity QTLs, and candidate gene testing in the L×S recombinant inbred mice. *J. Pharmacol. Exp. Ther.* **319**, 299–307. (doi:10.1124/jpet.106.103572)

Bennett, B., Downing, C., Carosone-Link, P., Ponicsan, H., Ruf, C. & Johnson, T. E. 2007 Quantitative trait locus mapping for acute functional tolerance to ethanol in the L×S recombinant inbred panel. *Alcohol. Clin. Exp. Res.* **31**, 200–8. (doi:10.1111/j.1530-0277.2006.00296.x)

Besheer, J., Lepoutre, V., Mole, B. & Hodge, C. W. 2006 GABA$_A$ receptor regulation of voluntary ethanol drinking requires PKC ε. *Synapse* **60**, 411–19. (doi:10.1002/syn. 20314)

Bice, P., Foroud, T., Bo, R., Castelluccio, P., Lumeng, L., Li, T.-K. & Carr, L. G. 1998 Genomic screen for QTLs underlying alcohol consumption in the P and NP rat lines. *Mamm. Genome* **9**, 949–55. (doi:10.1007/s003359900905)

Blomeyer, D., Treutlein, J., Esser, G., Schmidt, M. H., Schumann, G. & Laucht, M. 2008 Interaction between CRHR1 gene and stressful life events predicts adolescent heavy alcohol use. *Biol. Psychiatry* **63**, 146–51. (doi:10. 1016/j.biopsych.2007.04.026)

Bonsch, D., Lenz, B., Reulbach, U., Kornhuber, J. & Bleich, S. 2004a Homocysteine associated genomic DNA hypermethylation in patients with chronic alcoholism. *J. Neural Transm.* **111**, 1611–16. (doi:10.1007/s00702-004-0232-x)

Bonsch, D., Reulbach, U., Bayerlein, K., Hillemacher, T., Kornhuber, J. & Bleich, S. 2004b Elevated α synuclein mRNA levels are associated with craving in patients with alcoholism. *Biol. Psychiatry* **56**, 984–6. (doi:10.1016/ j.biopsych.2004.09.016)

Bonsch, D., Greifenberg, V., Bayerlein, K. et al. 2005a α -Synuclein protein levels are increased in alcoholic patients and are linked to craving. *Alcohol. Clin. Exp. Res.* **29**, 763–5. (doi:10.1097/01. ALC.00001643 60.43907.24)

Bonsch, D., Lenz, B., Kornhuber, J. & Bleich, S. 2005b DNA hypermethylation of the α synuclein promoter in patients with alcoholism. *Neuroreport* **16**, 167–70. (doi:10.1097/ 00001756-200502080-00020)

Bowers, B. J., Radcliffe, R. A., Smith, A. M., Miyamoto-Ditmon, J. & Wehner, J. M. 2006 Microarray analysis identifies cerebellar genes sensitive to chronic ethanol treatment in PKCγ mice. *Alcohol* **40**, 19–33. (doi:10. 1016/j.alcohol.2006.09.004)

Broadbent, J., Muccino, K. J. & Cunningham, C. L. 2002 Ethanol-induced conditioned taste aversion in 15 inbred mouse strains. *Behav. Neurosci.* **116**, 138–48. (doi:10. 1037/0735-7044.116.1.138)

Buck, K. J., Metten, P., Belknap, J. K. & Crabbe, J. C. 1997 Quantitative trait loci involved in genetic predisposition to acute alcohol withdrawal in mice. *J. Neurosci.* **17**, 3946–55.

Carr, L. G., Foroud, T., Bice, P. et al. 1998 A quantitative trait locus for alcohol consumption in selectively bred rat lines. *Alcohol. Clin. Exp. Res.* **22**, 884–7.

Carr, L. G., Kimpel, M. W., Liang, T., McClintick, J. N., McCall, K., Morse, M. & Edenberg, H. J. 2007 Identification of candidate genes for alcohol preference by expression profiling of congenic rat strains. *Alcohol. Clin. Exp. Res.* **31**, 1089–98. (doi:10.1111/j. 1530-0277. 2007.00397.x)

Chesler, E. J. et al. 2005 Complex trait analysis of gene expression uncovers polygenic and pleiotropic networks that modulate nervous system function. *Nat. Genet.* **37**, 233–42. (doi:10.1038/ng1518)

Chu, K., Koob, G. F., Cole, M., Zorrilla, E. P. & Roberts, A. J. 2007 Dependence-induced increases in ethanol self-administration in mice are blocked by the CRF$_1$ receptor antagonist antalarmin and by CRF$_1$ receptor knockout. *Pharmacol. Biochem. Behav.* **86**, 813–21. (doi:10.1016/ j.pbb. 2007.03.009)

Clarimon, J., Gray, R. R., Williams, L. N., Enoch, M. A., Robin, R. W., Albaugh, B., Singleton, A., Goldman, D. & Mulligan, C. J. 2007 Linkage disequilibrium and association analysis of α-synuclein and alcohol and drug dependence in two American Indian populations. *Alcohol. Clin. Exp. Res.* **31**, 546–54.

Colombo, G., Lobina, C., Carai, M. A. & Gessa, G. L. 2006 Phenotypic characterization of genetically selected Sardinian alcohol-preferring (sP) and -non-preferring (sNP) rats. *Addict. Biol.* **11**, 324–38. (doi:10.1111/j. 1369-1600.2006.00031.x)

Cowmeadow, R. B., Krishnan, H. R. & Atkinson, N. S. 2005 The slowpoke gene is necessary for rapid ethanol tolerance in *Drosophila*. *Alcohol. Clin. Exp. Res.* **29**, 1777–86. (doi:10.1097/01. alc.0000183232.56788.62)

Crabbe, J. C. & Morris, R. G. M. 2004 *Festina lente*: late night thoughts on high-throughput screening of mouse behavior. *Nat. Neurosci.* **7**, 1175–9. (doi:10.1038/ nn1343)

Crabbe, J. C., Phillips, T. J., Feller, D. J. et al. 1996 Elevated alcohol consumption in null mutant mice lacking 5-HT1B serotonin receptors. *Nat. Genet.* **14**, 98–101. (doi:10. 1038/ng0996-98)

Crabbe, J. C., Phillips, T. J., Harris, R. A., Arends, M. A. & Koob, G. F. 2006 Alcohol-related genes: contributions from studies with genetically engineered mice. *Addict. Biol.* **11**, 195–269. (doi:10.1111/j.1369-1600.2006.00038.x)

Crabbe, J. C., Metten, P., Rhodes, J. S. et al. 2009. A line of mice selected for drinking in the dark to intoxication. *Biol. Psychiat.* **65**, 662–670. (doi:10.1016/j.biopsych.2008.11.002)

Cunningham, C. L. & Phillips, T. J. 2003 Genetic basis of ethanol reward. In *Molecular biology of drug addiction* (ed. R. Maldonado), pp. 263–94. Totowa, NJ: Humana Press, Inc.

Cunningham, C. L., Henderson, C. M. & Bormann, N. M. 1998 Extinction of ethanol-induced conditioned place preference and conditioned place aversion: effects of naloxone. *Psychopharmacology (Berl.)* **139**, 62–70. (doi:10. 1007/s002130050690)

Dahl, J. P., Doyle, G. A., Oslin, D. W. et al. 2005 Lack of association between single nucleotide polymorphisms in the corticotropin releasing hormone receptor 1 (CRHR1) gene and alcohol dependence. *J. Psychiatr. Res.* **39**, 475–9. (doi: 10.1016/j.jpsychires.2004.12.004)

Downing, C., Carosone-Link, P., Bennett, B. & Johnson, T. 2006 QTL mapping for low-dose ethanol activation in the L×S recombinant inbred strains. *Alcohol. Clin. Exp. Res.* **30**, 1111–20. (doi:10.1111/j.1530-0277.2006.00137.x)

Enoch, M. A. & Goldman, D. 2001 The genetics of alcoholism and alcohol abuse. *Curr. Psychiatry Rep.* **3**, 144–51. (doi:10.1007/s11920-001-0012-3)

Falconer, D. S. & Mackay, T. F. C. 1996 *Introduction to quantitative genetics*, 4th edn. Harlow, UK: Longman.

Fehr, C., Shirley, R. L., Belknap, J. K., Crabbe, J. C. & Buck, K. J. 2002 Congenic mapping of alcohol and pentobarbital withdrawal liability loci to a<1 centimorgan interval of murine chromosome 4: identification of *Mpdz* as a candidate gene. *J. Neurosci.* **22**, 3730–8.

Finn, D. A., Ford, M. M., Wiren, K. M., Roselli, C. E. & Crabbe, J. C. 2004 The role of pregnane neurosteroids in ethanol withdrawal: behavioral genetic approaches. *Pharmacol. Therapeut.* **101**, 91–112. (doi:10.1016/j.pharmth era.2003.10.006)

Finn, D. A., Snelling, C., Fretwell, A. M. et al. J. 2007 Increased drinking during withdrawal from intermittent ethanol exposure is blocked by the CRF receptor antagonist D-Phe-CRF12-41. *Alcohol. Clin. Exp. Res.* **31**, 939–49. (doi:10.1111/j.1530-0277.2007.00379.x)

Flint, J., Valdar, W., Shifman, S. & Mott, R. 2005 Strategies for mapping and cloning quantitative trait genes in rodents. *Nat. Rev. Genet.* **6**, 271–86. (doi:10.1038/nrg1576)

Foroud, T. et al. 2007 Association of alcohol craving with α -synuclein (SNCA). *Alcohol. Clin. Exp. Res.* **31**, 537–45. (doi: 10.1111/j. 1530-0277.2007.00505.x)

Francis, D., Diorio, J., Liu, D. & Meaney, M. J. 1999 Nongenomic transmission across generations of maternal behavior and stress responses in the rat. *Science* **286**, 1155–8. (doi:10.1126/science.286.5442.1155)

Francis, D. D., Szegda, K., Campbell, G., Martin, W. D. & Insel, T. R. 2003 Epigenetic sources of behavioral differences in mice. *Nat. Neurosci.* **6**, 445–6.

Gelernter, J., Gueorguieva, R., Kranzler, H. R. et al. 2007 Opioid receptor gene (OPRM1, OPRK1, and OPRD1) variants and response to naltrexone treatment for alcohol dependence: results from the VA cooperative study. *Alcohol. Clin. Exp. Res.* **31**, 555–63.

Green, A. S. & Grahame, N. J. 2008 Ethanol drinking in rodents: is free-choice drinking related to the reinforcing effects of ethanol? *Alcohol* **42**, 1–11. (doi:10.1016/ j.alcohol.2007.10.005)

Grupe, A., Germer, S., Usuka, J. et al. 2001 In silico mapping of complex disease-related traits in mice. *Science* **292**, 1915–18. (doi:10.1126/science. 1058889)

Hamre, K. M., Goldowitz, D., Wilkinson, S. & Matthews, D. B. 2007 Screening for ENU-induced mutations in mice that result in aberrant ethanol-related phenotypes. *Behav. Neurosci.* **121**, 665–78. (doi:10.1037/0735-7044. 121.4.665)

Heilig, M. & Egli, M. 2006 Pharmacological treatment of alcohol dependence: target symptoms and target mechanisms. *Pharmacol. Ther.* **111**, 855–76. (doi:10. 1016/j.pharmthera.2006.02.001)

Hitzemann, R. et al. 2004 On the integration of alcohol-related quantitative trait loci and gene expression analyses. *Alcohol. Clin. Exp. Res.* **28**, 1437–48. (doi:10.1097/01.ALC.0000139827.86749.DA)

Hood, H. M., Metten, P., Crabbe, J. C. & Buck, K. J. 2006 Fine mapping of a sedative-hypnotic drug withdrawal locus on mouse chromosome 11. *Genes Brain Behav.* **5**, 1-10. (doi:10.1111/j.1601-183X.2005.00122.x)

Kakihana, R. 1979 Alcohol intoxication and withdrawal in inbred strains of mice: behavioral and endocrine studies. *Behav. Neural Biol.* **26**, 97–105. (doi:10.1016/S0163-1047(79)92933-9)

Kalant, H. 1998 Research on tolerance: what can we learn from history? *Alcohol. Clin. Exp. Res.* **22**, 67–76.

Kalant, H., LeBlanc, A. E. & Gibbins, R. J. 1971 Tolerance to, and dependence on, some non-opiate psychotropic drugs. *Pharmacol. Rev.* **23**, 135–91.

Kamdar, N. K., Miller, S. A., Syed, Y. M., Bhayana, R., Gupta, T. & Rhodes, J. S. 2007 Acute effects of naltrexone and GBR 12909 on ethanol drinking-in-the-dark in C57BL/6J mice. *Psychopharmacology* **192**, 207–17. (doi:10.1007/s00213-007-0711-5)

Kim, J. S. & Shukla, S. D. 2006 Acute *in vivo* effect of ethanol (binge drinking) on histone H3 modifications in rat tissues. *Alcohol Alcohol.* **41**, 126–32.

Kumar, A. et al. 2005 Chromatin remodeling is a key mechanism underlying cocaine-induced plasticity in striatum. *Neuron* **48**, 303–14. (doi:10.1016/j.neuron. 2005.09.023)

Lê, A. D., Israel, Y., Juzytsch, W., Quan, B. & Harding, S. 2001 Genetic selection for high and low alcohol consumption in a limited-access paradigm. *Alcohol. Clin. Exp. Res.* **25**, 1613–20. (doi:10.1111/j.1530-0277.2001. tb02168.x)

Letwin, N. E., Kafkafi, N., Benjamini, Y. et al. 2006 Combined application of behavior genetics and microarray analysis to identify regional expression themes and gene-behavior associations. *J. Neurosci.* **26**, 5277–87. (doi:10.1523/ JNEUROSCI.4602-05.2006)

Lewohl, J. M., Wang, L., Miles, M. F., Zhang, L., Dodd, P. R. & Harris, R. A. 2000 Gene expression in human alcoholism: microarray analysis of frontal cortex. *Alcohol. Clin. Exp. Res.* **24**, 1873–82. (doi:10.1111/j.1530-0277. 2000.tb01993.x)

Li, C. Y., Mao, X. & Wei, L. 2008 Genes and (common) pathways underlying drug addiction. *PLoS Comput. Biol.* **4**, e2. (doi:10.1371/journal.pcbi.0040002)

Liang, T. et al. 2003 α-Synuclein maps to a quantitative trait locus for alcohol preference and is differentially expressed in alcohol-preferring and -nonpreferring rats. *Proc. NatlAcad. Sci. USA* **100**,4690-4695. (doi:10.1073/pnas.0737182100)

Liao, G. et al. 2004 *In silico* genetics: identification of a functional element regulating H2-E α gene expression. *Science* **306**, 690–5. (doi:10.1126/science.1100636)

Liu, J., Lewohl, J. M., Harris, R. A. et al. D. 2006 Patterns of gene expression in the frontal cortex discriminate alcoholic from nonalcoholic individuals. *Neuropsychopharmacology* **31**, 1574–82. (doi:10.1038/sj.npp.1300947)

Logue, S. F., Swartz, R. J. & Wehner, J. M. 1998 Genetic correlation between performance on an appetitive-signaled nosepoke task and voluntary ethanol consumption. *Alcohol. Clin. Exp. Res.* **22**, 1912–20.

Lopez, M. F. & Becker, H. C. 2005 Effect of pattern and number of chronic ethanol exposures on subsequent voluntary ethanol intake in C57BL/6J mice. *Psychopharmacology* (*Berl.*) **181**, 688–96. (doi:10.1007/s0021 3-005-0026-3)

Lovinger, D. M. & Crabbe, J. C. 2005 Laboratory models of alcoholism: treatment target identification and insight into mechanisms. *Nat. Neurosci.* **8**, 1471–80. (doi:10.1038/ nn1581)

Lowery, E. G., Sparrow, A. M., Breese, G. R., Knapp, D. J. & Thiele, T. E. 2008 The CRF-1 receptor antagonist, CP-154,526, attenuates stress-induced increases in ethanol consumption by BALB/cJ mice. *Alcohol. Clin. Exp. Res.* **32**, 240–8.

Mahadev, K. & Vemuri, M. C. 1998 Effect of ethanol on chromatin and nonhistone nuclear proteins in rat brain. *Neurochem. Res.* **23**, 1179–84. (doi:10.1023/A:102077 8018149)

Mardones, J. & Segovia-Riquelme, N. 1983 Thirty-two years of selection of rats by ethanol preference: UChA and UChB strains. *Neurobehav. Toxicol. Teratol.* **5**, 171–8.

McClearn, G. E. 1979 Genetics and alcoholism simulacra. *Alcohol. Clin. Exp. Res.* **3**, 255–8. (doi:10.1111/j.1530-0277.1979.tb05310.x)

McClearn, G. E. & Rodgers, D. A. 1959 Differences in alcohol preference among inbred strains of mice. *Quart. J. Stud. Alcohol* **20**, 691–5.

Melo, J. A., Shendure, J., Pociask, K. & Silver, L. M. 1996 Identification of sex-specific quantitative trait loci controlling alcohol preference in C57BL/6 mice. *Nat. Genet.* **13**, 147–53. (doi:10.1038/ ng0696-147)

Metten, P. & Crabbe, J. C. 1996 Dependence and withdrawal. In *Pharmacological effects of ethanol on the nervous system* (eds R. A. Deitrich & V. G. Erwin), pp. 269–90. Boca Raton, FL: CRC Press.

Metten, P., Phillips, T. J., Crabbe, J. C. et al. 1998 High genetic susceptibility to ethanol withdrawal predicts low ethanol consumption. *Mamm. Genome* **9**, 983–90. (doi:10.1007/s003359900911)

Moore, E. M., Serio, K. M., Goldfarb, K. J., Stepanovska, S., Linsenbardt, D. N. & Boehm, S. L. 2007 GABAergic modulation of binge-like ethanol intake in C57BL/6J mice. *Pharmacol. Biochem. Behav.* **88**, 105–13. (doi:10. 1016/j.pbb.2007.07.011)

Mott, R., Talbot, C. J., Turri, M. G., Collins, A. C. & Flint, J. 2000 A method for fine mapping quantitative trait loci in outbred animal stocks. *Proc. Natl Acad. Sci. USA* **97**, 12649–54. (doi:10.1073/pnas.230304397)

Mulligan, M. K. et al. 2006 Toward understanding the genetics of alcohol drinking through transcriptome meta-analysis. *Proc. Natl Acad. Sci. USA* **103**, 6368–73. (doi:10.1073/pnas.0510188103)

Murphy, J. M., Stewart, R. B., Bell, R. L. et al. 2002 Phenotypic and genotypic characterization of the Indiana University rat lines selectively bred for high and low alcohol preference. *Behav. Genet.* **32**, 363–88. (doi:10. 1023/A:1020266306135)

Newton, P. M. & Messing, R. O. 2007 Increased sensitivity to the aversive effects of ethanol in PKCε null mice revealed by place conditioning. *Behav. Neurosci.* **121**, 439–42. (doi: 10.1037/0735-7044.121.2.439)

Ocaranza, P., Quintanilla, M. E., Tampier, L., Karahanian, E., Sapag, A. & Israel, Y. 2008 Gene therapy reduces ethanol intake in an animal model of alcohol dependence. *Alcohol. Clin. Exp. Res.* **32**, 52–7.

Olive, M. F., Mehmert, K. K., Messing, R. O. & Hodge, C. W. 2000 Reduced operant ethanol self-administration and *in vivo* mesolimbic dopamine responses to ethanol in PKCε-deficient mice. *Eur. J. Neurosci.* **12**, 4131–40. (doi: 10.1046/j.1460-9568.2000.00297.x)

Olive, M. F., Mehmert, K. K., Nannini, M. A., Camarini, R., Messing, R. O. & Hodge, C. W. 2001 Reduced ethanol withdrawal severity and altered withdrawal-induced *c-fos* expression in various brain regions of mice lacking protein kinase C-ε. *Neuroscience* **103**, 171–9. (doi:10.1016/ S0306-4522(00)00566-2)

Palmer, A. A. & Phillips, T. J. 2002 Effect of forward and reverse selection for ethanol-induced locomotor response on other measures of ethanol sensitivity. *Alcohol. Clin. Exp. Res.* **26**, 1322–9.

Pawlak, R., Melchor, J. P., Matys, T., Skrzypiec, A. E. & Strickland, S. 2005 Ethanol-withdrawal seizures are controlled by tissue plasminogen activator via modulation of NR2B-containing NMDA receptors. *Proc. Natl Acad. Sci. USA* **102**, 443–8. (doi:10.1073/pnas.0406454102)

Peirce, J. L. et al. 2006 How replicable are mRNA expression QTL? *Mamm. Genome* **17**, 643–56. (doi:10.1007/ s00335-005-0187-8)

Petkov, P. M. et al. 2004 An efficient SNP system for mouse genome scanning and elucidating strain relationships. *Genome Res.* **14**, 1806–11. (doi:10.1101/gr.2825804)

Phillips, T. J. & Belknap, J. K. 2002 Complex-trait genetics: emergence of multivariate strategies. *Nat. Rev. Neurosci.* **3**, 478–85.

Phillips, T. J. & Crabbe, J. C. 1991 Behavioral studies of genetic differences in alcohol action. In *The genetic basis of alcohol and drug actions* (eds J. C. Crabbe & R. A. Harris), pp. 25–104. New York, NY: Plenum Press.

Phillips, T. J., Crabbe, J. C., Metten, P. & Belknap, J. K. 1994 Localization of genes affecting alcohol drinking in mice. *Alcohol. Clin. Exp. Res.* **18**, 931–41. (doi:10.1111/j.1530-0277.1994.tb00062.x)

Phillips, T. J., Belknap, J. K., Buck, K. J. & Cunningham, C. L. 1998 Genes on mouse chromosomes 2 and 9 determine variation in ethanol consumption. *Mamm. Genome* **9**, 936–41. (doi:10.1007/ s003359900903)

Phillips, T. J., Broadbent, J., Burkhart-Kasch, S. et al. 2005 Genetic correlational analyses of ethanol reward and aversion phenotypes in short-term selected mouse lines bred for ethanol drinking or ethanol-induced conditioned taste aversion. *Behav. Neurosci.* **119**, 892–910. (doi:10.1037/0735-7044.119.4.892)

Qi, Z. H. et al. 2007 Protein kinase C ε regulates γ-aminobutyrate type A receptor sensitivity to ethanol and benzodiazepines through phosphorylation of γ^2 subunits. *J. Biol. Chem.* **282**, 33052–63. (doi:10.1074/jbc.M707233200)

Quintanilla, M. E., Israel, Y., Sapag, A. & Tampier, L. 2006 The UChA and UChB rat lines: metabolic and genetic differences influencing ethanol intake. *Addict. Biol.* **11**, 310–23. (doi:10.1111/j.1369-1600.2006.00030.x)

Reilly, M. T., Fehr, C. & Buck, K. J. 2001 Alcohol and gene expression in the central nervous system. In *Nutrient-gene interactions in health and disease* (eds N. Moussa-Moustaid & C. D. Berdanier), pp. 131–62. Boca Raton, FL: CRC Press.

Renthal, W. et al. 2007 Histone deacetylase 5 epigenetically controls behavioral adaptations to chronic emotional stimuli. *Neuron* **56**, 517–™29. (doi:10.1016/j.neuron. 2007.09.032)

Rhodes, J. S., Best, K., Belknap, J. K., Finn, D. A. & Crabbe, J. C. 2005 Evaluation of a simple model of ethanol drinking to intoxication in C57BL/6J mice. *Physiol. Behav.* **84**, 53–63. (doi:10.1016/j.physbeh.2004.10.007)

Rhodes, J. S., Ford, M. M., Yu, C.-H. et al. 2007 Mouse inbred strain differences in ethanol drinking to intoxication. *Genes Brain Behav.* **6**, 1–18. (doi:10.1111/j.1601-183X.2006. 00210.x)

Richardson, H. N., Zhao, Y., Fekete, E. M. et al. 2008 MPZP: a novel small molecule corticotropin-releasing factor type 1 receptor (CRF$_1$) antagonist. *Pharmacol. Biochem. Behav.* **88**, 497–510. (doi:10.1016/ j.pbb.2007.10.008)

Rodriguez, L. A., Plomin, R., Blizard, D. A., Jones, B. C. & McClearn, G. E. 1994 Alcohol acceptance, preference, and sensitivity in mice. I. Quantitative genetic analysis using B × D recombinant inbred strains. *Alcohol. Clin. Exp. Res.* **18**, 1416–22. (doi:10.1111/j.1530-0277.1994. tb01444.x)

Ryabinin, A. E., Yoneyama, N., Tanchuck, M. A., Mark, G. P. & Finn, D. A. 2008 Urocortin 1 micro-injection into the mouse lateral septum regulates the acquisition and expression of alcohol consumption. *Neuroscience* **151**, 780–90. (doi:10.1016/j.neuroscience.2007.11.014)

Scholz, H., Ramond, J., Singh, C. M. & Heberlein, U. 2000 Functional ethanol tolerance in Drosophila. *Neuron* **28**, 261–71. (doi:10.1016/S0896-6273(00)00101-X)

Sharpe, A. L., Tsivkovskaia, N. O. & Ryabinin, A. E. 2005 Ataxia and *c-Fos* expression in mice drinking ethanol in a limited access session. *Alcohol. Clin. Exp. Res.* 29, 1419–26. (doi:10.1097/01. alc.0000174746. 64499.83)

Shirley, R. L., Walter, N. A., Reilly, M. T., Fehr, C. & Buck, K. J. 2004 *Mpdz* is a quantitative trait gene for drug withdrawal seizures. *Nat. Neurosci.* **7**, 699–700. (doi: 10. 1038/nn1271)

Shram, M. J., Bahroos, M., Beleskey, J. I., Tampakeras, M., Lê, A. D. & Tomkins, D. M. 2004 Motor impairing effects of ethanol and diazepam in rats selectively bred for high and low ethanol consumption in a limited-access paradigm. *Alcohol. Clin. Exp. Res.* **28**, 1814–21. (doi:10. 1097/01. ALC.0000148105.79934.14)

Sillaber, I., Rammes, G., Zimmermann, S., Mahal, B. et al. 2002 Enhanced and delayed stress-induced alcohol drinking in mice lacking functional CRH1 receptors. *Science* **296**, 931–3. (doi:10.1126/science. 1069836)

Silver, L. M. 1995 *Mouse genetics*. New York, NY: Oxford University Press.

Sommer, W., Hyytia, P. & Kiianmaa, K. 2006 The alcohol-preferring AA and alcohol-avoiding ANA rats: neurobiology of the regulation of alcohol drinking. *Addict. Biol.* 11, 289–309. (doi:10.1111/j.1369-1600.2006.00037.x)

Sparta, D. R., Sparrow, A. M., Lowery, E. G., Fee, J. R., Knapp, D. J. & Thiele, T. E. 2008 Blockade of the corticotropin releasing factor type 1 receptor attenuates elevated ethanol drinking associated with drinking in the dark procedures. *Alcohol. Clin. Exp. Res.* **32**, 259–65.

Tabakoff, B., Saba, L., Kechris, K. et al. 2008 The genomic determinants of alcohol preference in mice. *Mamm. Genome.* **19**, 352–365.

Tarantino, L. M., McClearn, G. E., Rodriguez, L. A. & Plomin, R. 1998 Confirmation of quantitative trait loci for alcohol preference in mice. *Alcohol. Clin. Exp. Res.* **22**, 1099–105.

Thibault, C. et al. 2000 Expression profiling of neural cells reveals specific patterns of ethanol-responsive gene expression. *Mol. Pharmacol.* **58**, 1593–600.

Town, T., Schinka, J., Tan, J. & Mullan, M. 2000 The opioid receptor system and alcoholism: a genetic perspective. *Eur. J. Pharmacol.* **410**, 243–8. (doi:10.1016/S0014-2999(00)00818-9)

Treutlein, J. et al. 2006 Genetic association of the human corticotropin releasing hormone receptor 1 (CRHR1) with binge drinking and alcohol intake patterns in two independent samples. *Mol. Psychiatry* **11**, 594–602. (doi:10.1038/sj.mp.4001813)

Turek, V. F., Tsivkovskaia, N. O., Hyytia, P., Harding, S., Lê, A. D. & Ryabinin, A. E. 2005 Urocortin 1 expression in five pairs of rat lines selectively bred for differences in alcohol drinking. *Psychopharmacology (Berl.)* **181**, 511–17. (doi:10.1007/s00213-005-0011-x)

Valdar, W. et al. 2006 Genome-wide genetic association of complex traits in heterogeneous stock mice. *Nat. Genet.* **38**, 879–87. (doi:10.1038/ng1840)

Wahlsten, D. & Crabbe, J. C. 2007 Behavioral testing. In *The mouse in biomedical research*, vol. 3 (eds J. G. Fox, C. Newcomer, A. Smith, S. Barhold, F. Quimby & M. Davisson). Normative biology, immunology and husbandry, pp. 513–34. 2nd edn. Amsterdam, The Netherlands: Elsevier.

Wahlsten, D., Bachmanov, A., Finn, D. A. & Crabbe, J. C. 2006 Stability of inbred mouse strain differences in behavior and brain size between laboratories and across decades. *Proc. Natl Acad. Sci. USA* **103**, 16364–9. (doi:10.1073/pnas.0605342103)

Walker, S. J. & Grant, K. A. 2006 Peripheral blood α-synuclein mRNA levels are elevated in cynomolgus monkeys that chronically self-administer ethanol. *Alcohol* **38**, 1–4. (doi:10.1016/j.alcohol.2006.03.008)

Wang, Y., Krishnan, H. R., Ghezzi, A., Yin, J. C. & Atkinson, N. S. 2007 Drug-induced epigenetic changes produce drug tolerance. *PLoS. Biol.* **5**, 2342–53. (doi:10.1371/ journal.pbio.0050265)

Wilhelm, J., Bayerlein, K., Hillemacher, T. et al. 2006 Short-term cognition deficits during early alcohol withdrawal are associated with elevated plasma homocysteine levels in patients with alcoholism. *J. Neural Transm.* **113**, 357–63. (doi:10.1007/s00702-005-0333-1)

Wilhelm, C. J., Reeves, J. M., Phillips, T. J. & Mitchell, S. H. 2007 Mouse lines selected for alcohol consumption differ on certain measures of impulsivity. *Alcohol. Clin. Exp. Res.* **31**, 1839–45. (doi:10.1 111/j. 1530-0277.2007.00508.x)

Xu, Y., Ehringer, M., Yang, F. & Sikela, J. M. 2001 Comparison of global brain gene expression profiles between inbred long-sleep and inbred short-sleep mice by high-density gene array hybridization. *Alcohol. Clin. Exp. Res.* **25**, 810–18. (doi:10.1 111/j. 1530-0277.2001. tb02284.x)

11

Genetics of addictions: Strategies for addressing heterogeneity and polygenicity of substance use disorders

*Chloe C. Y. Wong, Toni-Kim Clarke, and Gunter Schumann**

Addictions are common psychiatric disorders that exert high cost to the individual and to society. Addictions are a result of the interplay of multiple genetic and environmental factors. They are characterized by phenotypic and genetic heterogeneity as well as polygenicity, implying a contribution of different neurobiological mechanisms to the clinical diagnosis. Therefore, treatments for most substance use disorders are often only partially effective, with a substantial proportion of patients failing to respond. To address heterogeneity and polygenicity, strategies have been developed to identify more homogenous subgroups of patients and to characterize genes contributing to their phenotype. These include genetic linkage and association studies as well as functional genetic analysis using endophenotyes and animal behavioural experimentation. Applying these strategies in a translational context aims at improving therapeutic response by the identification of subgroups of addiction patients for individualized, targeted treatment strategies.

This manuscript aims to discuss strategies addressing heterogeneity and polygenicity of substance use disorders by presenting results of recent research on genetic and environmental components of addiction. It will also introduce the European IMAGEN study, which aims to integrate methodical approaches discussed in order to identify the genetic and neurobiological basis of behavioural traits relevant for the development of addictions.

Keywords: Addictions; animal models; genetic; heterogeneity; neuroimaging; translational.

Drug addiction is characterized as a compulsion to take the substance with a narrowing of the behavioural repertoire toward excessive substance intake, and a loss of control in limiting intake (American Psychiatric Association 1994). Addictions are chronic, often relapsing common psychiatric disorders that exert tremendous cost on the individual and the society. According to the World Health Organisation (WHO), there is an estimate of 2 billion alcohol users, 1.3 billion tobacco users, and 185 million illicit drug users worldwide. The substantial social and economic costs of addiction are exemplified by the National Health Service of the United Kingdom, where £385 million is spent on drug treatment per year (http://www. homeoffice.gov.uk/). Despite the substantial sum of money spent on treatments for substance use disorder, effect sizes of all available therapies offered are typically modest with a substantial proportion of patients failing to respond. Advancement of understanding in the neurobiology and genetics of addiction is crucial for the future development of better and more effective interventions for addictive behaviour and substance use disorders. Elucidation of genetic factors underlying inter-individual differences in substance use behaviour will result in the individualization of therapies and targeting of specific clusters of patients using psychotherapeutic or pharmacological approaches, which include the prediction of therapeutic response based on pharmacogenetic profiles. The aim of this review is to evaluate the different approaches that have been employed to elucidate the genetics of addiction.

* g.schumann@iop.kcl.ac.uk

11.1 Heritability of substance use disorder

Addiction is a complex disorder and a genetic component has long been established as a contributor for inter-individual differences in vulnerability. The overall genetic influence for substance use disorders has proved to be substantial and heritabilities for most substance use disorders are estimated to be moderate to high. Family and adoption studies showed that biological offspring of alcoholics are three to five times more likely to develop alcohol dependence than individuals with no family history of alcoholism (Cotton 1979). Heritability for alcoholism is estimated to be between 50 and 60% and is comparable among male and female alcoholics (Heath et al. 1997; Kohnke 2007). Past studies demonstrated that genetic factors not only have influence on substance abuse, but also are involved in the different dimension of substance-taking behaviours (Schumann 2007). Heritabilities for substance initiation and use are generally lower than for problematic substance use, abuse, and dependence (McGue et al. 1992; True et al. 1997). A twin/sibling study in Colorado ($n = 1000$) found a modest to moderate heritability for alcohol initiation or quantity/frequency of alcohol use but a substantial heritability of 0.78 for alcohol use in adolescents (Rhee et al. 2003).

11.2 Substance use disorders are polygenic disorders with a complex inheritance pattern and result from interactions between the individual, the drug, and the environment

Substance use disorders are results of an interaction between drug, host, and environment. They are common, complex disorders that do not conform to a simple Mendelian transmission pattern and involve multiple genes and environment (G × E) interactions (Enoch & Goldman 1999; Goldman 1993). The complex genetic constitution is partly accounted for by heterogeneity and polygenicity, which are parallel mechanisms that are present to varying degrees in different substance use disorders (see Fig. 11.1). Heterogeneity assumes that a single or a few genetic variation(s) determine vulnerability and resiliency, but different alleles would lead to the same clinical presentation in different individuals (Goldman et al. 2005). The concept of polygenicity, on the other hand, assumes that a phenotype is a result of

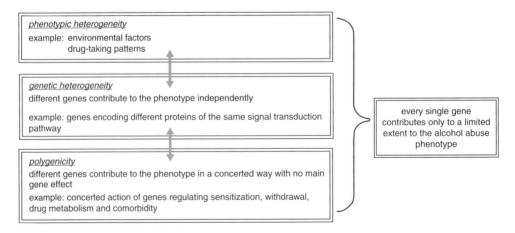

Fig. 11.1 Relationship between phenotypic heterogenetity, genetic heterogeneity, and polygenicty in alcohol use disorders.

simultaneous function of multiple genetic variants. In substance use disorders, polygenicity may include drugs-specific genes that contribute to different responses as well as common genes such as comorbidity-related genes and genes that alter environmental vulnerability (Schumann 2007).

11.3 Substance use disorders comprise a variety of behavioural and environmental characteristics that result in phenotypical heterogeneity

Phenotypic heterogeneity is extensive in the manifestation of alcoholism, with alcoholics differing in magnitudes such as age of onset of problems, alcohol symptoms, drinking history, and comorbid disorders (Dick & Foroud 2003). One of the approaches to reduce phenotypic heterogeneity is by classification of more genetically or neurobiologically homogenous phenotypes. Based on an adoption study and on a neurobiological learning model, alcoholism is distinguished into two subtypes of more genetically homogenous phenotypes (Cloninger 1987a, b). Type I alcoholism is characterized by late onset of alcohol problems and low inheritance, as well as a low degree of novelty seeking and psychological dependence, which is coupled with guilt and fear about alcoholism. Type II alcoholism is associated with early onset (prior to the age of 25), the presence of antisocial behaviour, elevated novelty seeking and reduced harm avoidance (Bau et al. 2001). This sub-typing of alcoholism into more homogenous groups has shown to reduce some phenotypic heterogeneity. However, identification of single genes that account for a large amount of variance within a phenotype still remains challenging. Therefore, geneticists have turned to endophenotypes as a way of dealing with the substantial heterogeneity involved in substance use disorder.

11.4 Endophenotypes characterize homogenous groups of individuals based on neurobiological criteria

Endophenotypes are defined as the measurable intermediates between an observed disorder and the biological processes responsible for the manifestation of that disorder (Gottesman & Gould 2003). As suggested by Gottesman and Gould, endophenotypes may be heritable intermediate phenotypes that are neurophysiological, biochemical, endocrinological, neuro-anatomical, cognitive, or neuropsychological. The deployment of endophenotypes in exploring the aetiology of disease is justified by being more homogenous in nature and provides simpler clues to genetic underpinning than the disease syndrome itself. Endophenotypes allow the identification of the 'downstream' traits of clinical phenotypes, as well as the 'upstream' effects of genes and are likely to be influenced by variation at fewer genes (see Fig. 11.2). By decomposing or deconstructing psychiatric diagnoses into their intermediate phenotypes, the complexity of genetic and phenotype analysis can be reduced. Although the concept of endophenotype in psychiatry has been developed 35 years ago (Gottesman & Shields 1973), technological advances have served to increase its relevance in recent years.

The search for endophenotypes of substance use disorder has been extensive in the past years with some fine successes. In alcoholism, several endophenotypes have been identified including the low-amplitude P300 event-related potential (ERP) robustly related to alcoholism and the observation of facial flushing syndrome predominantly in Southeast Asians (Enoch et al. 2003). The P300, also known as P3, is an evoked electroencephalographic (EEG) brain potential that is thought to index the physiologic correlate of attention allocation, basic

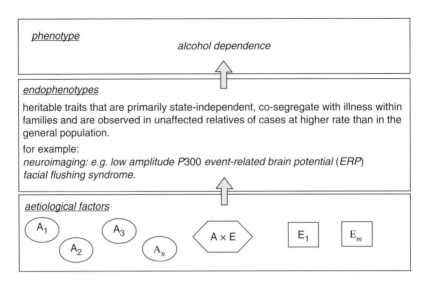

Fig. 11.2 Relationship between endophenotypes, disease (phenotype), and aetiological factors including genes, environment, and gene–environment interaction. A_1 and A_2 represent, respectively, the alcohol dehydrogenase 2 (*ADH2*) and aldehyde dehydrogenase 2 (*ALDH2*) polymorphisms that associated with reduced alcohol consumption in Southern Asians population. A_3 represents the association of *CHRM2* with low amplitude of P300 ERP. A_n, Additive genetic factors; A × E, gene-environment interaction; $E1_{-m}$, environmental factors.

information processing, and the activation and maintenance of working memory (Polich & Herbst 2000). Reduced amplitude of P300 was observed in the offspring of alcoholic families, regardless of whether the offspring are themselves alcoholics (Begleiter et al. 1984). The potential utility of P300 amplitude as an endophenotype of alcoholism was further endorsed by a carefully characterized study using data from the Collaborative Study on the Genetics of Alcoholism (COGA) that consists of more than 1,800 families, representing over 12,000 individuals (Hesselbrock et al. 2001). A reduced level of P300 amplitude was observed in alcoholics, unaffected relatives of alcoholics, and unaffected offspring of an alcoholic father, when compared correspondingly to non-alcoholics, unaffected relatives of controls, and offspring of controls. The use of electrophysiological data-based endophenotype has led to subsequent identification of a muscarinic cholinergic receptor gene, *CHRM2*, as gene associated with predisposition to alcohol dependence (Dick et al. 2006). Another useful example of endophenotype is the observation of the facial flushing syndrome mainly in Southeast Asians, which discourages alcohol intake. This observation not only led to the discovery of genetic variation of alcohol metabolising genes, alcohol dehydrogenase 2 and 3 genes (*ADH2,3*), and aldehyde dehydrogenase 1 and 2 genes (*ALDH1,2*). The reduced alcohol consumption in half of Southern Asians population was also in part explained by the presence of special functional variants of *ADH2* (Arg47His) and *ALDH2* (Glu487Lys), which lead to reduced metabolism of alcohol and thus confer a protective effect against development of alcoholism (Radel & Goldman 2001; Thomasson et al. 1991).

One of the technological advancements that greatly increases the use of endophenotypes in the assessment of G × E interaction in psychiatry is functional neuroimaging including functional magnetic resonance imaging (fMRI), positron emission tomography (PET), and magnetic encephalography (MEG). These technologies permit the measurement of information processing in discrete brain circuits that might not be immediately observable phenotypically but may be linked to the functional expression of disorder states (Hariri & Weinberger 2003). These unique properties of functional neuroimaging have been utilized in studies investigating G × E interactions. For example, the potential association between activation of specific brain regions to negative affective stimuli and selected genetic variations has been investigated extensively in fMRI studies. In these studies, brain activity is measured by metabolic activity represented by changes in blood flow in specific brain areas following a presentation of a stimulus (BOLD-response). These findings are analysed for association with genetic variations that typically are selected for a known biochemical effect on neurobiological pathways relevant for substance use disorders. An association of a serotonin transporter (*5HTT*) genotype *l/l* with increased amygdala activation during the presentation of aversive but not pleasant stimuli has been reported by several individual groups (Hariri et al. 2002; Heinz et al. 2005). Moreover, an additive effect of this *l/l* genotype, a A/G substitution of the *5HTT*, and a Val158Met polymorphism of the catechol-*O*-methyltransferase (*COMT*) gene have been reported to attribute for almost 40% of the inter-individual variance in the averaged BOLD response of amygdala, hippocampal, and limbic cortical regions elicited by unpleasant stimuli (Smolka et al. 2005, 2007). Findings from these genetic-neuroimaging studies demonstrate the great potential of functional brain imaging in assessing G × E interaction on the function of neuronal networks.

The use of endophenotypes in complex diseases has been supported by a recent study that compared the effect sizes of genes in complex diseases with those that have been discovered to influence intermediate phenotypes. As predicted, genes influencing endophenotypes demonstrated a greater effect size and thus endophenotypes are more powerful for discovering potential genes involved in regulation of brain activity (Goldman & Ducci 2007). These discoveries have prompted the development of integrated approaches to identify the genetic and neurobiological basis of behavioural traits relevant for the development of substance use. An example of such an integrated approach is the IMAGEN project (www.imagen-europe.com): Reinforcement-related behaviour in normal brain function and psychopathology is funded as part of the 6th framework programme of the European Commission. The goal of this study is to identify the genetic and neurobiological basis of traits that influences individual differences in brain responses to reward, impulsivity, and emotional cues in adolescents, and mediate risk for mental disorders with a major public health impact. Functional and structural genetic-neuroimaging study will be performed on a cohort of 2,000+ 14-year-old adolescents that are being recruited at 8 centres in the UK, Germany, France, and Ireland. Endophenotypes of risk for adolescent mental illness will be explored based on cognitive, behavioural, clinical, and neuroimaging data using 3T scanners. To determine the predictive value of intermediate phenotypes and genetics for the development of mental disorders, the cohort will be psychometrically assessed during recruitment and longitudinally at year 4 (age 16–18) of the project. Neuroimaging permits the measurement of specific brain functions implicated in the aetiology of mental disorders and link them to genetic variations and behavioural characteristics relevant to disease processes. In addition, DNA samples and phenotype database for the cohort will create a powerful resource for present and future genetic investigations. In this study, a whole-genome scan in humans will be performed and the results will be compared with transcriptional activation patterns of animals selected for extreme phenotypes of impulsivity and other relevant behavioural traits. Results obtained will be validated in 1,000 siblings from the Canadian Saguenay youth neuroimaging study. The IMAGEN study will help elucidate the neural basis of substance use disorders as well as environmental factors influencing pathological processes that contribute to addictions. It will, thus, lay the groundwork for development of treatments that target specific neurobiological mechanisms rather than heterogeneous categories of mental illness.

11.5 Gene × environment interactions: genetic variations mediate environmental influences on substance use disorders

Adoption studies have demonstrated that individuals that have the most susceptibility to alcohol abuse are those with both genetic and familial environmental risks, namely an alcohol-dependent biological parent and an alcoholic adoptive parent (Cadoret et al. 1986; Cloninger et al, 1981). Findings from past studies have revealed the association of multiple genetic and environmental factors with alcohol use disorders (see Fig. 11.3). A Finnish twin study of alcohol use amongst adolescents further exhibited the importance of G × E interaction in alcoholism by demonstrating a varied magnitude of genetic influences, with up to 5-fold differences, in different environments (Dick et al. 2001).

Social environment is a known influential factor for substance use disorders and environmental stress has long been established as one of the main external risk factors for alcohol abuse, including binge drinking and alcohol dependence (Aseltine & Gore 2000; Pohorecky 1991; Schmidt et al. 2000). Maternal stress, lack of normal parental care, and stressful life events as well as childhood physical maltreatment, delinquent peer groups, and head injury are some examples of environmental stress (Caspi & Moffitt 2006). Environmental stress is associated with the perpetuation of alcohol abuse, relapse, and aggravation of alcohol use disorder (Brady & Sonne 1999; Sinha 2001). Increased response to psychosocial stress and enhanced dampening effects of alcohol were observed in non-alcoholic sons of alcoholic fathers when compared to family history-negative subjects (Zimmermann et al. 2004).

11.6 Psychosocial stress is an important risk factor for substance use disorders and is mediated by genetic variations in the CRH system

The hypothalamic–pituitary–adrenal (HPA) axis is a fundamental neuroendocrine system that facilitates and regulates stress reaction (see Clarke et al. 2008). Upon activation of the HPA axis, a cascade of hormones including vasopressin, corticotrophin-releasing hormone (CRH), adrenocorticotropic hormone (ACTH), and glucocorticoids are secreted (Tsigos &

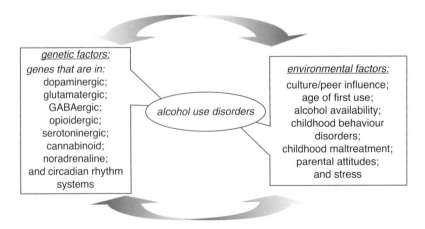

Fig. 11.3 Neurotransmitter systems and environmental factors that have been associated with alcohol use disorders.

Chrousos 2002). In a corticotrophin-releasing hormone receptor 1 (*CRHR1*)-knockout (KO) model, mice lacking a functional CRHR1 receptor demonstrated diminished stress response and the effect could not be compensated by other system or by the highly homologous CRHR2 receptor (Timpl et al. 1998). The critical role of *CRHR1* in mediating G × E interaction that affects drinking behaviour was illustrated by the identification of genetic variant in the promoter region of *CRHR1* in Marchigian-Sardian Preferring (msP) rats, genetically selected for alcohol preference (Hansson et al. 2006). This polymorphism of *CRHR1* results in higher expression of *CRHR1* in msP rats when compared to Wistar control rats and was associated with increased sensitivity to relapse into alcohol seeking induced by environmental stress. Recent human studies have also demonstrated interaction between genetic variants of *CRHR1* and environmental stress on alcohol drinking behaviour. Association of *CRHR1* with specific patterns of alcohol consumption was reported in two independent samples of alcohol-naïve adolescent and alcohol-dependent adult samples (Treutlein et al. 2006). Significant group differences between *CRHR1* genotypes were observed in binge drinking, lifetime prevalence of alcohol intake, and drunkenness in the adolescent samples, whilst an association of *CRHR1* with high amounts of drinking was demonstrated in the adult alcohol-dependent samples. The G × E interaction of *CRHR1* genotypes and environmental stress on alcohol consumption is further supported by a follow-up study demonstrating an association of polymorphism in *CRHR1* and stressful life events with heavy adolescent alcohol use (Blomeyer et al. 2008). Adolescents homozygous for the C allele of rs242938 drank higher maximum amounts of alcohol per occasion and showed greater lifetime rates of heavy drinking than individuals with the T allele in relation to negative life events. These results illustrated the potential importance of inter-individual differences in stress response on drug-taking behaviour. Further functional analyses of HPA axis genes will aid the characterization of molecular mechanisms in HPA axis regulation and define their role for substance use disorders.

As substance use disorders are complex, multifactorial disorders where a phenotype is likely to be the effect of multiple genetic variants with no main gene effect, identification of specific genes contributing to well-defined phenotypes of substance use disorders would facilitate the elucidation of underlying genes and deconstruction of the complex genetic network for substance use disorders. A number of gene identification strategies have been used in the study of alcoholism including both linkage and association studies. In whole genome linkage studies, the inheritance of polymorphic markers within families is used to identify chromosomal regions where susceptibility genes may reside. Linkage approaches to map chromosomal regions linked to alcohol use and dependence have been extensive with some substantial results, predominantly from the Collaborative study on the Genetics of Alcoholism (COGA). COGA is a large, family based study, whose goal is to detect and map susceptible genes for alcoholism and alcohol-related characteristics and behaviour (Dick et al. 2006). Increased susceptibility to alcohol use and dependence has been linked to regions on several chromosomes, including chromosomes 1, 2, 3, 7, and 8 (Edenberg & Foroud 2006). Two regions on chromosome 4p, in contrast, showed significant and suggestive linkage to non-alcoholic sibling pairs in the COGA study, which suggested a protective factor in these two regions of chromosome 4 (Reich et al. 1998). Regions that showed significant and suggestive linkage to chromosome 4p were close to the ADH gene cluster and the gamma-aminobutyric acid receptor A ($GABA_A$) gene cluster, respectively. Linkage findings on chromosome 4p have validated the role of genetic variation of ADH in conferring a protective effect against alcohol dependence. Subsequent analysis on the $GABA_A$ receptor gene cluster has resulted in the identification of a significant association between genetic variants of *GABRA2* with both alcohol dependence and brain oscillations in beta frequency range (Edenberg et al. 2004). In addition to the phenotype of alcohol dependence, several chromosomal regions have been linked to intermediate phenotypes, including a severity phenotype to chromosome 16, low level of response to alcohol to chromosome 1, 2, 9, and 21, and MAXDRINKS, a quantitative phenotype defined as the maximum number of drinks consumed in a 24-hour period to the *ADH* region of chromosome 4 (Foroud et al. 1998; Saccone et al. 2000; Schuckit et al. 2001).

Linkage analysis has been demonstrated to have limited power for the identification of common genetic variants that have modest effects on disease. A study examining the power of linkage studies in locating disease genes demonstrated that a sample size of about 700 affected sibling pairs (ASPs) was required for the detection of loci with high genotype relative risks ($g \geq 4$) and intermediate allele frequencies ($p = 0.05$–0.50). For loci with similar allele frequency ($p = 0.30$–40) but more modest relative risks ($g \leq 2$), a large sample size of around 3,000 ASPs would be needed for their detections. Association studies, in contrast, demonstrated adequate power in detecting genes of low relative risks in smaller sample size. Statistical evidence for loci with modest genotype relative risks ($g \leq 2$) and intermediate allele frequencies ($p = 0.10$–0.70) was provided by a sample size of around 700 ASPs in association study. Moreover, loci with intermediate allele frequencies ($p = 0.20$–0.70) but lower relative risks ($g \leq 1.5$) could be detected in association study by a sample size of about 1,000 ASPs (Risch 2000). Owing to the low sensitivity of linkage analysis, association studies have been used for the identification of variants in complex polygenic disorders that show no main gene effect. In association studies, correlations between genetic variants and trait differences on a population scale are assessed (Cardon & Bell 2001). Frequency of alleles or genotypes of a particular variant are compared between disease cases and controls. Any significant differences in allele frequencies between cases and controls are taken as evidence for involvement of an allele in disease susceptibility. Candidate gene association studies have some advantages over linkage studies, including a more straightforward sample collection process and a greater power to detect variants of modest effect size. However, findings from association studies are not always replicable and are prone to be the consequence of Type-I error.

11.7 Functional characterization of candidate genes using behavioural animal models is useful for dissecting genetic heterogeneity

Association analyses based on candidate genes derived from behavioural animal experiments, pharmacological data, neurobiological findings, or previously determined region of linkage have led to the identification of several susceptible genes for substance use disorders involving different neurotransmitter systems, such as dopamine, glutamate, GABA, opioids, CRH, noradrenaline, serotonin, cannabinoids, and circadian rhythm system. Detailed reviews of candidate genes for alcoholism have been published elsewhere (Dick & Fourud 2003; Gorwood et al. 2006). In this chapter, we will focus on specific candidate genes identified from our own work as well as a genetic variation where translational relevance for clinical application has been demonstrated: A functional polymorphism, A118G (Asn40Asp), of mu-opioid receptor gene (*OPRM1*) was associated with an attributable risk to alcohol dependence and greater feelings of reward during intravenous administration of alcohol to binge drinkers (Bart et al. 2005; Ray & Hutchison 2004). This same polymorphism in exon 1 of *OPRM1* has demonstrated to predict the clinical response to naltrexone in alcohol-dependent individuals

(Oslin et al. 2003). Under treatment of naltrexone, a competitive opioid receptor antagonist, individuals with one or two copies of the Asp40 allele showed significantly lower rates of relapse and a longer time to return to heavy drinking than those homozygous for the Asn40 allele. These findings on the effect of genetic variation of opioid receptor on alcoholism highlight the fundamental role of opioid system in alcohol reinforcement and provide an example for clinically relevant pharmacogenetic approaches to predict response to treatment.

Recent findings have provided evidence for the involvement of the glutamate system in acute and chronic effects of alcohol on the brain. The glutamatergic hypothesis suggests that alcohol consumption leads to enhanced glutamatergic activity in alcohol-dependent patients and the glutamate-induced hyperexcitability is uncovered during alcohol withdrawal (Gass & Olive 2008; Tsai & Coyle 1998). The hypothesis also suggests the contribution of augmented glutamatergic activity to craving and relapse behaviour as evidenced by the clinical use of anti-glutamatergic compounds such as acamprosate for relapse prevention (Spanagel & Kiefer 2008).

Alterations in different levels of glutamatergic neurotransmission, including presynaptic, synaptic, postsynaptic, and intracellular signalling, have been associated with drinking behaviour in animal models and biochemical experimentation (Vengeliene et al. 2008). Glutamate receptors are primary targets of alcohol action and a compensatory up-regulation of N-methyl-D-aspartate (NMDA) receptor subunits, mainly NR1, NR2A, and NR2B have been established in chronic alcohol exposure. This upregulation results in hyperexcitatory state in periods of acute and conditioned alcohol withdrawal (Gulya et al. 1991). The metabotropic Glutamate Receptor 5 (mGluR5), was shown to modulate alcohol self-administration and relapse behaviour in rodents (Backstrom et al. 2004; Cowen et al. 2005). Initiation of intracellular signalling pathway involving Calmodulin-dependent Kinase IV (CamKIV) and the transcription factor cAMP response element binding protein 1 (CREB) upon activation of NMDA receptors has been implicated in alcohol withdrawal and self-administration in alcohol preferring rats (Pandey et al. 2001, 2005). Glutamate-induced activation of CREB also occurs through a parallel pathway where mGluR5 and NMDA receptor signalling converges on Phosphatidyl Inositol 3 Kinase (PI3K) (Paul & Skolnick 2003). Alcohol sensitivity and self-administration in knockout models have been associated with neuronal nitric oxide synthase (nNOS) and GMP-kinase2, which are activated by PI3K (Crabbe et al. 2006; Spanagel et al. 2002; Werner et al. 2004). Synaptic concentration of glutamate is regulated by glutamate transporters such as glutamate transporter-1 (GLT-1) and glutamate aspartate transporter (GLAST), to name a few (Tanaka 2000). Elevated synaptic glutamate concentration and increased amount of alcohol intake was associated with decreased expression levels of GLAST in a recent animal study (Spanagel et al. 2005) (summarized in Fig. 11.4).

The contribution of glutamatergic transmission genes to alcohol-drinking behaviours is supported by a human genetic study, which investigates the association between variations of glutamatergic neurotransmission genes and alcohol dependence (Schumann et al. 2008). Ten glutamatergic neurotransmission genes were selected for their known alteration of alcohol drinking behaviour in animal models. These genes include GLAST, NMDA receptor subunits NR1, NR2A, and NR2B, mGluR5, nNOS, cGMP-kinaseII, CamKIV, and the regulatory subunit of PI3K and CREB. HaplotypeSNPs tagging functional domains were genotyped in two large independent samples of alcohol-dependent patients and one sample of adolescents. NR2A showed the highest relevance for human alcohol dependence (OR = 2.18), in particular, in patients with a positive family history, early onset of alcoholism and high maximum number of drinks in adults. NR2A was also associated with harmful

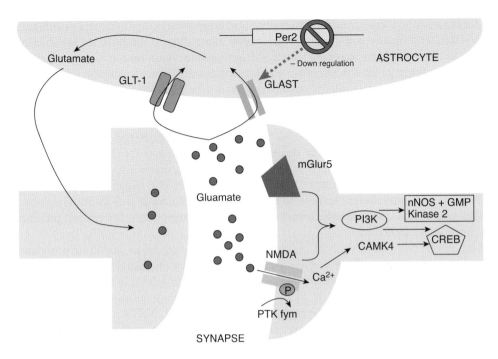

Fig. 11.4 Schematic summarising the role of the genes involved in glutamatergic neurotransmission and activation of subsequent intracellular signalling pathways. Glutamate transporter 1 (GLT-1), glutamate aspartate transporter (GLAST), nitric oxide synthase (NOS), phosphatidyl inositol-3 kinase (PI3K), N-methyl-D-aspartate receptor (NMDA), metabotropic glutamate receptor 5 (mGlur5), Calmodulin-dependent kinase IV (CAMKIV), cAMP response element binding protein 1 (CREB), Period2 (PER2), and protein tyrosine kinase fyn (PTK fyn).

drinking patterns in adolescents, suggesting a role of this gene, both in initiation and maintenance of alcohol dependence.

Phosphorylation of NR2A receptor is dependent on a src-like protein tyrosine kinase fyn (Fink & Gothert 1996; Masood et al. 1994). Interestingly, mice with a deleted fyn gene show enhanced alcohol sensitivity and lack of tolerance to the effects of alcohol (Miyakawa et al. 1997). The role of PTK fyn in human drinking behaviour was established by a study showing an association of a genetic variation of PTK fyn gene with alcohol dependence in two independent samples (Schumann et al. 2003).

Alcohol dependence has long been associated with disruptions of circadian rhythmicity, including sleep patterns, body temperature, blood pressure, and hormone secretion (Reppert & Weaver 2002). The regulation of circadian rhythm is dependent on the intertwined positive and negative regulatory loops involving the *Period (Per)*, *Cryptochrome (Cry)*, *Bmal1*, *Clock*, and *Rev-Erb*a genes (Leloup & Goldbeter 2003). Association of genetic variations in the clock gene *Per2* with alcohol-taking behaviour was demonstrated by a recent study where amount of alcohol consumption was shown to be associated with a haplotype in the *Per2* gene (Spanagel et al. 2005). This finding was complemented by animal study by the same group that showed a significant enhanced alcohol consumption and preference in *Per2*[Brdm1] mutant mice. The enhanced incentive motivation to consume more alcohol than control animals was explained by a hyperglutamatergic state in the brain reinforcement system of $Per2^{Brdm1}$ mutant mice due to a down-regulation of the glutamate transporter GLAST. Phenotypes of mutant mice were rescued by treatment of acamprosate, a drug that is thought to act primarily by dampening a hyper-glutamatergic state and use clinically for craving and relapse prevention in alcoholic patients. In this study, glutamate was shown to be an effector of Per2, thus providing a mechanistic hypothesis as to how circadian rhythm genes can influence addictive behaviour. The ascertainment of glutamate as a link between dysfunction of the Per2 gene and enhanced alcohol intake further bolsters the fundamental role of the glutamatergic system in alcohol-drinking behaviour.

The role of circadian rhythm system in drug addiction was first demonstrated in the fruit fly, *Drosophila melanogaster*. In flies mutant for circadian genes including *period, clock, cycle*, and *doubletime*, sensitization to repeated cocaine exposure, a phenomenon possibly related to drug craving (see article by Robinson & Berridge, this volume), was eliminated (Andretic et al. 1999). In mice, a hypersensitized response was observed in $Per2^{Brdm1}$ mice after a course of repeated cocaine administration, whereas behavioural sensitization is absent in $Per1^{Brdm1}$ mice (Abarca et al. 2002). These findings accentuate the contribution of circadian rhythm system in substance-taking behaviour.

11.8 Whole genome association analyses allow simultaneous identification of genes contributing to polygenicity of substance use disorders

While single candidate gene studies based on functional characterization of genes in animal models may effectively address genetic heterogeneity, successful identification of a candidate gene represents only a fraction of genetic risk factors in polygenic complex disorders like alcoholism (Hirschhorn & Daly 2005). With the limitations seen with linkage and candidate gene association studies, the potential advantage of genome-wide association (GWA) studies was forecast by Risch & Merikangas (1996). A GWA approach is defined as a study that surveys most of the genome for associated genetic variants, without the requirement of prior pathophysiological knowledge about the disease or any prediction of candidate genes. With the advancement of molecular genetic technologies, systematic association study of the whole genome can now be conducted using DNA chips or arrays. Application of the GWA approach in genetic studies of multifactorial complex disorders such as myocardial infarction, age-related macular degeneration, breast cancer, Crohn's disease, type 1 and 2 diabetes, and bipolar disorder has been extensive (Kingsmore et al. 2007). The systematic approach of GWA allows the identification of novel genes for traits of interest. Promising results have been demonstrated by a recent joint GWA study from the Wellcome Trust Case Control Consortium (WTCCC), which investigated seven major common disorders including bipolar disorder, coronary artery disease, hypertension, Crohn's disease, rheumatoid arthritis, type 1 diabetes, and type 2 diabetes (The Wellcome Trust Case Control Consortium 2007). Regarding addiction, some GWA studies have been performed for various substance use disorders, including dependency for alcohol, nicotine, methamphetamine, and heroin, with suggestion of some novel genes (Nielsen et al. 2008; Uhl et al. 2008). However, findings from these GWA studies should be treated with caution as sample sizes for some of these studies are small and no replication study has yet been conducted. Nevertheless, future well-characterized GWA studies with a large sample size will identify novel genes for substance use disorder, and thus provide a better understanding of the underlying mechanism for drug-taking behaviour.

11.9 Conclusion

In this article, we have described strategies for addressing the genetic structure of substance use disorders, which is characterized by phenotypic heterogeneity, including gene × environment interactions, genetic heterogeneity, and polygenicity. Endophenotypic characterization using functional neuroimaging, gene identification using both candidate and whole genome association analysis, and functional characterization of genes using behavioural animals are examples of strategies that have been employed thus far. While these approaches have demonstrated some success in the elucidation of substance use disorders, future research that implements a coordinated approach involving the integration of the various strategies described would offer great potential to better our understanding in the neurobiological basis of substance use disorders and behavioural traits associated with an increased susceptibility for addictions. Advancement of understanding in the genetics and neurobiological basis of addiction will result in the development of better and more effective interventions for addictive behaviour and substance use disorders.

References

Abarca, C., Albrecht, U., & Spanagel, R. 2002, Cocaine sensitization and reward are under the influence of circadian genes and rhythm, *Proc. Natl. Acad. Sci. USA*, **99**, 9026–30.

American Psychiatric Association. 1994, *Dignostic and statistical manual of mental disorders, IV edition (DSMIV)*. Washington, DC: APA.

Andretic, R., Chaney, S., & Hirsh, J. 1999, Requirement of circadian genes for cocaine sensitization in Drosophila, *Science*, **285**, 1066–8.

Aseltine, R. H., Jr. & Gore, S. L. 2000, The variable effects of stress on alcohol use from adolescence to early adulthood, *Subst. Use. Misuse*, **35**, 643–68.

Backstrom, P., Bachteler, D., Koch, S., Hyytia, P., & Spanagel, R. 2004, mGluR5 antagonist MPEP reduces ethanol-seeking and relapse behavior, *Neuropsychopharmacology*, **29**, 921–8.

Bart, G., Kreek, M. J., Ott, J., et al. 2005, Increased attributable risk related to a functional mu-opioid receptor gene polymorphism in association with alcohol dependence in central Sweden, *Neuropsychopharmacology*, **30**, 417–22.

Bau, C. H., Spode, A., Ponso, A. C., et al. 2001, Heterogeneity in early onset alcoholism suggests a third group of alcoholics, *Alcohol*, **23**, 9–13.

Begleiter, H., Porjesz, B., Bihari, B., & Kissin, B. 1984, Event-related brain potentials in boys at risk for alcoholism, *Science*, **225**, 1493–6.

Blomeyer, D., Treutlein, J., Esser, G., Schmidt, M. H., Schumann, G., & Laucht, M. 2008, Interaction between CRHR1 gene and stressful life events predicts adolescent heavy alcohol use, *Biol. Psychiatry*, **63**, 146–51.

Brady, K. T. & Sonne, S. C. 1999, The role of stress in alcohol use, alcoholism treatment, and relapse, *Alcohol Res. Health*, **23**, 263–71.

Cadoret, R. J., Troughton, E., O'Gorman, T. W., & Heywood, E. 1986, An adoption study of genetic and environmental factors in drug abuse, *Arch. Gen. Psychiatry*, **43**, 1131–6.

Cardon, L. R. & Bell, J. I. 2001, Association study designs for complex diseases, *Nat. Rev. Genet.*, **2**, 91–9.

Caspi, A. & Moffitt, T. E. 2006, Gene-environment interactions in psychiatry: joining forces with neuroscience, *Nat. Rev. Neurosci.*, **7**, 583–90.

Clarke, T. K., Treutlein, J., Zimmermann, U. S., et al. 2008, HPA-axis activity in alcoholism: examples for a gene-environment interaction, *Addict. Biol.*, **13**, 1–14.

Cloninger, C. R. 1987a, Neurogenetic adaptive mechanisms in alcoholism, *Science*, **236**, 410–16.

Cloninger, C. R. 1987b, A systematic method for clinical description and classification of personality variants. A proposal, *Arch. Gen. Psychiatry*, **44**, 573–88.

Cloninger, C. R., Bohman, M., & Sigvardsson, S. 1981, Inheritance of alcohol abuse. Cross-fostering analysis of adopted men, *Arch. Gen. Psychiatry*, **38**, 861–8.

Cotton, N. S. 1979, The familial incidence of alcoholism: a review, *J. Stud. Alcohol*, **40**, 89–116.

Cowen, M. S., Djouma, E., & Lawrence, A. J. 2005, The metabotropic glutamate 5 receptor antagonist 3-[(2-methyl-1,3-thiazol-4-yl)ethynyl]-pyridine reduces ethanol self-administration in multiple strains of alcohol-preferring rats and regulates olfactory glutamatergic systems, *J. Pharmacol. Exp. Ther.*, **315**, 590–600.

Crabbe, J. C., Phillips, T. J., Harris, R. A., Arends, M. A., & Koob, G. F. 2006, Alcohol-related genes: contributions from studies with genetically engineered mice, *Addict. Biol.*, **11**, 195–269.

Dick, D. M. & Foroud, T. 2003, Candidate genes for alcohol dependence: a review of genetic evidence from human studies, *Alcohol Clin. Exp. Res.*, **27**, 868–79.

Dick, D. M., Jones, K., Saccone, N., et al. 2006, Endophenotypes successfully lead to gene identification: results from the collaborative study on the genetics of alcoholism, *Behav. Genet.*, **36**, 112–126.

Dick, D. M., Rose, R. J., Viken, R. J., Kaprio, J., & Koskenvuo, M. 2001, Exploring gene-environment interactions: socioregional moderation of alcohol use, *J. Abnorm. Psychol.*, **110**, 625–32.

Edenberg, H. J., Dick, D. M., Xuei, X., et al. 2004, Variations in GABRA2, encoding the alpha 2 subunit of the GABA(A) receptor, are associated with alcohol dependence and with brain oscillations, *Am. J. Hum. Genet.*, **74**, 705–14.

Edenberg, H. J. & Foroud, T. 2006, The genetics of alcoholism: identifying specific genes through family studies, *Addict. Biol.*, **11**, 386–96.

Enoch, M. A. & Goldman, D. 1999, Genetics of alcoholism and substance abuse, *Psychiatr. Clin. North Am.*, **22**, 289–99, viii.

Enoch, M. A., Schuckit, M. A., Johnson, B. A., & Goldman, D. 2003, Genetics of alcoholism using intermediate phenotypes, *Alcohol Clin. Exp. Res.*, **27**, 169–76.

Fink, K. & Gothert, M. 1996, Both ethanol and ifenprodil inhibit NMDA-evoked release of various neurotransmitters at different, yet proportional potency: potential relation to NMDA receptor subunit composition, *Naunyn Schmiedebergs Arch. Pharmacol.*, **354**, 312–19.

Foroud, T., Bucholz, K. K., Edenberg, H. J., et al. 1998, Linkage of an alcoholism-related severity phenotype to chromosome 16, *Alcohol Clin. Exp. Res.*, **22**, 2035–42.

Gass, J. T. & Olive, M. F. 2008, Glutamatergic substrates of drug addiction and alcoholism, *Biochem. Pharmacol.*, **75**, 218–65.

Goldman, D. 1993, Recent developments in alcoholism: genetic transmission, *Recent Dev. Alcohol*, **11**, 231–48.

Goldman, D. & Ducci, F. 2007, Deconstruction of vulnerability to complex diseases: enhanced effect sizes and power of intermediate phenotypes, *ScientificWorldJournal*, **7**, 124–30.

Goldman, D., Oroszi, G., & Ducci, F. 2005, The genetics of addictions: uncovering the genes, *Nat. Rev. Genet.*, **6**, 521–32.

Gorwood, P., Schumann, G., Treutlein, J., & Ades, J. 2006, Pharmacogenetics of alcohol dependence. In: *Psychopharmacogenetics*. (Eds., P. Gorwood & M. Hamon) pp. 177–202. Heidelberg: Springer

Gottesman, I. I. & Gould, T. D. 2003, The endophenotype concept in psychiatry: etymology and strategic intentions, *Am. J. Psychiatry*, **160**, 636–45.

Gottesman, I. I. & Shields, J. 1973, Genetic theorizing and schizophrenia, *Br. J. Psychiatry*, **122**, 15–30.

Gulya, K., Grant, K. A., Valverius, P., Hoffman, P. L., & Tabakoff, B. 1991, Brain regional specificity and time-course of changes in the NMDA receptor-ionophore complex during ethanol withdrawal, *Brain Res.*, **547**, 129–34.

Hansson, A. C., Cippitelli, A., Sommer, W. H., et al. 2006, Variation at the rat Crhr1 locus and sensitivity to relapse into alcohol seeking induced by environmental stress, *Proc. Natl. Acad. Sci. USA*, **103**, 15236–41.

Hariri, A. R., Mattay, V. S., Tessitore, A., et al. 2002, Serotonin transporter genetic variation and the response of the human amygdala, *Science*, **297**, 400–3.

Hariri, A. R. & Weinberger, D. R. 2003, Imaging genomics, *Br. Med. Bull.*, **65**, 259–70.

Heath, A. C., Bucholz, K. K., Madden, P. A., et al. 1997, Genetic and environmental contributions to alcohol dependence risk in a national twin sample: consistency of findings in women and men, *Psychol. Med.*, **27**, 1381–96.

Heinz, A., Braus, D. F., Smolka, M. N., et al. 2005, Amygdala-prefrontal coupling depends on a genetic variation of the serotonin transporter, *Nat. Neurosci.*, **8**, 20–1.

Hesselbrock, V., Begleiter, H., Porjesz, B., O'Connor, S., & Bauer, L. 2001, P300 event-related potential amplitude as an endophenotype of alcoholism—evidence from the collaborative study on the genetics of alcoholism, *J. Biomed. Sci.*, **8**, 77–82.

Hirschhorn, J. N. & Daly, M. J. 2005, Genome-wide association studies for common diseases and complex traits, *Nat. Rev. Genet.*, **6**, 95–108.

Home Office. Ref Type: Internet Communication, 2007.

Kingsmore, S. F., Lindquist I. E., Mudge J., & Beavis W. D. 2007, Genome-wide association studies: progress in identifying genetic biomarkers in common, complex diseases, *Biomarker Insights*, **2**, 283–92.

Kohnke, M. D. In press, Approach to the genetics of alcoholism: A review based on pathophysiology, *Biochem. Pharmacol.*, p. doi:10.1016/j.bcp.2007.06.021.

Leloup, J. C. & Goldbeter, A. 2003, Toward a detailed computational model for the mammalian circadian clock, *Proc. Natl. Acad. Sci. USA*, **100**, 7051–6.

Masood, K., Wu, C., Brauneis, U., & Weight, F. F. 1994, Differential ethanol sensitivity of recombinant N-methyl-D-aspartate receptor subunits, *Mol. Pharmacol.*, **45**, 324–9.

McGue, M., Pickens, R. W., & Svikis, D. S. 1992, Sex and age effects on the inheritance of alcohol problems: a twin study, *J. Abnorm. Psychol.*, **101**, 3–17.

Miyakawa, T., Yagi, T., Kitazawa, H., et al. 1997, Fyn-kinase as a determinant of ethanol sensitivity: relation to NMDA-receptor function, *Science*, **278**, 698–701.

Nielsen, D. A., Ji, F., Yuferov, V., et al. 2008, Genotype patterns that contribute to increased risk for or protection from developing heroin addiction, *Mol. Psychiatry*, **13**, 417–28.

Oslin, D. W., Berrettini, W., Kranzler, H. R., et al. 2003, A functional polymorphism of the mu-opioid receptor gene is associated with naltrexone response in alcohol-dependent patients, *Neuropsychopharmacology*, **28**, 1546–52.

Pandey, S. C., Roy, A., & Mittal, N. 2001, Effects of chronic ethanol intake and its withdrawal on the expression and phosphorylation of the creb gene transcription factor in rat cortex, *J. Pharmacol. Exp. Ther.*, **296**, 857–868.

Pandey, S. C., Zhang, H., Roy, A., & Xu, T. 2005, Deficits in amygdaloid cAMP-responsive element-binding protein signaling play a role in genetic predisposition to anxiety and alcoholism, *J. Clin. Invest.*, **115**, 2762–73.

Paul, I. A. & Skolnick, P. 2003, Glutamate and depression: clinical and preclinical studies, *Ann. N.Y. Acad. Sci.*, **1003**, 250–72.

Pohorecky, L. A. 1991, Stress and alcohol interaction: an update of human research, *Alcohol Clin. Exp. Res.*, **15**, 438–59.

Polich, J. & Herbst, K. L. 2000, P300 as a clinical assay: rationale, evaluation, and findings, *Int. J. Psychophysiol.*, **38**, 3–19.

Radel, M. & Goldman, D. 2001, Pharmacogenetics of alcohol response and alcoholism: the interplay of genes and environmental factors in thresholds for alcoholism, *Drug Metab. Dispos.*, **29**, 489–494.

Ray, L. A. & Hutchison, K. E. 2004, A polymorphism of the mu-opioid receptor gene (OPRM1) and sensitivity to the effects of alcohol in humans, *Alcohol Clin. Exp. Res.*, **28**, 1789–95.

Reich, T., Edenberg, H. J., Goate, A., et al. 1998, Genome-wide search for genes affecting the risk for alcohol dependence, *Am. J. Med. Genet.*, **81**, 207–15.

Reppert, S. M. & Weaver, D. R. 2002, Coordination of circadian timing in mammals, *Nature*, **418**, 935–41.

Rhee, S. H., Hewitt, J. K., Young, S. E., Corley, R. P., Crowley, T. J., & Stallings, M. C. 2003, Genetic and environmental influences on substance initiation, use, and problem use in adolescents, *Arch. Gen. Psychiatry*, **60**, 1256–64.

Risch, N. & Merikangas, K. 1996, The future of genetic studies of complex human diseases, *Science*, **273**, 1516–17.

Risch, N. J. 2000, Searching for genetic determinants in the new millennium, *Nature*, **405**, 847–56.

Saccone, N. L., Kwon, J. M., Corbett, J., et al. 2000, A genome screen of maximum number of drinks as an alcoholism phenotype, *Am. J. Med. Genet.*, **96**, 632–637.

Schmidt, L. G., Dufeu, P., Kuhn, S., Smolka, M., & Rommelspacher, H. 2000, Transition to alcohol dependence: clinical and neurobiological considerations, *Compr. Psychiatry*, **41**, 90–4.

Schuckit, M. A., Edenberg, H. J., Kalmijn, J., et al. 2001, A genome-wide search for genes that relate to a low level of response to alcohol, *Alcohol Clin. Exp. Res.*, **25**, 323–9.

Schumann, G. 2007, Okey Lecture 2006: identifying the neurobiological mechanisms of addictive behaviour, *Addiction*, **102**, 1689–1695.

Schumann, G., Johann, M., Frank, J., et al. 2008, Systematic analysis of glutamatergic neurotransmission genes in alcohol dependence and adolescent risk drinking behaviour, *Arch. Gen. Psychiatry*, **65**, 826–38.

Schumann, G., Rujescu, D., Kissling, C., et al. 2003, Analysis of genetic variations of protein tyrosine kinase fyn and their association with alcohol dependence in two independent cohorts, *Biol. Psychiatry*, **54**, 1422–6.

Sinha, R. 2001, How does stress increase risk of drug abuse and relapse? *Psychopharmacology (Berl)*, **158**, 343–59.

Smolka, M. N., Buhler, M., Schumann, G., et al. 2007, Gene-gene effects on central processing of aversive stimuli, *Mol. Psychiatry*, **12**, 307–17.

Smolka, M. N., Schumann, G., Wrase, J., et al. 2005, Catechol-O-methyltransferase val158met genotype affects processing of emotional stimuli in the amygdala and prefrontal cortex, *J. Neurosci.*, **25**, 836–42.

Spanagel, R. & Kiefer, F. 2008, Drugs for relapse prevention of alcoholism—10 years of progress. *Trends Phramcol Sci.*, [Epub ahead of print]

Spanagel, R., Pendyala, G., Abarca, C., et al. 2005, The clock gene Per2 influences the glutamatergic system and modulates alcohol consumption, *Nat. Med.*, **11**, 35–42.

Spanagel, R., Siegmund, S., Cowen, M., et al. 2002, The neuronal nitric oxide synthase gene is critically involved in neurobehavioral effects of alcohol, *J. Neurosci.*, **22**, 8676–83.

Tanaka, K. 2000, Functions of glutamate transporters in the brain, *Neurosci. Res.*, **37**, 15–19.

The Wellcome Trust Case Control Consortium 2007, Genome-wide association study of 14,000 cases of seven common diseases and 3,000 shared controls, *Nature*, **447**, 661–78.

Thomasson, H. R., Edenberg, H. J., Crabb, D. W., et al. 1991, Alcohol and aldehyde dehydrogenase genotypes and alcoholism in Chinese men, *Am. J. Hum. Genet.*, **48**, 677–81.

Timpl, P., Spanagel, R., Sillaber, I., et al. 1998, Impaired stress response and reduced anxiety in mice lacking a functional corticotropin-releasing hormone receptor 1, *Nat. Genet.*, **19**, 162–6.

Treutlein, J., Kissling, C., Frank, J., et al. 2006, Genetic association of the human corticotropin releasing hormone receptor 1 (CRHR1) with binge drinking and alcohol intake patterns in two independent samples, *Mol. Psychiatry*, **11**, 594–602.

True, W. R., Heath, A. C., Scherrer, J. F., et al. 1997, Genetic and environmental contributions to smoking, *Addiction*, **92**, 1277–87.

Tsai, G. & Coyle, J. T. 1998, The role of glutamatergic neurotransmission in the pathophysiology of alcoholism, *Annu. Rev. Med.*, **49**, 173–84.

Tsigos, C. & Chrousos, G. P. 2002, Hypothalamic–pituitary–adrenal axis, neuroendocrine factors and stress, *J. Psychosom. Res.*, **53**, 865–71.

Uhl, G. R., Drgon, T., Johnson, C., et al. 2008, Higher order addiction molecular genetics: convergent data from genome-wide association in humans and mice, *Biochem. Pharmacol.*, **75**, 98–111.

Vengeliene, V., Bilbao, A., Molander, A., & Spanagel, R. 2008, Neuropharmacology of alcohol addiction. *Brit. J. Pharmacol.*, Epub ahead of print.

Werner, C., Raivich, G., Cowen, M., et al. 2004, Importance of NO/cGMP signalling via cGMP-dependent protein kinase II for controlling emotionality and neurobehavioural effects of alcohol, *Eur. J. Neurosci.*, **20**, 3498–506.

Zimmermann, U., Spring, K., Kunz-Ebrecht, S. R., Uhr, M., Wittchen, H. U., & Holsboer, F. 2004, Effect of ethanol on hypothalamic–pituitary–adrenal system response to psychosocial stress in sons of alcohol-dependent fathers, *Neuropsychopharmacology*, **29**, 1156–65.

12

Characterizing organism × environment interactions in non-human primate models of addiction: PET imaging studies of dopamine D2 receptors

Michael A. Nader,* Paul W. Czoty, Robert W. Gould, and Natallia V. Riddick

Animal models have provided valuable information related to trait and state variables associated with vulnerability to drug addiction. Our brain imaging studies in monkeys have implicated D2 receptors in cocaine addiction. For example, an inverse relationship between D2 receptor availability and rates of cocaine self-administration has been documented. Moreover, environmental variables, such as those associated with formation of the social hierarchy, can impact receptor availability and sensitivity to the abuse-related effects of cocaine. Similarly, both D2 receptor availability and cocaine self-administration can be altered by chronic drug administration and by fluctuations in hormone levels. In addition, cocaine self-administration can be altered in an orderly fashion by environmental manipulation such as acting as an intruder into an unfamiliar social group, which can shift the cocaine dose–response curve to the left in subordinate monkeys and to the right in dominant animals, suggesting an interaction between social variables and acute stressors. Conversely, irrespective of social rank, acute environmental enrichment, such as increasing the size of the living space, shifts the cocaine dose–response curve to the right. These findings highlight a pervasive influence of the environment in modifying the reinforcing effects of cocaine and strongly implicate brain D2 receptors.

Key Words: Dopamine (DA); D2 receptors; cocaine self-administration; social behaviour; animal models; non-human primates.

12.1 Introduction

Drug abuse continues to be a major public health problem worldwide (WHO 2004). In the United States, approximately 2.9 million persons aged 12 or older used an illicit drug for the first time in 2005, with recent estimates of 2.4 million Americans confirming current cocaine use (SAMHSA 2006). Within the European Union, lifetime experience with cocaine for 15–24-year-old males was reported at 5–13% (WHO 2004). In 2001, 56% of all countries reporting on cocaine trends reported increases; in Europe, the number was 67% (WHO 2004). At present there are no approved pharmacological treatments for cocaine addiction, although several novel avenues are being considered (O'Brien 2005; Elkashef et al. 2007). The overarching goal of the research program described in this review is to examine behavioural, pharmacological, and neurochemical correlates of vulnerability, maintenance, and relapse to cocaine addiction in non-human primate models. This research strategy holds the premise that a better understanding of these variables may lead to improved treatment strategies for cocaine addiction.

* mnader@wfubmc.edu

As pointed out by James Mills in 1965, '[A]ny disease—including drug addiction—depends for its spread on the three necessities: a susceptible individual, an infecting substance, and an environment where the two can meet'. More recently, these 'necessities' have been described in terms of the 'agent', the 'host', and the 'context' (O'Brien 2006). In this review, we will describe how these three variables are considered in the development of novel treatment strategies for cocaine abuse. While we focus on cocaine, it is our hypothesis that these strategies, which emphasize the social context and environmental conditions, are relevant for all drugs of abuse.

12.2 The agent

Cocaine is an indirect-acting monoamine agonist, which binds with approximately equal affinity to dopamine (DA), serotonin (5-HT), and norepinephrine (NE) transporters (Ritz et al. 1987; Woolverton & Johnson 1992). The vast majority of studies on the mechanisms of action mediating the high abuse liability of cocaine focus on the DA system. Briefly, DA cells from the ventral tegmental area project to structures within the striatum, including the nucleus accumbens, and project to the cortex (Haber & McFarland 1999); these pathways have been implicated in all rewarding behaviours (Di Chiara & Imperato 1988). DA released into the synapse is primarily removed by active uptake by the DA transporter (DAT). Cocaine acts by blocking the transporter and elevating the levels of extracellular DA, which produces its downstream effects by binding to two superfamilies of DA receptors: D1- and D2-like receptors (Sibley et al. 1993). The imaging work described in this review will focus on D2-like receptors and imaging tools, [^{11}C]raclopride and [^{18}F]fluoroclebopride (FCP), that do not differentiate among the subtypes of the D2-superfamily (Mach et al. 1993). Also of relevance is whether the D2 PET ligands interact with pre- or post-synaptic D2-like receptors. On the basis of lesioning work (Chalon et al. 1999), we hypothesize that changes in D2 receptor availability are primarily due to changes in post-synaptic D2 receptor function (Nader & Czoty 2005). Also of relevance is the recent work that has differentiated two states of the D2 receptor: D2^{high} and D2^{low} (Seeman et al. 2002, 2003). DA binds primarily to the high affinity state of the receptor as assessed *in vitro* (i.e. D2^{high}). However, the relevance of these states to *in vivo* function has not been fully elucidated. Interestingly, it has been shown in rats that cocaine increased the proportion of D2^{high} receptors *in vitro* (Briand et al. 2008); however, this occurred under conditions in which total number of D2 receptors did not change. Most PET imaging studies have used radiotracers that cannot differentiate the high- and low-affinity states of the D2 receptor, although more selective agents are being developed (Graff-Guerrero et al. 2008; Willeit et al. 2008). As described throughout this chapter, the parallel findings from human and non-human primate *in vivo* imaging techniques allow for translational research into mechanisms mediating cocaine reinforcement and the identification of effective treatment strategies.

Research into the pharmacodynamics and pharmacokinetics of cocaine that leads to its high abuse potential has enhanced our understanding of the DA system and reward mechanisms. Using techniques such as *in vivo* microdialysis in animals surgically implanted with cannulae targeting various brain structures, cocaine has been shown to elevate levels of extracellular DA in areas of the brain that are believed to mediate reinforcement (Bradberry 2000; Czoty et al. 2002; Howell and Wilcox 2002). In humans, using non-invasive brain imaging techniques such as positron emission tomography (PET), the relationship between elevating DA and subjective drug effects was examined (Volkow et al. 1999). In that study, investigators administered [^{11}C]raclopride, which binds to post-synaptic DA D2 receptors, and measured the displacement of that radiotracer by DA in non-drug abusing individuals. Because cocaine could not be administered to these individuals for ethical reasons, the investigators utilized another indirect-acting DA agonist, methylphenidate, which has reinforcing effects in animals and in humans (Johanson & Schuster 1975; Volkow et al. 1999). There was an orderly relationship between the ability of methylphenidate to elevate DA and displace [^{11}C]raclopride from D2-like receptors and the intensity of the subjective reports of 'high'. Importantly, in the subjects that did not report a 'high', methylphenidate did not elevate DA.

Finally, despite the clear relevance of specific actions of cocaine at neurobiological target sites, it is important to point out that it is our premise that the prominent abuse-related effects of cocaine are not simply explained by pharmacological interactions between drug and receptor. There are clearly profound differences in the behavioural effects of cocaine when administered non-contingently by the investigator vs. self-administered by the animal (Dworkin et al. 1995; Stefanski et al. 1999; Bradberry 2000). Moreover, as described in detail below, the schedule of cocaine availability can have profound effects on the CNS consequences of cocaine exposure.

12.3 The host

The studies described below used non-human primates, specifically, rhesus monkeys (*Macaca mulatta*) or cynomolgus monkeys (*M. fascicularis*). Along with baboons, these Old World monkeys are the most closely phylogenetically related species to humans that can be used in biomedical research. Thus, our ability to accurately generalize from laboratory animal models to human drug abuse is enhanced by using monkeys as subjects; this is particularly important for imaging studies (Nader & Czoty 2008). There are documented differences between monkey and rodent dopaminergic systems (Berger et al. 1991; Joel & Weiner 2000), including differences in DA affinity at D1- and D2-like receptors (Weed et al. 1998), as well as evidence of species differences in cocaine-induced changes in brain function (Lyons et al. 1996) and in the behavioural effects of indirect-acting DA agonists including cocaine (Lile et al. 2003; Roberts et al. 1999). There are also data indicating that many drugs, including drugs of abuse, have similar pharmacokinetic profiles in monkeys and humans that differ in rodents (Banks et al. 2007; Weerts et al. 2007 for review).

Monkeys also allow for the investigation of social variables in cocaine abuse (Morgan et al. 2002; Czoty et al. 2005); these studies provide a unique translational component to our research. The social hierarchy (i.e. the social ranks of each of the four monkeys in a group) is determined by recording winners of fights between the monkeys (Kaplan et al. 1982). The first-ranking ('dominant') monkey is defined as the monkey that wins fights against the other three monkeys. The second ranking monkey wins all fights except against the first ranking monkey, and so on. The monkey that loses fights with all others in the pen is designated the lowest-ranking ('subordinate') monkey.

Sex is a host factor that has been largely overlooked in drug abuse research. While the majority of our research has focused on male subjects, there is growing evidence for sex differences in behaviour, pharmacology, and neurochemical actions of abused drugs (Lynch et al. 2002; Lynch 2006; Terner & de Wit 2006). Importantly, these reported sex differences extend beyond drug abuse to include most psychiatric disorders including schizophrenia, Parkinson's disease, and obsessive-compulsive disorder (Seeman 1996; Wieck et al. 2003). In female subjects, there is evidence that menstrual cycle phase can alter sensitivity to drugs of abuse (Terner & de Wit 2006). Female macaques have an approximately 28-day menstrual cycle, with fluctuations in oestrogen and progesterone resembling those of women (Jewitt & Dukelow 1972; Appt 2004), making them ideal for studying conditions related to women's health. Although not discussed in this paper, studies related to prenatal drug exposure would also benefit from the use of non-human primates. For example, the gestation period in macaques is approximately 6 months, which is close to human gestation and much longer than rodent models (Sandberg & Olsen 1991).

Of relevance to the topic of this review, we recently investigated how menstrual cycle phase influenced measures of DA D2 receptor availability in female cynomolgus monkeys (Czoty et al. 2008). As will be described below, there appears to be a relationship between D2 receptor availability and reinforcing effects of cocaine. Thus, if menstrual cycle phase influences D2 receptor levels, this may be a primary mechanism for differences in abuse-related effects of cocaine (or other abused drugs) in women tested at different times of the month (Sofuoglu et al. 1999). Three PET imaging studies in women have investigated D2 receptor availability as a function of menstrual cycle; three different outcomes were reported. Wong et al. (1988) reported a trend toward lower radiotracer uptake in the striatum of women tested in the follicular versus luteal phase. In a more recent study, they found lower D2 receptor measures in the putamen (but not caudate nucleus or ventral striatum) in women in the luteal vs. follicular phase (Munro et al. 2006). Finally, Nordstrom et al. (1998) found no evidence of menstrual-cycle dependent variations in D2 receptor availability in the putamen in five women. Several factors could account for these disparate results including the stress level and the drug history of the women. Importantly, these factors can be controlled in animal studies. In seven experimentally naïve, normally cycling female cynomolgus monkeys, we found that D2 receptor availability was significantly (~13%) lower in the follicular phase compared to the same monkeys studied during the luteal phase (Czoty et al., 2008). Such an outcome supports differences in sensitivity to drug effects at various stages of the menstrual cycle and underscores the importance of the hormonal milieu as a host factor that may influence the effects of abused drugs. Moreover, these data suggest that studies in female subjects should minimize the influence of menstrual cycle fluctuations by taking measurements in the same menstrual cycle phase when conducting longitudinal studies. In addition, these results suggest that sensitivity to the abuse-related effects of psychostimulants may vary with menstrual cycle phase. Supporting this hypothesis, Mello et al. (2007) reported that a low cocaine dose was a stronger reinforcer during follicular versus luteal phase in monkeys self-administering cocaine under a progressive-ratio schedule of reinforcement and the majority of studies in humans report greater subjective effects of cocaine and amphetamine during the follicular phase (for review see, Terner & de Wit, 2006).

In addition to generating hypotheses regarding cocaine sensitivity across the menstrual cycle, results of these studies, when combined with similar data collected in male monkeys, may provide insight into sex differences in cocaine abuse. Although a greater proportion of cocaine abusers are men (SAMHSA 2006), specific sex differences and the neurobiological and sociocultural factors that produce them have not been fully elucidated (Wagner & Anthony 2007), and studies of sex differences in drug self-administration in laboratory animals have produced inconsistent results (for review see, Lynch et al. 2002). Few preclinical studies have examined neurobiological differences between male and female humans and animals that may account for sex differences in sensitivity to cocaine. In individually housed, drug-naive male cynomolgus monkeys (Czoty et al. 2005), D2 receptor availability in the caudate nucleus and putamen was lower than was observed in females in either the follicular or luteal phase (Czoty et al. 2008). These findings suggest sex differences in the availability of striatal D2 receptors in drug-naive non-human primates, with D2 availability in males more similar to females studied during the follicular phase. By extension, they suggest that sensitivity to psychostimulants will be higher in males than in females, but that females will be more similar to males during the follicular phase, and least sensitive during the luteal phase. Comparisons between our previous results in males and female monkeys are somewhat complicated by use of different PET cameras. However, the primary dependent variable, distribution volume ratio (DVR), is a relative measure (obtained by dividing radiotracer binding in regions of interest by binding in the cerebellum, an area devoid of D2 receptors), increasing the likelihood that the measures are comparable across cameras. Moreover, in previous PET studies of male and female cynomolgus monkeys using the same PET camera, basal ganglia DVRs were similar across sexes (Grant et al. 1998; Morgan et al. 2002). Studies such as these highlight the suitability of monkeys for long-term brain imaging studies that can reveal ways that host factors can influence sensitivity to cocaine.

12.4 The context

In our studies, we view the 'context' as encompassing all environmental stimuli, experimental history, and social status. For this paper, we will limit the context to a brief description of models used to assess cocaine reinforcement and to non-human primate social behaviour. When describing models of drug self-administration with respect to the schedule of reinforcement, an important distinction should be made between reinforcing 'effects' and reinforcing 'strength'. A reinforcing effect simply means that responding leading to drug presentation occurs at higher rates than responding leading to vehicle presentation. For every drug that has reinforcing effects, the shape of the dose–response curve approximates an inverted U-shape. That is, there is an ascending limb characterized by dose-dependent increases in responding, a dose that results in peak rates of responding and a descending limb in which increases in dose result in lower rates of responding (Zernig 2004). Because several factors influence the shape of the curve, it is impossible to compare dose–response curves from different drugs and make statements related to which drug is 'more reinforcing' (Woolverton & Nader 1990). However, other schedules can be used to make assessments related to reinforcing strength; these will be described in more detail below. The main point to highlight is that different schedules of reinforcement have features that render them suitable for answering different questions about the behavioural effects of cocaine. For example, questions related to the relative importance of drug seeking (i.e. simply self-administering cocaine) vs. total cocaine intake in producing changes in the brain can be assessed by studying different schedules of cocaine self-administration. Such a distinction is of clear relevance when considering treatment options for drug abuse—does it matter how much drug a patient has taken or how long (s)he has been abusing the drug? Volkow et al. (1999) found that levels of DA D2 receptor availability as measured with PET were more dependent on the duration of cocaine use than on the amount of drug used prior to the study. This finding suggested that the behaviours leading to drug procurement, independent of the pharmacology of cocaine, could contribute to the reported changes in DA receptor availability in cocaine abusers and supported the hypothesis that the environment can have profound effects on the brain.

The use of non-human primates, PET imaging, and different schedules of reinforcement provided an opportunity to directly assess the importance of drug seeking vs. total cocaine intake (Czoty et al. 2007a, b). To directly test this hypothesis, 12 experimentally naïve rhesus monkeys received baseline PET scans using the D2 receptor ligand [^{18}F]FCP. Six of these monkeys were then trained to self-administer cocaine under a second-order schedule, a very lean schedule of reinforcement in which drug seeking was maintained by the presentation of conditioned stimuli throughout the 60-min session until cocaine was finally administered (Katz 1980). Under the final schedule parameters, the first response after 3 min (FI 3-min) produced a stimulus change (S) associated with cocaine reinforcement and the tenth-completed FI (i.e. fixed-ratio 10) resulted in cocaine presentation (designated FR 10 [FI 3-min:S]). Sessions ended after 2 cocaine injections (0.1 mg/kg/injection). Thus, these animals had an extensive drug-seeking history, but very low levels of cocaine intake. The second group of six monkeys was trained to respond under an FR 30 schedule of cocaine presentation. Conditions for this group were arranged to model 'binge' access—monkeys could receive up to 30 injections of 0.2 mg/kg cocaine twice per day, two days per week. Thus, relative to the other group of monkeys, this set of subjects received much more cocaine but drug seeking was only two days per week. We found that binge access to cocaine resulted in significant reductions in D2 receptor availability at every time point, while 'drug seeking' under the second-order schedule did not significantly affect D2 receptor availability over 1 year. These findings suggest that the reductions in D2 availability seen in humans were due primarily to the direct effects of cocaine on DA receptor levels.

12.5 Organism × environment interactions—Part 1

Acquisition of drug reinforcement is influenced by characteristics of the individual (i.e. trait variables) as well as features of the environment (e.g. state variables). One of the first studies of the relationship of trait variables to sensitivity to drug reinforcement was provided by Piazza et al. (1989), in which two groups of rats were differentiated based on locomotor activity in an open-field apparatus as high-responders (HR) or low-responders (LR). Rats were implanted with indwelling intravenous catheters, and given access to low doses of D-amphetamine under an FR schedule. HR rats acquired D-amphetamine self-administration at lower doses than LR rats. The use of this simple schedule allowed for characterization of vulnerability based on an inherent behavioural characteristic, namely, locomotor activity in an open field.

   More recently, laboratory animal studies have examined behaviours related to 'impulsivity', a trait shown to be high in cocaine abusers (Moeller et al. 2002). Rats characterized as more impulsive acquired cocaine self-administration more rapidly than less impulsive rats (Dalley et al. 2007). Perry et al. (2005) addressed whether impulsivity precedes drug abuse. In that study, rats were trained on a delay discounting procedure in which responding on one lever under an FR 1 contingency resulted in the immediate delivery of one food pellet, while responding on another lever under an FR 1 contingency resulted in the delivery of three food pellets after a variable delay. If the rat chose the immediate option, the delay value decreased on the next trial for the alternative; if the delay option was chosen, the delay value increased on the next trial. A mean adjusted delay (MAD) value was calculated for each rat by averaging all delay values across trials. As described by Perry et al. (2005), the MAD served as a quantitative measure of the extent to which each rat discounted delayed food reinforcers. Higher MAD values, representing longer delays, were indicative of low impulsivity, while smaller MAD values indicated more impulsive behaviour. The rats were divided into two groups, high and low impulsiveness (HiI and LoI, respectively) based on MAD values. When cocaine acquisition was studied, HiI animals acquired self-administration more rapidly and at higher levels than LoI rats. Taken together, these findings support the hypothesis that there are behavioural traits that predispose individuals to drug abuse and these can be examined using animal models.

Our group has studied trait variables and gene–environment interactions in relation to drug abuse in non-human primates for over a decade. Much of our research has been conducted in cocaine-naïve monkeys prior to being exposed to cocaine in order to address gaps in the clinical data—prospective questions that cannot be answered in humans due to ethical concerns. For example, as described above, cocaine abusers have lower levels of D2 receptor availability than control subjects (Volkow et al. 1990, 1993; Martinez et al. 2004) and non-drug abusers with lower basal levels of D2 receptor availability found methylpheni- date more reinforcing (Volkow et al. 1999). It is not known whether low D2 levels observed in cocaine abusers were the result of cocaine use or a pre-existing feature that conferred vulnerability to the reinforcing effect of cocaine. The question is whether D2 receptor avail- ability is a trait marker for vulnerability to cocaine abuse. We have addressed this question in two ways. First, we correlated basal D2 receptor availability in cocaine-naïve monkeys with subsequent rates of cocaine self-administration. Second, we studied changes in D2 receptor availability in initially cocaine-naïve monkeys over 1 year of cocaine access to determine if cocaine reinforcement decreased levels (Nader et al. 2006). A summary of the findings is shown in Fig. 12.1. Initially, cocaine-naive monkeys were scanned with the D2 receptor ligand [18F]FCP and then trained to respond under an FI 3-min schedule of food presentation. When responding was stable, each monkey was surgically implanted with an indwelling venous catheter, a dose of cocaine (0.2 mg/kg/injection) was substituted for food, and response rates were recorded. An important point is that there was no training under the cocaine self-administration paradigm—the monkeys were simply exposed to the drug and response rates recorded. We found an inverse relationship between baseline D2 receptor availability and rates of cocaine self-administration (Fig. 12.1A). Monkeys with low D2 receptor levels self-administered cocaine at higher rates compared to monkeys with high D2 receptor availability. These findings are very similar to the observations by Volkow et al. (1999) using non-drug abusers and methylphenidate. We also found that, over a 1-year period in which cocaine intake increased steadily, D2 receptor availability decreased irre- spective of what the initial levels of D2 receptor availability were for each monkey (Fig. 12.1B). Thus, it appears that low D2 receptor availability makes an individual more vulner- able to cocaine reinforcement *and* continued exposure to cocaine further decreases those levels (Nader et al. 2002, 2006).

The above findings clearly support the idea that there are biological trait variables, in this case D2 receptor availability, that influence vulnerability to cocaine abuse. We have also examined the impact of environmental variables on D2 receptor availability and whether these effects influenced vulnerability to cocaine reinforcement. Earlier work from our group demonstrated a relationship between D2 receptor availability and social rank in female monkeys, such that subordinate monkeys had lower D2 receptor levels than dominant monkeys (Grant et al. 1998). We next assessed whether D2 receptor availability was a trait variable that predicted social rank. For these studies, we used 20 experimentally naïve and individually housed male cynomolgus monkeys. After baseline PET scans using [18F]FCP were conducted, monkeys were placed in social groups of 4 monkeys per pen and after 3 months were rescanned with [18F]FCP (Morgan et al., 2002). D2 receptor availability was not a trait marker for eventual social rank. After 3 months of social housing, we observed the same effect that was reported by Grant and colleagues (1998) in female monkeys that had been living together for over 3 years—subordinate monkeys had lower D2 receptor availability compared to dominant monkeys. However, it came about in a manner opposite to

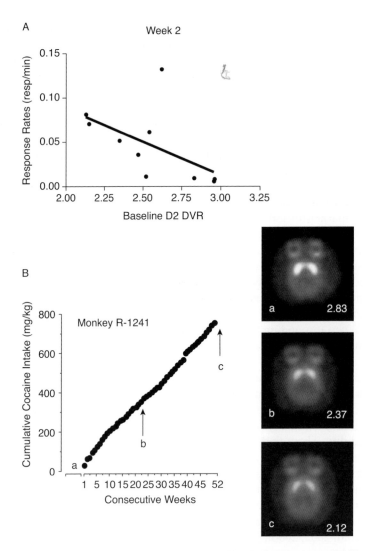

Fig. 12.1 (See also Plate 6) (**A**) Correlation between baseline D2 receptor availability and rates of cocaine self-administration in male rhesus monkeys. (**B**) Representative data from one monkey (R-1241) showing cumulative cocaine intake and associated changes in D2 receptor availability. From Nader et al. (2006).

what we had expected. We had hypothesized that the lower D2 receptor levels in subordinate compared to dominant monkeys arose as the result of chronic social stress that is unequivocally experienced by subordinate monkeys (Kaplan et al. 1982; Shively & Kaplan 1984). However, the over 20% difference between dominant and subordinate monkeys in our study was due to a significant *increase* in D2 receptor availability in dominant monkeys, whereas subordinates, on average, did not change. These increases in D2 measures were in the same direction as reported in rodent studies demonstrating the influence of environmental enrichment on DA function, including increased D2 receptor densities (Bowling et al. 1993; Rilke et al. 1995; Hall et al. 1998). On the basis of these rodent studies and our findings that there was an inverse relationship between D2 receptor availability and cocaine self-administration, we hypothesized that the subordinate monkeys would self-administer more cocaine than the dominant monkeys. Our hypothesis was borne out (Morgan et al. 2002). In fact, cocaine was not a reinforcer in the dominant monkeys when self-administration was assessed under an FR 50 schedule of reinforcement (see Nader & Czoty 2005 for additional discussion).

We also examined other behaviours that we hypothesized could be trait variables predictive of social rank. In our initial study (Morgan et al. 2000), locomotor activity predicted eventual social rank, in that eventual subordinate monkeys had higher locomotor scores compared to eventual dominant monkeys; interestingly, this was not extended to female monkeys (Riddick et al., 2009). Most recently, we have extended our measures to include behaviours deemed to assess impulsivity in an effort to extend more recent work in rodents (Perry et al. 2005; Dalley et al. 2007). In a group of experimentally naïve and individually housed female cynomolgus monkeys, we used a measure of novel object reactivity to assess impulsivity in each animal prior to being socially housed (Riddick et al., 2009). Monkeys that would eventually become subordinate had a significantly shorter average latency to touch the novel object compared to eventual dominant female monkeys. Shorter latency is hypothesized to represent greater impulsivity. In male monkeys who had been housed socially for several years, the latencies of monkeys who had been dominant were significantly longer than those who had been subordinate, further supporting an association between social rank and temperament (Czoty et al., under review). Whether the more impulsive female monkeys are also more vulnerable to self-administer cocaine, as was reported in rodents by Perry et al. (2005) and Dalley et al. (2007), is currently being evaluated.

12.6 Organism × environment interactions—Part 2

In our socially housed male monkeys, we have extended earlier work in an effort to further enhance our homologous model of the human condition. These experiments primarily focus on changing environmental conditions. For example, we found that the protective effect associated with being the dominant monkey can be attenuated by continual exposure to cocaine (Czoty et al. 2004). That is, while there were differences in rates of self-administration when initially exposed to the FR 50 schedule (Morgan et al. 2002), repeated exposure to cocaine over a 1-year period resulted in cocaine becoming a reinforcer in dominant monkeys (see example in Fig. 12.2A). After several months to years of cocaine self-administration, neither response rates nor D2 receptor availability were different in dominant compared to subordinate monkeys (Czoty et al. 2004). As mentioned above, simple schedules do not provide information related to reinforcing strength. Thus, we examined whether there would be differences between social ranks under conditions in which cocaine was available in the context of an alternative, non-drug reinforcer (Czoty et al. 2005). We found that subordinate monkeys were significantly more sensitive to the reinforcing effects of cocaine using this procedure, such that they would choose a lower dose of cocaine over food compared to dominant monkeys (Fig. 12.2B). These findings highlight several important facets of organismal and environmental interactions. These data support the observations that measures of reinforcing strength provide different information related to cocaine self-administration than measures of reinforcing effects. In addition, these findings indicate that after years of living in these stable groups, the influence of the social context was still apparent.

A question that is frequently asked is 'what if circumstances change and a dominant monkey becomes subordinate and a subordinate monkey becomes dominant'? To address this question, we rearranged groups such that one pen consisted of four previously dominant

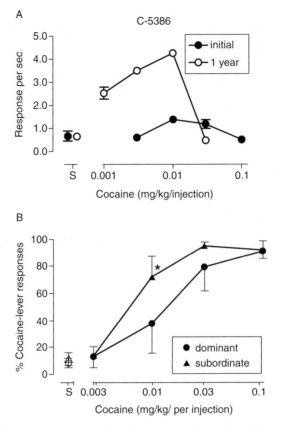

Fig. 12.2(A) Cocaine dose–response curve in a dominant male monkey. Closed symbols were taken shortly after social hierarchies became stable (from Morgan et al. 2002); open symbols are the re-determined cocaine dose–response curve after approximately 1 year of self-administration (from Czoty et al. 2004). **(B)** Cocaine-food choice data from dominant and subordinate monkeys (Czoty et al. 2005). These data were acquired after the data shown in panel A.

(#1-ranked) monkeys and another pen was made up of four previously subordinate (#4-ranked) monkeys. Additional pens were composed of intermediate (#2- and #3-ranked) monkeys and experimentally naïve monkeys (Czoty et al., in preparation). After 3 months of social housing under these new conditions, PET studies were conducted and cocaine self-administration was examined under the concurrent schedule of reinforcement with food as the alternative. The relationship between new social rank and D2 receptor availability was not evident—that is, the newly dominant monkeys did not have significantly higher levels of D2 receptor availability compared to newly subordinate monkeys. (Note, some of the dominant monkeys were previously subordinate and some of the subordinate monkeys were once dominant). In addition, there were no systematic differences in cocaine choice between the monkeys. Additional studies using other measures, including novel object reactivity, noted that previous rank was more predictive of outcome than current rank. There is a long and extensive literature on behavioural and pharmacological history influencing behaviour and drug effects (Barrett et al. 1989), and these studies extend those findings to include a history of social interactions.

Another example of organism × environment interaction involves the use of socially housed monkeys to examine drug-induced changes in social behaviour and the consequence of those effects on subsequent cocaine self-administration. There is an extensive literature on the interaction of social rank with drug effects in non-human primates (Martin et al. 1990; Smith & Byrd 1985; reviewed by Miczek et al. 2004). For example, Miczek and colleagues (Miczek & Gold 1983a; Miczek & Yoshimura 1982) have shown that the effects of alcohol, amphetamine, or cocaine can be influenced by social rank and environmental context. In one study (Winslow & Miczek 1985), low to intermediate doses of alcohol produced increases in aggression by dominant monkeys, but no effect on aggression by subordinate animals. However, co-administration of alcohol and testosterone to subordinate monkeys resulted in increases in aggression. Crowley and colleagues (1974, 1992) examined the effects of a number of abused drugs on the social behaviour of macaques. Methamphetamine produced pronounced increases in locomotion and stereotypies, and declines in food-foraging behaviour and aggression. In a low-ranking monkey, high doses of methamphetamine produced such profound increases in submissive behaviours that the amount of aggression directed from the (untreated) dominant monkeys towards the drug-treated animal increased. Of all the studies examining the effects of drugs on social behaviour, this result is one of the few descriptions of the behaviour of the untreated monkeys. We undertook a study to further investigate this interaction, with the hypothesis that if reinforcing doses of cocaine resulted in increased aggression and changes in social rank, that the frequency of cocaine self-administration in that individual would increase in subsequent experimental sessions.

Monkeys lived in stable social groups of three and social rank was determined in each pen as described above. For these studies, only one monkey in the social group was given access to cocaine (saline, 0.01–0.1 mg/kg/injection) under an FR 50 schedule of reinforcement, while the remaining monkeys in the pen had access to food presentation under an FR 50 schedule; conditions remained in effect for five consecutive sessions. When the session was completed, monkeys were returned to their social groups, and agonistic and submissive behaviours were recorded over a 15 min period. All monkeys (dominant, intermediate, and subordinate) were studied at all cocaine doses. Social interactions did not affect response rates or cocaine intake for any monkey. However, cocaine-induced changes in social behaviour were dependent on the rank of the monkey. Irrespective of which animal in the pen self-administered cocaine, the #1 and #2 ranked monkeys showed increases in aggression; the subordinate monkey never demonstrated any aggression during the course of the study. These data indicate that social rank is the most important determinant of cocaine-induced changes in social behaviour. One possible reason that self-administration was insensitive to the consequences of social behaviour is that cocaine access was not scheduled until nearly 24 h after the social interaction. Current studies are examining the consequences of cocaine-induced changes in social behaviour on cocaine self-administration that are more closely associated in time.

12.7 Conclusions

The goal of this review was to highlight several important factors that mediate drug abuse using animal models. All animal models are, as a minimum, predictive of some clinical outcome. Animal models of drug self-administration are perhaps the most reliable animal model of a human condition available to researchers (see Griffiths et al. 1980). When social behaviour of non-human primates and cocaine self-administration are included, these models are homologous models of human drug abuse. We described studies that investigated behavioural and neuropharmacological variables that have been identified as trait variables to a vulnerable phenotype. We also described situations in which social and environmental conditions produced changes that increased or decreased vulnerability to drug abuse.

When considering models of drug addiction, researchers have focused on factors that can increase or decrease drug self-administration. For example, we have known for some time that stress can increase vulnerability to self-administer cocaine. Perhaps more clinically significant is the understanding that environmental enrichment can attenuate the reinforcing effects of drugs. Not only has it been shown that alternative non-drug reinforcers can decrease vulnerability (Carroll et al. 1989) and maintenance of cocaine self-administration (Nader and Woolverton, 1991, 1992), but experience with these alternative reinforcers, frequently referred to as environmental enrichment, can profoundly decrease cocaine reinforcement. As a final example for this review, we highlight two preliminary studies that have documented these divergent effects on cocaine reinforcement in socially housed monkeys. Acute stressors, such as being an intruder into a pen of other monkeys (see Miczek & Gold 1983b; Miczek & Tidey 1989), can affect the reinforcing strength of cocaine. Although data are preliminary, it appears that the effects of being an intruder in an established social group are different depending on the social rank of the intruder. When a subordinate monkey is an intruder to a well-established pen of four socially housed male monkeys, the subordinate animal's cocaine dose–response curve is likely to shift to the left, while the same intruder manipulation with a dominant monkey can result in rightward shifts in the cocaine dose–response curve. On the other end of the continuum, placing monkeys (irrespective of social rank) into larger enclosures with novel objects for three days prior to studying self-administration resulted in shifts to the right in the cocaine dose–response curve, such that doses that were chosen over food prior to the enrichment condition were no longer reinforcing. These findings suggest that environmental enrichment, even to monkeys that have been exposed to chronic stressors such as subordinate animals, can produce powerful effects on the likelihood of drug self-administration. These findings are consistent with human studies showing that alternative reinforcers and environmental enrichment can increase the duration of abstinence from cocaine (Higgins 1997). The research described in this review has consistently shown that the environment can have profound effects on drug use and that there are neurobiological changes that accompany these effects. We believe the combination of environmental enrichment and pharmacotherapy will be most effective in treating cocaine addiction.

Acknowledgements

We thank D. Morgan, K.A. Grant, L.J. Porrino, R.H. Mach, J.R. Kaplan, and H.D. Gage for their long-standing collaborations and contributions to this research and Susan Nader, Tonya Calhoun, Mikki Sandridge, Michelle Icenhower, and Nicholas Garrett for excellent technical assistance throughout these research projects. Research from our laboratory and preparation of this manuscript was supported in part by NIDA grants DA 10584, DA 17763, DA 14637, DA 25120, DA 21658, and DA 06634.

References

Appt, S.E. 2004. Usefulness of the monkey model to investigate the role soy in postmenopausal women's health. *ILAR J.* **45**, 200–11.

Banks, M.L., Sprague, J.E., Kisor, D.F., Czoty, P.W., Nichols, D.E. & Nader, M.A. 2007. Ambient temperature effects on 3,4-methylenedioxymethamphetamine (MDMA)-induced thermodysregulation and pharmacokinetics in male monkeys. *Drug Disposition Metab.* **35**, 1840–5.

Barrett, J.E., Glowa, J.R. & Nader, M.A. 1989. Behavioral and pharmacological history as determinants of tolerance and sensitization-like phenomena in drug action. In *Psychoactive Drugs*, Goudie, A.J. & Emmett-Oglesby, M.W. (eds), pp. 181–219, Clifton, NJ: Humana Press.

Berger, B., Gaspar, P. & Verney, C. 1991. Dopaminergic innervation of the cerebral cortex: unexpected differences between rodents and primates. *Trends Neurosci.* **14**, 21–7.

Bowling, S.L., Rowlett, J.K. & Bardo, M.T. 1993. The effect of environmental enrichment on amphetamine-stimulated locomotor activity, dopamine synthesis and dopamine release. *Neuropsychopharmacology* **32**, 885–93.

Bradberry, C.W. 2000. Acute and chronic dopamine dynamics in a nonhuman primate model of recreational cocaine use. *J. Neurosci.* **20**, 7109–15.

Briand, L.A., Flagel, S.B., Seeman, P. & Robinson, T.E. 2008. Cocaine self-administration produces a persistent increase in dopamine D2^{High} receptors. *Eur. Neuropsychopharmacol.* **18**, 551–6.

Carroll, M.E., Lac, S.T. & Nygaard, S.L. 1989. A concurrently available nondrug reinforcer prevents the acquisition or decreases the maintenance of cocaine-reinforced behavior. *Psychopharmacology* **97**, 23–9.

Chalon, S., Edmond, P., Bodard, S. et al. 1999. Time course of changes in striatal dopamine transporters and D2 receptors with specific iodinated markers in a rat model of Parkinson's disease. *Synapse* **31**, 134–9.

Crowley, T.J., Mikulich, S.K., Williams, E.A., Zerbe, G.O. & Ingersoll, N.C. 1992. Cocaine, social behavior, and alcohol-solution drinking in monkeys. *Drug Alcohol Dep.* **29**, 205–23.

Crowley, T.J., Stynes, A.J., Hydinger, M. & Kaufman, I.C. 1974. Ethanol, methamphetamine, pentobarbital, morphine, and monkey social behavior. *Arch. Gen. Psychiatry* **31**, 829–38.

Czoty, P.W., Gage, H.D., Nader, S.H., et al. 2007a. Acquisition of cocaine self-administration does not alter dopamine D2 receptor or transporter availability in rhesus monkeys. *J. Addiction Med.* **1**, 33–9.

Czoty, P.W., Ginsburg, B.C. & Howell, L.L. 2002. Serotonergic attenuation of the reinforcing and neurochemical effects of cocaine in squirrel monkeys. *J. Pharmacol. Exp. Ther.* **300**, 831–7.

Czoty, P.W., McCabe, C. & Nader, M.A. 2005. Assessment of the reinforcing strength of cocaine in socially housed monkeys using a choice procedure. *J. Pharmacol. Exp. Ther.* **312**, 96–102.

Czoty, P.W., Morgan, D., Shannon, E.E., Gage, H.D. & Nader, M.A. 2004. Characterization of dopamine D1 and D2 receptor function in socially housed cynomolgus monkeys self-administering cocaine. *Psychopharmacology* **174**, 381–8.

Czoty, P.W., Reboussin, B.A., Calhoun, T.L., Nader, S.H. & Nader, M.A. 2007b. Long-term cocaine self-administration under fixed-ratio and second-order schedules in monkeys. *Psychopharmacology* **131**, 287–95.

Czoty, P.W., Riddick, N.V., Gage, H.D. et al. 2009. Effect of menstrual cycle phase on dopamine D2 receptor availability in female cynomolgus monkeys. *Neuropsychopharmacology*. **34**, 548–54.

Dalley, J.W., Fryer, T.D., Brichard, L. et al. 2007. Nucleus accumbens D2/3 receptors predict trait impulsivity and cocaine reinforcement. *Science* **315**, 1267–70.

Di Chiara, G. & Imperato, A. 1988. Drugs abused by humans preferentially increase synaptic dopamine concentrations in the mesolimbic system of freely moving rats. *Proc. Natl. Acad. Sci.* **85**, 5274–8.

Dworkin, S.I., Mirkis, S. & Smith, J.E. 1995. Response-dependent versus response-independent presentation of cocaine: differences in the lethal effects of the drug. *Psychopharmacology* **117**, 262–6.

Elkashef, A., Biswas, J., Acri, J.B. & Vocci, F. 2007. Biotechnology and the treatment of addictive disorders. *BioDrugs* **21**, 259–67.

Graff-Guerrero, A., Willeit, M., Ginovart, N. et al. 2008. Brain region binding of the new D$_{2/3}$ agonist [^{11}C]-(+)-PHNO and the D$_{2/3}$ antagonist [^{11}C]raclopride in healthy humans. *Hum. Brain Mapp.* **29**, 400–10.

Grant, K.A., Shively, C.A., Nader, M.A. et al. 1998. Effect of social status on striatal dopamine D2 receptor binding characteristics in cynomolgus monkeys assessed with positron emission tomography. *Synapse* **29**, 80–3.

Griffiths, R.R., Bigelow, G.E. & Henningfield, J.E. 1980. Similarities in animal and human drug-taking behavior. In *Advances in Substance Abuse*, Vol. 1, Mello, N.K. (ed), pp. 1–90, Greenwich, CN: JAI Press.

Haber, S.N. & McFarland, N.R. 1999. The concept of the ventral striatum in nonhuman primates. *Ann. N.Y. Acad. Sci.* **877**, 33–48.

Hall, F.S., Wilkinson, L.S., Humby, T. et al. 1998. Isolation rearing in rats: pre- and postsynaptic changes in striatal dopaminergic systems. *Pharmacol. Biochem. Behav.* **58**, 859–72.

Higgins, S.T. 1997. The influence of alternative reinforcers on cocaine use and abuse: a brief review. *Pharmacol. Biochem. Behav.* **57**, 419–27.

Howell, L.L. & Wilcox, K.M. 2002. Functional imaging and neurochemical correlates of stimulant self-administration in primates. *Psychopharmacology* **163**, 352–61.

Jewitt, D.A. & Dukelow, W.R. 1972. Cyclicity and gestation length of Macaca fascicularis. *Primates* **13**, 327–30.

Joel, D. & Weiner, I. 2000. The connections of dopaminergic system with the striatum in rats and primates: an analysis with respect to the functional and compartmental organization of the striatum. *Neuroscience* **96**, 451–74.

Johanson, C.E. & Schuster, C.R. 1975. A choice procedure for drug reinforcers: cocaine and methylphenidate in the rhesus monkey. *J. Pharmacol. Exp. Ther.* **193**, 676–88.

Kaplan, J.R., Manuck, S.B., Clarkson, T.B., Lusso, F.M. & Taub, D.M. 1982. Social status, environment, and atherosclerosis in cynomolgus monkeys. *Arterosclerosis* **2**, 359–68.

Katz, J.L. 1980. Second-order schedules of intramuscular cocaine injection in the squirrel monkey: comparisons with food presentation and effects of D-amphetamine and promazine. *J. Pharmacol. Exp. Ther.* **212**, 405–11.

Lile, J.A., Wang, Z., Woolverton, W.L. et al. 2003. The reinforcing efficacy of psychostimulants in rhesus monkeys: the role of pharmacokinetics and pharmacodynamics. *J. Pharmacol. Exp. Ther.* **307**, 356–66.

Lynch, W.J. 2006. Sex differences in vulnerability to drug self-administration. *Exp. Clin. Psychopharmacol.* **14**, 34–41.

Lynch, W.J., Roth, M.E. & Carroll, M.E. 2002. Biological basis of sex differences in drug abuse: preclinical and clinical studies. *Psychopharmacology* **164**, 121–37.

Lyons, D., Friedman, D.P., Nader, M.A. & Porrino, L.J. 1996. Cocaine alters cerebral metabolism within the ventral striatum and limbic cortex of monkeys. *J. Neurosci.* **16**, 1230–8.

Mach, R.H., Luedtke, R.R., Unsworth, C.D. et al. 1993. ^{18}F-Labeled radioligands for studying the dopamine D_2 receptor with positron emission tomography. *J. Med. Chem.* **36**, 3707–20.

Martin, S.P., Smith, E.O. & Byrd, L.D. 1990. Effects of dominance rank on *d*-amphetamine-induced increases in aggression. *Pharmacol. Biochem. Behav.* **37**, 493–6.

Martinez, D., Broft, A., Foltin, R.W. et al. 2004. Cocaine dependence and D2 receptor availability in the functional subdivisions of the striatum: relationship with cocaine-seeking behavior. *Neuropsychopharmacology* **29**, 1190–202.

Mello, N.K., Knudson, I.M. & Mendelson, J.H. 2007. Sex and menstrual cycle effects on progressive ratio measures of cocaine self-administration in rhesus monkeys. *Neuropsychopharmacology* **32**, 1956–66.

Miczek, K.A., Covington, H.E., Nikulina, E. & Hammer, R.P. 2004. Aggression and defeat: persistant effects on cocaine self-administration and gene expression in peptidergic and aminergic mesocorticolimbic circuits. *Neurosci. Biobehav. Rev.* **27**, 787–802.

Miczek, K.A. & Gold, L.H. 1983a. D-Amphetamine in squirrel monkeys of different social status: Effects on social and agonistic behavior, locomotion, and stereotypies. *Psychopharmacology* **81**, 183–190.

Miczek, K.A. & Gold, L.H. 1983b. Ethological analysis of amphetamine action on social behavior in squirrel monkeys (Saimiri sciureus). In *Ethopharmacology: Primate Models of Neuropsychiatric Disorders*, Miczek, K.A. (ed.), pp. 137–55, New York, NY: Alan R. Liss.

Miczek, K.A. & Tidey, J.W. 1989. Amphetamines: aggressive and social behavior. In *Pharmacology and Toxicology of Amphetamine and Related Designer Drugs, NIDA Research Monograph No. 94*, Asghar, K. & De Souza, E. (eds), pp. 68–100, Washington, DC: U.S. Government Printing Office.

Miczek, K.A. & Yoshimura, H. 1982. Disruption of primate social behavior by D-amphetamine and cocaine: differential antagonism by antipsychotics. *Psychopharmacology* **76**, 163–71.

Mills, J. 1965. Needle park. Life Magazine, March 5.

Moeller, F.G., Dougherty, D.M., Barratt, E.S. et al. 2002. Increased impulsivity in cocaine dependent subjects independent of antisocial personality disorder and aggression. *Drug Alc. Dep.* **68**, 105–11.

Morgan, D., Grant, K.A., Gage, H.D. et al. 2002. Social dominance in monkeys: dopamine D$_2$ receptors and cocaine self-administration. *Nature Neurosci.* **5**, 169–74.

Morgan, D., Grant, K.A., Prioleau, O.A., Nader, S.H., Kaplan, J.R. & Nader, M.A. 2000. Predictors of social status in cynomolgus monkeys (*macaca fascicularis*) after group formation. *Am. J. Primatol.* **52**, 115–31.

Munro, C.A., McCaul, M.E., Wong, D.F. et al. 2006. Sex differences in striatal dopamine release in healthy adults. *Biol Psychiatry* **59**, 966–74.

Nader, M.A. & Czoty, P.W. 2005. PET imaging of dopamine D2 receptors in monkeys: genetic predisposition vs. environmental modulation. *Am. J. Psychiatry* **162**, 1473–82.

Nader, M.A. & Czoty, P.W. 2008. Brain imaging in nonhuman primates: insights into drug addiction. *ILAR* **49**, 89–102.

Nader, M.A., Daunais, J.B., Moore, T. et al. 2002. Effects of cocaine self-administration on striatal dopamine systems in rhesus monkeys: initial and chronic exposure. *Neuropsychopharmacology* **27**, 35–46.

Nader, M.A., Morgan, D., Gage, H.D. et al. 2006. PET imaging of dopamine D2 receptors during chronic cocaine self-administration in monkeys. *Nature Neurosci.* **9**, 1050–6.

Nader, M.A. & Woolverton, W.L. 1991. Effects of increasing the magnitude of an alternative reinforcer on drug choice in a discrete-trials choice procedure. *Psychopharmacology* **105**, 169–174.

Nader, M.A. & Woolverton, W.L. 1992. Effects of increasing response requirement on choice between cocaine and food in rhesus monkeys. *Psychopharmacology* **108**, 295–300.

Nordstrom, A.L., Olsson, H. & Halldin, C. 1998. A PET study of D2 dopamine receptor density at different phases of the menstrual cycle. *Psychiatry Res.* **83**, 1–6.

O'Brien, C.P. 2005. Anticraving medications for relapse prevention: a possible new class of psychoactive medications. *Am. J. Psychiatry* **162**, 1423–31.

O'Brien, C.P. 2006. Drug addiction and drug abuse. In *Goodman and Gilman's The Pharmacological Basis of Therapeutics*, Brunton, L., Lazo, J.S. & Parker, K.L. (eds), Chapter 23, pp. 607–27, New York, NY: McGraw-Hill.

Perry, J.L., Larson, E.B., German, J.P., Madden, G.J. & Carroll, M.E. 2005. Impulsivity (delay discounting) as a predictor of acquisition of IV cocaine self-administration in female rats. *Psychopharmacology* **178**, 193–201.

Piazza, P.V., Deminiere, J.M., Le Moal, M. & Simon, H. 1989. Factors that predict individual vulnerability to amphetamine self-administration. *Science* **245**, 1511–13.

Riddick, N.R., Czoty, P.W., Gage, H.D. et al. 2009. Behavioral and neurobiological characteristics influencing social hierarchy formation in female cynomolgus monkeys. *Neuroscience* **158**, 1257–65.

Rilke, O., May, T., Oehler, J. & Wolffgramm, J. 1995. Influences of housing conditions and ethanol intake on binding characteristics of D$_2$, 5-HT$_{1A}$, and benzodiazepine receptors of rats. *Pharmacol. Biochem. Behav.* **52**, 23–8.

Ritz, M.C., Lamb, R.J., Goldberg, S.R. & Kuhar, M.J. 1987. Cocaine receptors on dopamine transporters are related to self-administration of cocaine. *Science* **237**, 1219–23.

Roberts, D.C.S., Phelan, R., Hodges, L.M. et al. 1999. Self-administration of cocaine analogs by rats. *Psychopharmacology* **144**, 389–97.

SAMHSA: Substance Abuse and Mental Health Services Administration. 2006. *Results from the 2005 National Survey on Drug Use and Health: National Findings* (Office of Applied Studies, NSDUH Series H-30, DHHS Publication No. SMA 06-4194). Rockville, MD.

Sandberg, J.A. & Olsen, G.D. 1991. Cocaine pharmacokinetics in the pregnant guinea pig. *J. Pharmacol. Exp. Ther.* **258**, 447–82.

Seeman, M.V. 1996. Schizophrenia, gender, and affect. *Can. J. Psychiatry* **41**, 263–4.

Seeman, P., Tallerico, T. & Ko, F. 2003. Dopamine displaces [3H]domperidone from high-affinity sites of the dopamine D2 receptor but not [3H]raclopride or [3H]spiperone in isotonic medium: implications for human positron emission tomography. *Synapse* **49**, 209–15.

Seeman, P., Tallerico, T., Ko, F., Tenn, C. & Kapur, S. 2002. Amphetamine-sensitized animals show a marked increase in dopamine D2 high receptors occupied by endogenous dopamine, even in the absence of acute challenges. *Synapse* **46**, 235–9.

Shively, C. & Kaplan, J.R. 1984. Effects of social factors on adrenal weight and related physiology in *Macaca fascicularis*. *Physiol. Behav.* **33**, 777–82.

Sibley, D.R., Monsma, F.J. Jr. & Shen, Y. 1993. Molecular neurobiology of dopaminergic receptors. *Int. Rev. Neurobiol.* **35**, 391–415.

Smith, E.O. & Byrd, L.D. 1985. D-Amphetamine induced changes in social interaction patterns. *Pharmacol. Biochem. Behav.* **22**, 135–9.

Sofuoglu, M., Dudish-Poulsen, S., Nelson, D., Pentel, P.R. & Hatsukami, D.K. 1999. Sex and menstrual cycle differences in the subjective effects from smoked cocaine in humans. *Exp. Clin. Psychopharmacol.* **7**, 274–83.

Stefanski, R., Ladenheim, B., Lee, S.H., Cadet, J.L. & Goldberg, S.R. 1999. Neuroadaptations in the dopaminergic system after active self-administration but not after passive administration of methamphetamine. *Eur. J. Pharmacol.* **371**, 123–35.

Terner, J.M. & de Wit, H. 2006. Menstrual cucle phase and responses to drugs of abuse in humans. *Drug Alcohol Depend.* **84**, 1–13.

Volkow, N.D., Fowler, J.S., Wang, G.J. et al. 1993. Decreased dopamine D2 receptor availability is associated with reduced frontal metabolism in cocaine abusers. *Synapse* **14**, 169–77.

Volkow, N.D., Fowler, J.S., Wolf, A.P. et al. 1990. Effects of chronic cocaine abuse on postsynaptic dopamine receptors. *Am. J. Psychiatry* **147**, 719–24.

Volkow, N.D., Wang, G.-J., Fowler, J.S. et al. 1999. Blockade of striatal dopamine transporters by intravenous methylphenidate is not sufficient to induce self-reports of 'high.' *J. Pharmacol. Exp. Ther.* **288**, 14–20.

Wagner, F.A. & Anthony, J.C. 2007. Male-female differences in the risk of progression from first use to dependence upon cannabis, cocaine and alcohol. *Drug Alcohol Depend.* **86**, 191–8.

Weed, M.R., Woolverton, W.L. & Paul, I. A. 1998. Dopamine D1 and D2 receptor sensitivities of phenyl-benzazepines in rhesus monkey striata. *Eur. J. Pharmacol.* **361**, 129–42.

Weerts, E.M., Fantegrossi, W.E. & Goodwin, A.K. 2007. The value of nonhuman primates in drug abuse research. *Exp. Clin. Psychopharmacol.* **15**, 309–27.

WHO. 2004. '*Neuroscience of Psychoactive Substance Use and Dependence*'. World Health Organization, Geneva, Switzerland.

Wieck, A., Davies, R.A., Hirst, A.D. et al. 2003. Menstrual cycle effects on hypothalamic dopamine receptor function in women with a history of puerperal bipolar disorder. *J. Psychopharmacol.* **17**, 204–9.

Willeit, M., Ginovart, N., Graff, A. et al. 2008. First human evidence of D-amphetamine induced displacement of a $D_{2/3}$ agonist radioligand: A [^{11}C]-(+)-PHNO positron emission tomography study. *Neuropsychopharmacology* **33**, 279–89.

Winslow, J.T. & Miczek, K.A. 1985. Social status as determinant of alcohol effects on aggressive behavior in squirrel monkeys (Saimiri sciureus). *Psychopharmacology* **85**, 167–72.

Wong, D.F., Broussolle, E.P., Wand, G. et al. 1988. In vivo measurement of dopamine receptors in human brain by positron emission tomography. Age and sex differences. *Ann. N.Y. Acad. Sci.* **515**, 203–14.

Woolverton, W.L. & Johnson, K.M. 1992. Neurobiology of Cocaine Abuse. *Trends Pharmacol. Sci.* **13**, 193–200.

Woolverton, W.L. & Nader, M.A. 1990. Experimental evaluation of the reinforcing effects of drugs. In *Testing and Evaluation of Drugs of Abuse*, Adler, M.W. & Cowan, A. (eds.), pp. 165–92, New York: Wiley-Liss.

Zernig, G., Wakonigg, G., Madlung, E., Haring, C. & Saria, A. 2004. Do vertical shifts in dose-response rate-relationships in operant conditioning procedures indicate 'sensitization' to 'drug wanting'? *Psychopharmacology* **171**, 352–63.

13

Context-induced relapse to drug seeking: A review

Hans S. Crombag, Jennifer M. Bossert, Eisuke Koya, and Yavin Shaham*

In humans, exposure to environmental contexts previously associated with drug intake often provokes relapse to drug use, but the mechanisms mediating this relapse are unknown. Based on early studies by Bouton & Bolles on context-induced 'renewal' of learned behaviours, we developed a procedure to study context-induced relapse to drug seeking. In this procedure, rats are first trained to self-administer drug in one context. Next, drug-reinforced lever responding is extinguished in a different (non-drug) context. Subsequently, context-induced reinstatement of drug seeking is assessed by re-exposing rats to the drug-associated context. Using variations of this procedure, we and others reported reliable context-induced reinstatement in rats with a history of heroin, cocaine, heroin–cocaine combination, alcohol and nicotine self-administration. Here, we first discuss potential psychological mechanisms of context-induced reinstatement, including excitatory and inhibitory Pavlovian conditioning, and occasion setting. We then summarize results from pharmacological and neuroanatomical studies on the role of several neurotransmitter systems (dopamine, glutamate, serotónin, and opioids) and brain areas (ventral tegmental area, accumbens shell, dorsal striatum, basolateral amygdala, prefrontal cortex, dorsal hippocampus, and lateral hypothalamus) in context-induced reinstatement. We conclude by discussing the clinical implications of rat studies on context-induced reinstatement of drug seeking.

Key Words: Conditioned cues; drug self-administration; extinction; reinstatement; renewal; relapse.

13.1 Introduction

The seminal studies of Wikler (1973) and subsequent investigations (O'Brien et al. 1992) indicate that environmental contexts previously associated with drug intake can provoke *relapse* to drug use in humans. Despite this evidence, the role of contextual cues in preclinical models of relapse to drug use has until recently been largely ignored (Shalev et al. 2002). This issue is important for understanding drug relapse, because contexts strongly influence extinction and resumption of learned behaviours (Bouton 2002).

We adapted an ABA renewal procedure (Bouton & Bolles 1979) to study the role of the drug environmental context in *reinstatement* of drug seeking (Crombag & Shaham 2002). In this procedure, rats are first trained to self-administer drugs in one context (A); each drug infusion is paired with an explicit *discrete drug cue* (a light cue or a compound tone-light cue). Next, drug-reinforced lever responding in the presence of the discrete drug cue is extinguished in a different (non-drug) context (B), which is distinct from the drug-associated context in its tactile, visual, auditory, and olfactory or circadian (time of day) features.

Subsequently, context-induced reinstatement of drug seeking is assessed by re-exposing rats to the drug-associated (A) context. During the reinstatement tests under *extinction* conditions, responding on the previously *active lever* leads to contingent presentations of the discrete drug cue but not the drug. Using variations of this procedure, we and others found context-induced reinstatement of heroin (Bossert et al. 2004, 2006, 2007), cocaine (Crombag et al. 2002a; Fuchs et al. 2005–2007; Kearns & Weiss 2007; Fletcher et al. 2008;

* yshaham@intra.nida.nih.gov

Hamlin et al. 2008), speedball (Crombag & Shaham 2002), alcohol (Burattini et al. 2006; Zironi et al. 2006; Hamlin et al. 2007; Marinelli et al. 2007; Chaudhri et al. 2008), and nicotine (Diergaarde et al. 2008) seeking (Fig. 13.1). In these studies, the magnitude of lever (or nose-poke) responding during tests for context-induced reinstatement after extinction was similar to that observed on the first extinction session. Thus, an attractive feature of our 'adapted' renewal procedure is its reliability across different training conditions, context manipulations, test conditions, and drug classes, making it suitable for studying context-induced reinstatement of drug seeking.

Here we summarize recent results (2002–2008) by us and others on psychological, pharmacological, and neuroanatomical mechanisms of context-induced reinstatement of drug seeking in rats. We also briefly discuss clinical implications. Table 13.1 provides a glossary of terms, which appear in italics in the text.

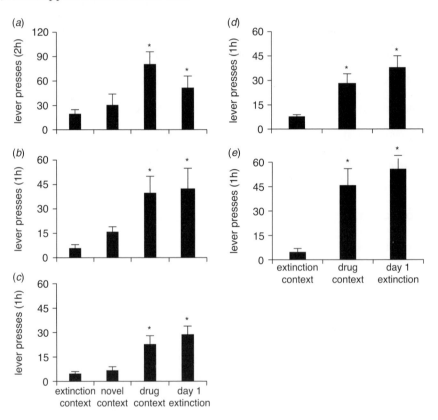

Fig. 13.1 Context-induced reinstatement of drug seeking. Data are mean G s.e.m. number of non-reinforced lever or nose-poke responses on the previously active manipulandum (previously paired with drug delivery) during tests for context-induced reinstatement of drug seeking; non-reinforced responses on the previously active manipulandum serve as the operational measure of drug seeking during testing. The rats were previously trained to self-administer (*a*) speedball (a heroin–cocaine combination), (*b*) heroin, (*c*) nicotine, (*d*) cocaine, or (*e*) alcohol. The rats were trained in one context (drug context). Next, lever or nose-poke responding in the presence of a discrete cue was extinguished in a second non-drug context (extinction context). The rats were then tested either in the drug context or in the extinction context. For comparison purposes, the mean±s.e.m. number of non-reinforced responding during the first extinction session is also depicted. Data were adapted from Crombag & Shaham (2002), Bossertetal. (2004), Marinellietal. (2007), Diergaarde et al. (2008), and Hamlin et al. (2008) for (*a-e*), respectively. *Different from the extinction context, $p<0.05$.

Table 13.1 Glossary of terminology.

Active lever. Responses on this lever lead to drug infusions during drug self-administration training. During
 extinction training and tests for reinstatement, responses on this lever are not reinforced by the drug. In
 studies using the reinstatement procedure, non-reinforced responding on the active lever during testing serves
 as the operational measure of reinstatement of drug-taking behaviour (often refers to as reinstatement of drug
 seeking; Shaham et al. 2003).

Conditioned reinforcer. A previously neutral stimulus (tone and light), which has acquired reinforcing effects
 through its prior association with a primary or unconditioned reinforcer (food, drug; Mackintosh 1974).

Context. Refers to a configuration of diffuse cues providing the background setting of learning. Investigations
 on context effects in learning indicate that many stimuli can function as contexts, including external cues such
 as smells and physical environments, interceptive drug states, mood, or hormonal states and time of day
 (Bouton 1993).

Discrete drug cue. A neutral stimulus (e.g. light, tone, sound of infusion pump) that during self-administration
 training becomes a conditioned reinforcer following repeated temporal pairing with drug infusions and effects
 (Goldberg 1976). In studies on discrete-cue-induced reinstatement, rats are trained to self-administer a drug;
 each reward delivery is temporally paired with a discrete cue (e.g. tone and light). Lever pressing is then
 extinguished in the absence of the discrete cue. During reinstatement testing, exposure to the discrete cue,
 which is earned contingently by responding on the drug-associated lever, reinstates drug seeking (See 2002).

Discriminative drug cue. An environmental stimulus that after discrimination training signals whether
 instrumental performance is reinforced. During training this stimulus, termed the S + (or S^D), is presented just
 before the drug becomes available or throughout the period of self-administration; a different stimulus, termed
 the S$^-$ (or S$^\Delta$), is presented when the drug is not available on alternate days or sessions. Investigators have used
 discrimination procedures to study the role of discriminative drug cues on reinstatement of drug seeking
 (McFarland & Ettenberg 1997; Ciccocioppo et al. 2001).

Extinction. The decrease in the frequency or intensity of learned responses after the removal of the unconditioned
 stimulus (e.g. food, drug) that has reinforced the learning (Catania 1992).

Excitatory conditioning. A form of Pavlovian conditioning during which pairing of a neutral stimulus (a conditioned
 stimulus, CS) with reinforcement results in the CS eliciting a conditioned response that often resembles the
 unconditioned response (Pavlov 1927).

Inhibitory conditioning. A Pavlovian CS becomes inhibitory when the probability that the unconditioned stimulus
 (US) will occur in the presence of the CS is lesser than the probability that the US will occur in the absence of
 the CS (Rescorla 1969).

Occasion setter. In Pavlovian conditioning, occasion setter cues signal whether another conditioned cue (CS) is
 to be reinforced or not reinforced. In contrast to traditional excitatory of inhibitory Pavlovian CSs, occasion
 setter cues typically do not affect behaviour directly but modulate behaviour elicited by other Pavlovian CSs
 (Holland 1992).

Pavlovian-instrumental transfer (PIT). Refers to the ability of a Pavlovian conditioned stimulus (CS) to influence
 instrumental (operant) responding (e.g. lever pressing) for reinforcement. In the PIT procedure, a rat learns to
 lever press for a reinforcer; the rat also learns in different sessions a Pavlovian association between the CS and
 the reinforcer. Subsequently, lever pressing is assessed in extinction tests in the presence or absence of the
 Pavlovian CS; the CS is presented non-contingently during esting. Altered responding in the presence of the
 CS is referred to as Pavlovian-instrumental transfer and is thought to reflect he general motivating effect of
 the Pavlovian cue (Lovibond 1983).

Reinstatement. In the learning literature, reinstatement refers to the recovery of a learned response (e.g. lever-
 pressing behaviour) that occurs when a subject is exposed non-contingently to the unconditioned stimulus
 (e.g. food) after extinction. In studies of reinstatement of drug seeking, reinstatement typically refers to the
 resumption of drug seeking after extinction following exposure to drugs (de Wit & Stewart 1981; Self et al.
 1996; Spealman et al. 1999), different types of drug cues (Meil & See 1996; Weiss et al. 2000; Crombag &
 Shaham 2002), or different stressors (Shaham & Stewart 1995; Shalev et al. 2001; Shepard et al. 2004).

Relapse. A term used to describe the resumption of drug-taking behaviour during periods of self-imposed or
 forced abstinence in humans.

Renewal. Refers to the recovery of extinguished conditioned behaviour, which can occur when the context is
 changed after extinction; renewal often occurs when the subject returns to the learning (training) environment
 after extinction of the conditioned response in a different environment (Bouton & Swartzentruber 1991).

13.2 Psychological mechanisms of context-induced reinstatement

In discussing psychological mechanisms of context-induced reinstatement, it is important to highlight a procedural difference in the published studies which has implications for the underlying mechanisms. Based on Bouton & Bolles' (1979) work, our original intention was to test the ability of the drug-associated context to renew the rat's conditioned response to discrete injection-paired cues after extinction (Crombag & Shaham 2002). Thus, drug infusions during self-administration training were explicitly paired with a discrete light cue, and during extinction training and reinstatement tests, this cue is presented contingent on lever responding. By contrast, in Fuchs et al. studies, explicit drug-paired cues were not presented during acquisition, extinction, and reinstatement tests (Fuchs et al. 2005). This procedural difference is important, because the presence or absence of discrete drug-paired cues during training, extinction, and reinstatement can determine whether contexts directly induce drug seeking by acquiring Pavlovian conditioned stimulus (CS) properties, or indirectly by modulating the effects of discrete infusion cues on drug seeking by serving as *occasion setters* (Rescorla et al. 1985; Holland 1992). Although these two mechanisms are not mutually exclusive (contexts may serve as both traditional Pavlovian CSs and occasion setters), they probably involve different neurobiological substrates (Holland & Bouton 1999).

13.2.1 Excitatory Pavlovian conditioning

One account of context-induced reinstatement is that contexts cause reinstatement by functioning as traditional excitatory Pavlovian CSs. According to this view, because contexts reliably signal drug availability during training, they acquire excitatory conditioned stimulus (CS+) properties, and as extinction occurs in a different context, drug-associated contexts retain their motivational properties and reinstate drug seeking. In agreement with this notion, Fuchs et al. (2005) reported that contexts reinstate cocaine seeking in the absence of any explicit discrete cocaine-paired cues.

An excitatory Pavlovian conditioning mechanism potentially involved in context-induced reinstatement is *Pavlovian-to-instrumental transfer* (PIT). PIT is inferred from the observations that discrete Pavlovian CSs, previously paired with reward in a non-operant setting, increase non-reinforced instrumental responding for the same reward (Mackintosh 1974; Lovibond 1983). Results from PIT studies are often interpreted to suggest that appetitive Pavlovian CSs become endowed with incentive motivational properties that directly potentiate instrumental goal-directed behaviours (Berridge 2004). There is evidence that psychostimulants enhance PIT in rats trained to lever press for sucrose (Wyvell & Berridge 2000). However, the degree to which PIT contributes to drug relapse remains unknown, because non-contingent presentations of drug-paired discrete cues fail to reinstate cocaine seeking (Grimm et al. 2000; Kruzich et al. 2001). These studies, however, were not designed to assess PIT and, even in non-drug settings, PIT is often difficult to reproduce because this phenomenon is critically dependent on subtle experimental parameters (Lovibond 1981; Crombag et al. 2008). Thus, the degree to which PIT contributes to context-induced reinstatement is a subject for future research.

13.2.2 Inhibitory Pavlovian conditioning

Context-induced reinstatement may also occur because contextual stimuli acquire conditioned inhibitory properties (Rescorla et al. 1985). As context (B) is explicitly paired with non-reinforcement during extinction in the ABA renewal condition, contextual cues may acquire inhibitory CS properties, which actively inhibit drug seeking. On test day, rats are removed from the inhibitory control of context B, resulting in reinstatement of drug seeking in the drug (A) context. Consistent with this view, exposure to a third (novel) context in an ABC condition often reinstates instrumental performance (Gunther et al. 1998). These findings may suggest that the critical manipulation to renew drug seeking is removal from the inhibitory influence of the extinction context, rather than re-exposure to the excitatory influence of the drug context. However, renewal of conditioned responses in the ABC condition is often much weaker than that observed in the ABA condition (Bouton 2002), and ABC renewal has yet to be demonstrated in a drug setting. Thus, in our view it seems unlikely that inhibitory Pavlovian conditioning processes alone can fully account for context-induced reinstatement of drug seeking.

13.2.3 Contexts as occasion setters

Contexts may reinstate drug seeking indirectly by functioning as occasion setters (Holland 1992). According to this view, contexts function as retrieval cues in cases where the meaning of the discrete drug-infusion cues (the CSs) is ambiguous, because these cues have been paired with drug taking in one context and no drug (extinction) in a different context (CS → drug AND CS → no drug). Because the occurrence of drug versus no drug is reliably signalled by contextual cues, responding to the discrete cues is determined by whether the background context retrieves the conditioning (training) or the extinction experience (Bouton 2002).

The notion that contexts serve as retrieval cues to 'disambiguate' the meaning and impact of other discrete cues is in line with the phenomenon of occasion setting that was extensively studied by Holland and colleagues while exploring the nature of feature-positive and feature-negative discrimination learning (for review, see Holland 1992). In feature-positive discrimination procedures, one cue (a target CS) is sometimes followed by a reinforcing unconditioned stimulus (UCS) and sometimes not, depending on the presence or absence of another cue called feature cue. Thus, if feature cue A is present, the target CS is reinforced, but if feature cue A is absent, the target CS is not reinforced. In feature-negative discriminations, these contingencies are reversed such that the target CS is reinforced in the absence of feature cue A, while the presence of the feature cue signals non-reinforcement.

Holland and colleagues (1992) reported that feature-positive and feature-negative discrimination procedures often result in the feature cue acquiring occasion setter properties, leading to powerful modulating effects on behaviours induced by the target CS, in the absence of detectable direct conditioned excitatory or inhibitory effects by the feature cue itself. Based on these studies, they concluded that stimuli are more likely to acquire 'occasion setting' properties when the stimulus elements are presented sequentially (Feature cue followed by the CS) rather than simultaneously, and that these occasion setting effects depend on the modulation of direct discrete CS-UCS associations (Holland 1992). Importantly, several authors argued that contextual cues, owing to their temporal nature and associative relationship with other stimuli (i.e. preceding and predicting *when* discrete stimuli are followed by reward), often act in ways similar to that of feature-positive or feature-negative occasion setters (Holland 1992; Bouton 1993; Pearce & Bouton 2001), and evidence for this notion was provided by Swartzentruber (1991).

Finally, Kearns & Weiss (2007) assessed whether cocaine-associated contexts reinstate (renew) drug seeking by serving as *discriminative drug cues.* They reported that exposure to the cocaine context selectively reinstates the ability of a discriminative tone cue to control nose-poke responding after extinction of the tone's discriminated response in a non-drug context. These data are consistent with the notion that occasion setting properties of contexts contribute to context-induced reinstatement by modulating the conditioned responses to other drug cues.

13.2.4 Conclusions

We outlined several potential mechanisms by which contexts could affect relapse to drug seeking. At present, little empirical evidence exists to determine which of these different learning mechanisms are more likely to contribute to context-induced reinstatement of drug seeking. Additionally, the mechanisms described above (direct excitatory and inhibitory Pavlovian conditioning, and occasion setting) are not mutually exclusive and thus may operate simultaneously to mediate context-induced reinstatement. Studies on the different psychological mechanisms of context-induced reinstatement are important, because they can have implications for relapse prevention in humans. For example, one of the cardinal features of occasion setting cues, which distinguishes them from traditional Pavlovian CSs, is that extended exposure to these cues alone (extinction) has little effect on their ability to affect responding to discrete CSs (Holland 1992). Thus, if contexts modulate drug seeking by serving as occasion setters, extinction-based therapeutic approaches (cue-exposure therapies) may be of little consequence in preventing context-induced relapse.

13.3 Pharmacology and neuroanatomy of context-induced reinstatement

Results from pharmacological and neuroanatomical studies on context-induced reinstatement of drug seeking are summarized in Tables 13.2–4. In these studies, the effects of pharmacological agents on context-induced reinstatement were observed at doses that had minimal effects on extinction responding in non-drug or novel contexts, inactive lever or nose-poke hole responding, or operant responding for non-drug rewards.

Table 13.2 Effect of systemic injections of pharmacological agents on context-induced reinstatement of drug seeking.

	Cocaine	Heroin	Alcohol	Nicotine
Dopamine D_1 receptor antagonist: SCH 23390	Crombag et al. (2002a)	Bossert et al. (2007)	Hamlin et al. (2007)	
Dopamine D_2 receptor Antagonist: raclopride	Crombag et al. (2002a)			
Glutamate mGluR$_{2/3}$ agonist: LY379268		Bossert et al. (2004)		
Preferential mu-opiate receptor antagonist: naltrexone			Burattini et al. (2006) and Marinelli et al. (2007)	
Serotonin 5H-T$_{2C}$ receptor agonist: Ro 60-0175	Fletcher et al. (2008)			
CB1 receptor antagonist: SR141716A				Diergaarde et al. (2008)

Table 13.3 Effect of intracranial injections of pharmacological agents on context-induced reinstatement of drug seeking. (BLA, basolateral amygdala; CPu, caudate putamen; DH, dorsal hippocampus; PFC, prefrontal cortex; VTA, ventral tegmental area.)

	Cocaine	Heroin	Anatomical specificity
VTA: LY379268 accumbens shell: LY379268, SCH 23390		Bossert et al. (2004) Bossert et al. (2006, 2007)	No effect in substantia nigra no effect in accumbens core (SCH 23390) and CPu (LY379268)
DH: tetrodotoxin	Fuchs et al. (2005)		No effect in trunk of somatosensory cortex
BLA: tetrodotoxin	Fuchs et al. (2005)		No effect in barrel field of somatosensory cortex
Dorsal medial PFC: tetrodotoxin	Fuchs et al. (2005)		No effect in ventral medial PFC
Dorsolateral CPu: muscimol+ baclofen	Fuchs et al. (2006)		No effect in somatosensory cortex
BLA–DH disconnection: muscimol +baclofen	Fuchs et al. (2007)		*Note:* contralateral but not ipsilateral injections were effective
BLA-dorsal medial PFC disconnection: muscimol+ baclofen	Fuchs et al. (2007)		*Note:* both contralateral and ipsilateral injections were effective

Table 13.4 Summary of Fos immediate early gene neuroanatomical mapping studies on context-induced reinstatement of drug seeking. (Under 'cocaine' or 'alcohol', we list brain sites where there are significant differences in Fos expression between groups of rats exposed to the training context (ABA) versus the distinct (ABB) or recent (AAA) extinction context. Under 'anatomical specificity', we provide a partial list of brain sites where group differences in Fos expression were not observed. BLA, basolateral amygdala; BNST, bed nucleus of stria terminalis; CPu, caudate putamen; PFC, prefrontal cortex; VTA, ventral tegmental area.)

	Cocaine	Alcohol	Anatomical specificity
Marinelli et al. (2007); *c-fos* mRNA		BLA Lateral amygdala Hippocampus CA3 area (non-significant trend in CA1 and CA2)	accumbens core and shell CPu Septum BNST VTA Central amygdala
Hamlin et al. (2007); Fos protein		BLA Lateral hypothalamus Ventral accumbens shell	Accumbens core and rostral pole Accumbens dorsomedial shell Dorsomedial and perifornical Hypothalamus Ventral and dorsal medial PFC VTA Substantia nigra
Hamlin et al. (2008); Fos protein	BLA lateral hypothalamus ventral medial PFC		Dorsal medial PFC Accumbens core and shell CPu Central amygdala Lateral amygdala BNST Dorsomedial and perifornical Hypothalamus VTA Substantia nigra

13.3.1 Role of dopamine and glutamate

Dopamine and glutamate transmissions in ventral tegmental area (VTA) and its projection areas—accumbens and dorsal medial prefrontal cortex (PFC)—contribute to the reinstatement of drug seeking (Kalivas & McFarland 2003; Bossert et al. 2005; Schmidt et al. 2005). Based on these studies, we initially assessed the effect of systemic injections of SCH 23390 or raclopride (dopamine D_1- and D_2-family receptor antagonists) or of LY379268, a group II metabotropic glutamate receptor (mGluR$_{2/3}$), which decreases evoked glutamate release, on context-induced reinstatement. We found that SCH 23390 or raclopride injections attenuate context-induced reinstatement of cocaine seeking (Crombag et al. 2002a), and that SCH 23390 or LY379268 injections attenuate context-induced reinstatement of heroin seeking (Bossert et al. 2004, 2007). Hamlin et al. (2006, 2007) reported that systemic SCH 23390 injections attenuate context-induced reinstatement of alcohol and sucrose seeking.

The VTA and accumbens shell contribute to the effect of systemic injections of SCH 23390 and LY379268 on context-induced reinstatement. We found that medial and lateral accumbens shell (but not core) SCH 23390 injections attenuate context-induced reinstatement of heroin seeking (Bossert et al. 2007). These findings are consistent with those of Hamlin et al. (2007): context-induced reinstatement of alcohol seeking is associated with increased Fos (a neuronal activity marker) expression in accumbens shell, an effect reversed by systemic SCH 23390 injections. Additionally, we found that VTA and medial accumbens shell injections of LY379268 attenuate context-induced reinstatement of heroin seeking (Bossert et al. 2004, 2006). These effects were anatomically specific: substantia nigra and caudate-putamen LY379268 injections were ineffective, and the effective LY379268 dose in accumbens core was 10 times higher than the effective dose in medial accumbens shell.

Because accumbens shell SCH 23390 injections attenuate context-induced reinstatement, the effect of LY379268 injections in VTA on context-induced reinstatement is probably due to decreases in VTA dopamine transmission; this would result in decreases in accumbens shell dopamine release, and consequently decreased stimulation of local D_1-family receptors. In VTA, dopamine transmission is controlled in part by excitatory glutamate projections from several brain areas (Geisler et al. 2007), and based on electrophysiological and anatomical studies (Manzoni & Williams 1999; Rouse et al. 2000), LY379268 VTA injections should activate local presynaptic inhibitory mGluR$_2$, resulting in decreased glutamate transmission, which leads to decreased dopamine transmission.

The effect of accumbens shell LY379268 injections on context-induced reinstatement may also be due to decreased glutamate and dopamine transmission. In accumbens, agonist activation of mGluR$_{2/3}$ receptors decreases glutamate transmission (Xi et al. 2002) via presynaptic mechanisms (Manzoni et al. 1997). Additionally, local perfusion of LY379268 decreases dopamine levels in accumbens shell (Greenslade & Mitchell 2004). Based on findings that accumbens neuronal activity is dependent on glutamate and dopamine D_1 receptor-mediated transmission (O'Donnell 2003), we propose that local dopamine–glutamate interaction mediates context-induced reinstatement. Below, we speculate on the nature of this interaction (see Fig. 13.2).

Under normal conditions, accumbens neurons exhibit negative resting membrane potentials, referred to as a 'down-state'. Excitatory glutamate inputs from PFC, hippocampus, and amygdala (Voorn et al. 2004) can drive quiescent down-state neurons into an 'up-state' and action-potential neuronal firing can occur (Wilson & Kawaguchi 1996). Once neurons are in the up-state, additional neuronal excitation is provided by dopamine-mediated D_1 receptor activation, which further enhances the up-state (O'Donnell 2003). LY379268 decreases glutamate release, while SCH 23390 blocks D_1-family receptors; each of these effects can

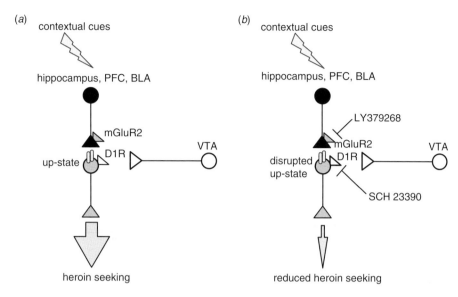

Fig. 13.2 A model of dopamine-glutamate interaction in the accumbens shell that mediates context-induced reinstatement of heroin seeking. (*a*) Exposure to heroin-associated contexts activates both dopamine and glutamate neurons that project to accumbens shell. Glutamate activation of shell medium spiny neurons increases the number of up-state neurons, which is further potentiated via D_1 receptor (D1R) activation by dopamine, resulting in the activation of downstream targets, which leads to the reinstatement of drug seeking. (*b*) Blockade of either glutamate transmission in accumbens shell by LY379268 (an agonist of inhibitory $mGluR_2$ located on presynaptic glutamatergic neurons) or dopamine transmission by SCH 23390 (an antagonist of postsynaptic D_1 receptors) prevents context-induced transition to the neuronal up-state, resulting in decreased activity of accumbens shell medium spiny output neurons, which in turn leads to the inhibition of context-induced reinstatement of heroin seeking. *White,* dopamine neurons; *black,* glutamate neurons; *gray,* medium spiny accumbens projection neurons.

interfere with the up-state excitation of accumbens medium spiny neurons. We propose that exposure to drug contexts activates both dopamine and glutamate neurons that project to accumbens shell. Glutamate activation of shell medium spiny neurons causes a shift from a down-state to an up-state, which is further enhanced via dopamine-mediated D_1 receptor activation, resulting in the activation of downstream targets (Meredith 1999), and consequently to drug seeking. Within this framework, accumbens shell injections of LY379268 or SCH 23390 prevent context-induced transition to the neuronal up-state, resulting in decreased activity of shell medium spiny output neurons, which in turn leads to attenuation of context-induced reinstatement.

13.3.2 Role of opioid, serotonin and endocannabinoid systems

The preferential mu-opioid receptor antagonist naltrexone attenuates reinstatement of alcohol seeking induced by alcohol priming (Le et al. 1999), and discrete (Liu & Weiss 2002) and discriminative (Katner & Weiss 1999) alcohol cues. Burattini et al. (2006) and Marinelli et al. (2007) reported that systemic injections of naltrexone decrease context-induced reinstatement of alcohol seeking. Marinelli et al. (2007) also found that systemic naltrexone injections decrease context-induced increases in *c-fos* mRNA expression in basolateral amygdala (BLA) and dorsal hippocampus, suggesting a potential role of mu-opioid receptors in these brain areas in this reinstatement. This suggestion should be confirmed in future studies on the effect of site-specific injections of mu-opiate receptor antagonists on context-induced reinstatement.

Systemic injections of Ro 60-0175 (an agonist of 5-HT_{2C} serotonin receptors) or SR141716A (an antagonist of cannabinoid receptor 1, CB1) decrease drug priming- and discrete cue-induced reinstatement of drug seeking (Grottick et al. 2000; De Vries et al. 2001, 2003; Burbassi & Cervo 2008). Based on these studies, Fletcher et al. (2008) examined the effect of systemic injections of Ro 60-0175 on context-induced reinstatement of cocaine seeking, and Diergaarde et al. (2008) examined the effect of systemic injections of SR141716A on context-induced reinstatement of nicotine seeking. They found that these injections decrease context-induced reinstatement. A question for future research from the findings with Ro 60-0175 and SR141716A is which brain sites mediate their effects on this reinstatement.

13.3.2 Role of BLA, dorsal medial PFC, dorsal hippocampus, dorsal striatum and lateral hypothalamus

Using reversible inactivation methods, Fuchs, See and colleagues provided evidence for a role of BLA, dorsal medial PFC, dorsal hippocampus and dorsolateral striatum in context-induced reinstatement of cocaine seeking. Fuchs et al. (2005) found that tetrodotoxin (a sodium channel blocker) injections into BLA, dorsal hippocampus and dorsal medial (but not ventral medial) PFC attenuate context-induced reinstatement. An issue to consider in interpreting these data is that tetrodotoxin inactivates both cell bodies in the target area and fibers of passage. Thus, tetrodotoxin's behavioural effects may be due to inactivation of fibers that pass through the target area rather than inactivation of cell bodies in the target area. Fuchs et al. (2006) also reported that inactivation of dorsolateral striatum by a mixture of GABAa and GABAb agonists (muscimol + baclofen, which inactivate cell bodies but not fibers of passage) attenuates context-induced reinstatement of cocaine seeking.

Fuchs et al. (2007) used an asymmetric lesion/inactivation procedure to assess whether a BLA-dorsal medial PFC pathway or a BLA–dorsal hippocampus pathway interacts sequentially to control context-induced reinstatement of cocaine seeking. In this procedure, the role a neuronal pathway plays in a given behaviour is inferred from the observation that lesion (permanent or reversible) or receptor blockade of one brain site in one hemisphere together with lesion/receptor blockade of a second brain site in the contralateral hemisphere disrupts the behaviour of interest (Gaffan et al. 1993; Di Ciano & Everitt 2004). Because most learned behaviours can be maintained by an intact single hemisphere (but see Christakou et al. (2005) for data inconsistent with this view), and most neuronal projections are ipsilateral, a main requirement for interpreting results from 'disconnection' studies is that the target behaviour remains largely intact after ipsilateral lesion/inactivation of the two brain sites (Setlow et al. 2002). Fuchs et al. found that while contralateral but not ipsilateral inactivation (muscimol + baclofen) of the BLA–dorsal hippocampus attenuates context-induced reinstatement, both contralateral and ipsilateral inactivation of BLA-dorsal medial PFC decrease this reinstatement.

These findings potentially suggest that a serial interaction between BLA and dorsal hippocampus, but not BLA and dorsal medial PFC, mediates context-induced reinstatement. However, before accepting this conclusion, several issues should be considered, especially regarding the similar effects of ipsilateral and contralateral BLA–dorsal medial PFC inactivation. Anatomical studies indicate strong reciprocal connections between the BLA and PFC (McDonald 1998; Pitkanen 2000), including bilateral PFC projections to amygdala (McDonald et al. 1996). Electrophysiology data also suggest that conditioned neuronal responses in PFC depend on amygdala input (Grace 2006). Based on these anatomical and electrophysiology findings, the similar effects of ipsilateral and contralateral BLA-PFC inactivation on context-induced reinstatement may not reflect independence of BLA and PFC in the control of context-induced reinstatement, but rather occur because BLA-PFC unilateral input is not sufficient to maintain normal responding for contexts during reinstatement testing.

In agreement with the results of Fuchs et al., studies using the neuronal activity marker Fos suggest that BLA and dorsal hippocampus neuronal activities contribute to context-induced reinstatement. In both alcohol- and cocaine-trained rats, context-induced reinstatement is associated with selective Fos (or *c-fos*) induction in BLA (Hamlin et al. 2007, 2008; Marinelli et al. 2007). Context-induced reinstatement of alcohol seeking is also associated with consistent (though modest) increases in *c-fos* in dorsal hippocampal areas (Marinelli et al. 2007). However, the findings of Hamlin et al. (2008) that context-induced reinstatement of cocaine seeking is associated with Fos induction in ventral medial but not dorsal medial PFC are inconsistent with the results of Fuchs et al. (2005) that tetrodotoxin inactivation of the dorsal medial but not ventral medial PFC attenuates this reinstatement. However, findings with Fos should be interpreted with caution. For example, the accumbens mediates many behavioural effects of cocaine, yet acute cocaine injections have minimal effect on accumbens Fos induction (Crombag et al. 2002b; Hope et al. 2006). Also, while our data suggest a role of VTA in context-induced reinstatement, this reinstatement is not associated with Fos induction in this brain area (Table 13.4).

An interesting finding emerging from the studies of Hamlin et al. is the association between context-induced reinstatement and Fos induction in lateral hypothalamus. This is a consistent finding that occurs not only in cocaine- and alcohol-trained rats, but also in sucrose-trained rats (Hamlin et al. 2006), suggesting a general role of lateral hypothalamus in context-induced reward seeking. Hamlin et al. (2008) also attempted to determine the afferent areas to lateral hypothalamus that are recruited during tests for context-induced reinstatement. This was achieved by injecting the retrograde tracer cholera toxin into lateral hypothalamus prior to cocaine self-administration training, and subsequently double-labelling the cholera toxin-labelled neurons in the target areas (e.g. PFC, accumbens, VTA) with Fos (induced during reinstatement testing). Surprisingly, very little double-labelling of Fos-cholera toxin was found in the projection areas, suggesting that context-induced lateral hypothalamus neuronal activity is largely independent of neuronal activity in VTA, accumbens and PFC. This unexpected finding suggests that the role of lateral hypothalamus in context-induced reinstatement is independent of the role of VTA, accumbens shell and dorsal medial PFC in this reinstatement. However, based on the limitations of interpreting Fos mapping studies mentioned above, it is important to further test this interesting hypothesis in studies using the disconnection approach.

13.3.4 Conclusions

Studies using systemic drug injections indicate a role of D_1- and D_2-family, $mGluR_{2/3}$, mu-opioid, $5\text{-}HT_{2C}$ and CB1 receptors in context-induced reinstatement of drug seeking. Our studies indicate that dopamine and glutamate transmissions in VTA and accumbens shell mediate context-induced reinstatement (Fig. 13.2). From a circuitry perspective, questions for future research are the sources of the glutamatergic projections to the VTA and accumbens shell that are activated during the tests for context-induced reinstatement, and the accumbens shell downstream brain sites involved in this reinstatement. There is also evidence for a role of the dorsal hippocampus, BLA, dorsal striatum and dorsal medial PFC in context-induced reinstatement. A question for future research is the neurotransmitters involved in this reinstatement in these brain areas. Fos mapping studies suggest a role of lateral hypothalamus in context-induced reinstatement of drug seeking. However, these data are correlational and should be confirmed in studies using local drug injections.

An unresolved issue for future research, which has begun to be addressed by the laboratories of McNally and Fuchs, is which brain pathways mediate context-induced reinstatement. Fuchs's studies led to the surprising result, based on limited anatomical connectivity (Pitkanen 2000), that a serial interaction between BLA and dorsal hippocampus contributes to context-induced reinstatement. McNally's studies potentially suggest that lateral hypothalamus' role in context-induced reinstatement is independent of its afferents from VTA, accumbens shell and PFC. Another issue for future research, which has begun to be addressed by McNally laboratory, is whether similar or different neuronal mechanisms underlie context-induced reinstatement across drug classes. The studies by Hamilin, McNally and colleagues suggest that these mechanisms are not identical. For example, context-induced reinstatement of cocaine seeking, but not alcohol seeking, is associated with Fos induction in ventral medial PFC, while context-induced reinstatement of alcohol seeking, but not cocaine seeking, is associated with the activation of hypocretin (orexin) neurons in lateral hypothalamus (Hamlin et al. 2007, 2008).

13.4 Clinical implications

We reviewed studies on context-induced reinstatement of drug seeking in rats. We suggest that to the degree that our preclinical model is relevant to understanding human drug relapse (Epstein et al. 2006), the results of the studies reviewed may have implications for the understanding of the psychological processes underlying this relapse. The reliable effect of context exposure on reinstatement after extinction of the response to the discrete cues in a different context can explain results from 'cue exposure' studies demonstrating that most human drug users relapse when they return to their home environment after successful extinction of the physiological and psychological responses to drug-associated discrete cues in the clinic (Carter & Tiffany 1999). More generally, the phenomenon of context-induced reinstatement in laboratory rats can also explain in part why many drug addicts who after having successfully undergone inpatient detoxification (with or without cue-exposure therapy) return to drug use upon returningto their home environment (Hunt et al. 1971). Finally, the studies reviewed, together with previous studies using non-drug reinforcers (Bouton 2002), may have implications for behavioural treatment of drug addiction. We suggest that for drug addiction interventions to succeed, it is critical that contextual cues are considered, and that treatment strategies aimed at extinguishing the complex association between contextual cues, discrete cues and drug-taking behaviour may improve long-term drug abstinence. In this regard, two recent studies in rats self-administering alcohol or cocaine suggest alternative strategies that could be more effective at altering contextual influences on relapse to drug seeking. These include exposure to alternative reinforcers during extinction (Kearns & Weiss 2007), and extinction in multiple contexts (Chaudhri et al. 2008).

Part of the research described in this review was supported by the Intramural Research Program of the National Institute on Drug Abuse. We thank Taco De Vries, Gavan McNally and Peter Marinelli for providing data depicted in Fig. 13.1.

References

Berridge, K. C. 2004 Motivation concepts in behavioral neuroscience. *Physiol. Behav.* **81**, 179–209. (doi:10.1016/ j.physbeh.2004.02.004)

Bossert, J. M., Liu, S. Y., Lu, L. & Shaham, Y. 2004 A role of ventral tegmental area glutamate in contextual cue-induced relapse to heroin seeking. *J. Neurosci.* **24**, 10 726–10 730. (doi:10.1523/ JNEUROSCI.3207–04.2004)

Bossert, J. M., Ghitza, U. E., Lu, L., Epstein, D. H. & Shaham, Y. 2005 Neurobiology of relapse to heroin and cocaine seeking: an update and clinical implications. *Eur. J. Pharmacol.* **526**, 36–50. (doi:10.1016/j.ejphar. 2005.09.030)

Bossert, J. M., Gray, S. M., Lu, L. & Shaham, Y. 2006 Activation of group II metabotropic glutamate receptors in the nucleus accumbens shell attenuates context-induced relapse to heroin seeking. *Neuropsychopharmacology* **31**, 2197–209. (doi:10.1038/sj.npp.1300977)

Bossert, J. M., Poles, G. C., Wihbey, K. A., Koya, E. & Shaham, Y. 2007 Differential effects of blockade of dopamine D₁-family receptors in nucleus accumbens core or shell on reinstatement of heroin seeking induced by contextual and discrete cues. *J. Neurosci.* **27**, 12655–163. (doi:10.1523/ JNEUROSCI.3926–07.2007)

Bouton, M. E. 1993 Context, time, and memory retrieval in the interference paradigms of Pavlovian learning. *Psychol. Bull.* **114**, 80–99. (doi:10.1037/0033–2909.114.1.80)

Bouton, M. E. 2002 Context, ambiguity, and unlearning: sources of relapse after behavioral extinction. *Biol. Psychiatry* **52**, 976–86. (doi:10.1016/S0006–3223(02) 01546–9)

Bouton, M. E. & Bolles, R. C. 1979 Contextual control of the extinction of conditioned fear. *Learn. Motiv.* **10**, 445–66. (doi:10.1016/0023–9690(79)90057–2)

Bouton, M. E. & Swartzentruber, D. 1991 Sources of relapse after extinction in Pavlovian and instrumental learning. *Clin. Psychol. Rev.* **11**, 123–40. (doi:10.1016/0272–7358(91)90091–8)

Burattini, C., Gill, T. M., Aicardi, G. & Janak, P. H. 2006 The ethanol self-administration context as a reinstatement cue: acute effects of naltrexone. *Neuroscience* **139**, 877–87. (doi:10.1016/j. neuroscience.2006.01.009)

Burbassi, S. & Cervo, L. 2008 Stimulation of serotonin2C receptors influences cocaine-seeking behavior in response to drug-associated stimuli in rats. *Psychopharmacology* **196**, 15–27. (doi:10.1007/ s00213–007–0916–7)

Carter, B. L. & Tiffany, S. T. 1999 Meta-analysis of cue-reactivity in addiction research. *Addiction* **94**, 327–40. (doi:10.1046/j.1360–0443.1999.9433273.x)

Catania, C. A. 1992 *Learning,* 3rd edn. Englewood Cliffs, NJ: Prentice-Hall.

Chaudhri, N., Sahuque, L. L. & Janak, P. H. 2008 Context-induced relapse of conditioned behavioral responding to ethanol cues in rats. *Biol. Psychiatry* **64**, 203–10. (doi:10.1016/j.biopsych. 2008.03.007)

Christakou, A., Robbins, T. W. & Everitt, B. J. 2005 Prolonged neglect following unilateral disruption of a prefrontal cortical-dorsal striatal system. *Eur. J. Neurosci.* **21**, 782–92. (doi:10.1111/ j.1460–9568.2005.03892.x)

Ciccocioppo, R., Sanna, P. P. & Weiss, F. 2001 Cocaine-predictive stimulus induces drug-seeking behavior and neural activation in limbic brain regions after multiple months of abstinence: reversal by D(1) antagonists. *Proc. Natl Acad. Sci. USA* **98**, 1976–81. (doi:10.1073/pnas. 98.4.1976)

Crombag, H. S. & Shaham, Y. 2002 Renewal of drug seeking by contextual cues after prolonged extinction in rats. *Behav. Neurosci.* **116**, 169–73. (doi:10.1037/0735–7044. 116.1.169)

Crombag, H., Grimm, J. W. & Shaham, Y 2002a Effect of dopamine receptor antagonists on renewal of cocaine seeking by reexposure to drug–associated contextual cues. *Neuropsychopharmacology* **27**, 1007–16. (doi:10.1016/ S0893–133X(02)00356–1)

Crombag, H. S., Jedynak, J. P., Redmond, K., Robinson, T. E. & Hope, B. T. 2002b Locomotor sensitization to cocaine is associated with increased Fos expression in the accumbens, but not in the caudate. *Behav. Brain Res.* **136**, 455–62. (doi:10.1016/S0166–4328(02)00196–1)

Crombag, H. S., Galarce, E. M. & Holland, P. C. 2008 Pavlovian influences on goal-directed behavior in mice: the role of cue-reinforcer temporal relations. *Learn. Mem* **15**, 299–303. (doi:10.1101/lm.762508)

De Vries, T. J., Shaham, Y., Homberg, J. R. et al. 2001 A cannabinoid mechanism in relapse to cocaine seeking. *Nat. Med.* **7**, 1151–4. (doi:10.1038/nm1001–1151)

De Vries, T. J., Homberg, J. R., Binnekade, R., Raaso, H. & Schoffelmeer, A. N. 2003 Cannabinoid modulation of the reinforcing and motivational properties of heroin and heroin-associated cues in rats. *Psychopharmacology* **168**, 164–9. (doi:10.1007/s00213–003–1422–1)

de Wit, H. & Stewart, J. 1981 Reinstatement of cocaine-reinforced responding in the rat. *Psychopharmacology* **75**, 134–43. (doi:10.1007/BF00432175)

Di Ciano, P. & Everitt, B. J. 2004 Direct interactions between the basolateral amygdala and nucleus accumbens core underlie cocaine-seeking behavior by rats. *J. Neurosci.* **24**, 7167–73. (doi:10.1523/JNEUROSCI. 1581–04.2004)

Diergaarde, L., de Vries, W., Raasø, H., Schoffelmeer, A. N. M. & de Vries, T. J. 2008. Contextual renewal of nicotine seeking in rats and its suppression by the cannabinoid-1 receptor antagonist Rimonabant (SR141716A). (doi:10. 1016/j.neuropharm.2008.06.003)

Epstein, D. H., Preston, K. L., Stewart, J. & Shaham, Y. 2006 Toward a model of drug relapse: an assessment of the validity of the reinstatement procedure. *Psychopharmacology* **189**, 1–16. (doi:10.1007/s00213–006–0529–6)

Fletcher, P. J., Rizos, Z., Sinyard, J., Tampakeras, M. & Higgins, G. A. 2008 The 5–HT(2C) receptor agonist Ro60–0175 reduces cocaine self-administration and reinstatement induced by the stressor yohimbine, and contextual cues. *Neuropsychopharmacology* **33**, 1402–12. (doi:10.1038/sj.npp. 1301509)

Fuchs, R. A., Evans, K. A., Ledford, C. C. et al. 2005 The role of the dorsomedial prefrontal cortex, basolateral amygdala, and dorsal hippocampus in contextual reinstatement of cocaine seeking in rats. *Neuropsychopharmacology* **30**, 296–309. (doi: 10.1038/sj.npp.1300579)

Fuchs, R. A., Branham, R. K. & See, R. E. 2006 Different neural substrates mediate cocaine seeking after abstinence versus extinction training: a critical role for the dorso-lateral caudate-putamen. *J. Neurosci.* **26**, 3584–8. (doi:10.1523/JNEUROSCI.5146–05.2006)

Fuchs, R. A., Eaddy, J. L., Su, Z. I. & Bell, G. H. 2007 Interactions of the basolateral amygdala with the dorsal hippocampus and dorsomedial prefrontal cortex regulate drug context-induced reinstatement of cocaine–seeking in rats. *Eur. J. Neurosci.* **26**, 487–98. (doi:10.1111/j.1460–9568.2007.05674.x)

Gaffan, D., Murray, E. A. & Fabre-Thorpe, M. 1993 Interaction of the amygdala with the frontal lobe in reward memory. *Eur. J. Neurosci.* **5**, 968–75. (doi:10.1111/ j.1460–9568.1993.tb00948.x)

Geisler, S., Derst, C., Veh, R. W. & Zahm, D. S. 2007 Glutamatergic afferents of the ventral tegmental area in the rat. *J. Neurosci.* **27**, 5730–43. (doi:10.1523/JNEUR–OSCI.0012–07.2007)

Goldberg, S. R. 1976 Stimuli associated with drug injections as events that control behavior. *Pharmacol. Rev.* **27**, 325–40.

Grace, A. A. 2006 Disruption of cortical-limbic interaction as a substrate for comorbidity. *Neurotox. Res.* **10**, 93–101.

Greenslade, R. G. & Mitchell, S. N. 2004 Selective action of (-)-2-oxa-4-aminobicyclo [3.1.0]hexane-4,6-dicarboxylate (LY379268), a group II metabotropic glutamate receptor agonist, on basal and phencyclidine-induced dopamine release in the nucleus accumbens shell. *Neuropharmacology* **47**, 1–8. (doi:10.1016/j.neuropharm. 2004.02.015)

Grimm, J. W., Kruzich, P. J. & See, R. E. 2000 Contingent access to stimuli associated with cocaine self-administration is required for reinstatement of drug-seeking behavior. *Psychobiology* **28**, 383–6.

Grottick, A. J., Fletcher, P. J. & Higgins, G. A. 2000 Studies to investigate the role of 5-HT$_{2C}$ receptors on cocaine and food maintained behaviour. *J. Pharmacol. Exp. Ther.* **295**, 1183–91.

Gunther, L. M., Denniston, J. C. & Miller, R. R. 1998 Conducting exposure treatment in multiple contexts can prevent relapse. *Behav. Res. Ther.* **36**, 75–91. (doi:10. 1016/S0005-7967(97)10019–5)

Hamlin, A. S., Blatchford, K. E. & McNally, G. P. 2006 Renewal of an extinguished instrumental response: neural correlates and the role of D$_1$ dopamine receptors. *Neuroscience* **143**, 25–38. (doi:10.1016/j.neuroscience. 2006.07.035)

Hamlin, A. S., Newby, J. & McNally, G. P. 2007 The neural correlates and role of D$_1$ dopamine receptors in renewal of extinguished alcohol-seeking. *Neuroscience* **146**, 525–36. (doi:10.1016/j. neuroscience.2007.01.063)

Hamlin, A. S., Clemens, K. J. & McNally, G. P. 2008 Renewal of extinguished cocaine–seeking. *Neuroscience* **151**, 659–70. (doi:10.1016/j.neuroscience.2007.11.018)

Holland, P. C. 1992 Occasion setting in Pavlovian conditioning. In *The psychology of learning and motivation* (ed. D. L. Medlin), pp. 69–125. San Diego, CA: Academic Press.

Holland, P. C. & Bouton, M. E. 1999 Hippocampus and context in classical conditioning. *Curr. Opin. Neurobiol.* **9**, 195–202. (doi:10.1016/S0959–4388(99)80027–0)

Hope, B. T., Simmons, D. E., Mitchell, T. B., Kreuter, J. D. & Mattson, B. J. 2006 Cocaine-induced locomotor activity and Fos expression in nucleus accumbens are sensitized for 6 months after repeated cocaine administration outside the home cage. *Eur. J. Neurosci.* **24**, 867–75. (doi:10. 1111/j. 1460–9568.2006.04969.x)

Hunt, W. A., Barnett, L. W. & Branch, L. G. 1971 Relapse rates in addiciton programs. *J. Clin. Psychol* **27**, 455–56. (doi:10.1002/1097–4679(197110)27:4 <455::AID–JCLP2 270270412>3.0.CO;2–R)

Kalivas, P. W. & McFarland, K. 2003 Brain circuitry and the reinstatement of cocaine-seeking behavior. *Psychopharmacology* **168**, 44–56. (doi:10.1007/s00213–003–1393–2)

Katner, S. N. & Weiss, F. 1999 Ethanol-associated olfactory stimuli reinstate ethanol-seeking behavior after extinction and modify extracellular dopamine levels in the nucleus accumbens. *Alcohol Clin. Exp. Res.* **23**, 1751–60.

Kearns, D. N. & Weiss, S. J. 2007 Contextual renewal of cocaine seeking in rats and its attenuation by the conditioned effects of an alternative reinforcer. *Drug Alcohol Depend.* **90**, 193–202. (doi:10.1016/j. drugalcdep. 2007.03.006)

Kruzich, P. J., Congleton, K. M. & See, R. E. 2001 Conditioned reinstatement of drug-seeking behavior with a discrete compound stimulus classically conditioned with intravenous cocaine. *Behav. Neurosci.* **115**, 1086–92. (doi:10.1037/0735–7044.115.5.1086)

Le, A. D., Poulos, C. X., Harding, S., Watchus, W., Juzytsch, W & Shaham, Y. 1999 Effects of naltrexone and fluoxetine on alcohol self-administration and reinstatement of alcohol seeking induced by priming injections of alcohol and exposure to stress in rats. *Neuropsychopharmacology* **21**, 435–44. (doi:10.1016/S0893–133X(99)00024–X)

Liu, X. & Weiss, F. 2002 Additive effect of stress and drug cues on reinstatement of ethanol seeking: exacerbation by history of dependence and role of concurrent activation of corticotropin-releasing factor and opioid mechanisms. *J. Neurosci.* **22**, 7856–61.

Lovibond, P. F. 1981 Appetitive Pavlovian-instrumental interactions: effects of inter-stimulus interval and baseline reinforcement conditions. *Q. J. Exp. Psychol. B* **33**, 257–69.

Lovibond, P. F. 1983 Facilitation of instrumental behavior by a Pavlovian appetitive conditioned stimulus. *J. Exp. Psychol. Anim. Behav. Process.* **9**, 225–47. (doi:10.1037/ 0097–7403.9.3.225)

Mackintosh, N. J. 1974 *The psychology of animal learning.* London, UK: Academic Press.

Manzoni, O. J. & Williams, J. T. 1999 Presynaptic regulation of glutamate release in the ventral tegmental area during morphine withdrawal. *J. Neurosci.* **19**, 6629–36.

Manzoni, O., Michel, J. M. & Bockaert, J. 1997 Metabotropic glutamate receptors in the rat nucleus accumbens. *Eur. J. Neurosci.* **9**, 1514–23. (doi:10.1111/j.1460–9568. 1997.tb01506.x)

Marinelli, P. W., Funk, D., Juzytsch, W., Li, Z. & Le, A. D. 2007 Effects of opioid receptor blockade on the renewal of alcohol seeking induced by context: relationship to *c-fos* mRNA expression. *Eur. J. Neurosci.* **26**, 2815–23. (doi: 10.1111/j.1460–9568.2007.05898.x)

McDonald, A. J. 1998 Cortical pathways to the mammalian amygdala. *Prog. Neurobiol.* **55**, 257–332. (doi:10.1016/ S0301–0082(98)00003–3)

McDonald, A. J., Mascagni, F. & Guo, L. 1996 Projections of the medial and lateral prefrontal cortices to the amygdala: a *Phaseolus vulgaris* leucoagglutinin study in the rat. *Neuroscience* **71**, 55–75. (doi:10.1016/0306–4522(95)00417–3)

McFarland, K. & Ettenberg, A. 1997 Reinstatement of drug-seeking behavior produced by heroin-predictive environmental stimuli. *Psychopharmacology* **131**, 86–92. (doi: 10.1007/s002130050269)

Meil, W. M. & See, R. E. 1996 Conditioned cued recovery of responding following prolonged with-
    drawal from self-administered cocaine in rats: an animal model of relapse. *Behav. Pharmacol.* **7**,
    754–63.
Meredith, G. E. 1999 The synaptic framework for chemical signaling in nucleus accumbens. *Ann. N. Y.
    Acad. Sci.* **877**, 140–56. (doi:10.1111/j.1749–6632.1999.tb09266.x)
O'Brien, C. P., Childress, A. R., Mclellan, T. A. & Ehrman, R. 1992 Classical conditioning in drug
    dependent humans. *Ann. N. Y. Acad. Sci.* **654**, 400–15. (doi: 10. 1111/j.1749–6632.1992.tb25984.x)
O'Donnell, P. 2003 Dopamine gating of forebrain neural ensembles. *Eur. J. Neurosci.* **17**, 429–35.
    (doi:10.1046/ j. 1460–9568.2003.02463.x)
Pavlov, I. P. 1927 *Conditioned reflexes.* Oxford, UK: Oxford University Press.
Pearce, J. & Bouton, M. E. 2001 Theories of associative learning in animals. *Annu. Rev. Psychol.* **52**,
    111–39. (doi:10.1146/annurev.psych.52.1.111)
Pitkanen, A. 2000 Connectivity of the rat amygdaloid complex. In *The amygdala: a functional analysis*
    (ed. J. P. Aggleton), pp. 31–115. Oxford, UK: Oxford University Press.
Rescorla, R. A. 1969 Conditioned inhibition of fear resulting from negative CS–US contingencies.
    J. Comp. Physiol. Psychol. **67**,504–9. (doi:10.1037/h0027313)
Rescorla, R. A., Durlach, P. J. & Grau, J. W. 1985 Contextual learning in Pavlovian conditioning.
    In *Context and learning* (eds P. Balsam & A. Tomie), pp. 23–56. Hillsdale, NJ: Erlbaum.
Rouse, S. T., Marino, M. J., Bradley, S. R., Awad, H., Wittmann, M. & Conn, P. J. 2000 Distribution
    and roles of metabotropic glutamate receptors in the basal ganglia motor circuit: implications for
    treatment of Parkinson's disease and related disorders. *Pharmacol. Ther.* **88**, 427–35. (doi:10.1016/
    S0163–7258(00)00098–X)
Schmidt, H. D., Anderson, S. M., Famous, K. R., Kumaresan, V. & Pierce, R. C. 2005 Anatomy and
    pharmacology of cocaine priming-induced reinstatement of drug seeking. *Eur. J. Pharmacol.* **526**,
    65–76. (doi:10. 1016/j.ejphar.2005.09.068)
See, R. E. 2002 Neural substrates of conditioned-cued relapse to drug-seeking behavior. *Pharmacol.
    Biochem. Behav.* **71**, 517–29. (doi:10.1016/S0091–3057(01)00682–7)
Self, D. W., Barnhart, W. J., Lehman, D. A. & Nestler, E. J. 1996 Opposite modulation of cocaine-
    seeking behavior by D_1- and D_2-like dopamine receptor agonists. *Science* **271**, 1586–9. (doi:10.1126/
    science.271.5255.1586)
Setlow, B., Holland, P. C. & Gallagher, M. 2002 Disconnection of the basolateral amygdala complex
    and nucleus accumbens impairs appetitive Pavlovian second-order conditioned responses. *Behav.
    Neurosci.* **116**, 267–75. (doi: 10.1037/0735–7044.116.2.267)
Shaham, Y. & Stewart, J. 1995 Stress reinstates heroin self-administration behavior in drug-free
    animals: an effect mimicking heroin, not withdrawal. *Psychopharmacology* **119**,334–41.(doi:10.1007/
    BF02246300)
Shaham, Y., Shalev, U., Lu, L., De Wit, H. & Stewart, J. 2003 The reinstatement model of drug
    relapse: history, methodology and major findings. *Psychopharmacology* **168**, 3–20. (doi: 10.1007/
    s00213–002–1224–x)
Shalev, U., Yap, J. & Shaham, Y 2001 Leptin attenuates food deprivation-induced relapse to heroin
    seeking. *J. Neurosci.* **21**, RC129.
Shalev, U., Grimm, J. W. & Shaham, Y 2002 Neurobiology of relapse to heroin and cocaine seeking:
    a review. *Pharmacol. Rev.* **54**, 1–42. (doi:10.1124/pr.54.1.1)
Shepard, J. D., Bossert, J. M., Liu, S. Y & Shaham, Y 2004 The anxiogenic drug yohimbine reinstates
    methamphetamine seeking in a rat model of drug relapse. *Biol. Psychiatry* **55**, 1082–9. (doi:10.1016/j.
    biopsych.2004.02.032)
Spealman, R. D., Barrett-Larimore, R. L., Rowlett, J. K., Platt, D. M. & Khroyan, T. V. 1999
    Pharmacological and environmental determinants of relapse to cocaine-seeking behavior.
    Pharmacol. Biochem. Behav. **64**, 327–36. (doi: 10. 1016/S0091–3057(99)00049–0)
Swartzentruber, D. 1991 Blocking between occasion setters and contextual stimuli. *J. Exp. Psychol.
    Anim. Behav. Processes* **17**, 163–73. (doi:10.1037/0097–7403.17.2.163)
Voorn, P., Vanderschuren, L. J., Groenewegen, H. J., Robbins, T. W. & Pennartz, C. M. 2004 Putting a
    spin on the dorsal-ventral divide of the striatum. *Trends Neurosci.* **27**, 468–74. (doi:10.1016/j.
    tins.2004.06.006)

Weiss, F., Maldonado-Vlaar, C. S., Parsons, L. H., Kerr, T. M., Smit, D. L. & Ben-Shahar, O. 2000 Control of cocaine-seeking behavior by drug-associated stimuli in rats: effects on recovery of extinguished operant-responding and extracellular dopamine levels in amygdala and nucleus accumbens. *Proc. Natl Acad. Sci. USA* **97**, 4321–6. (doi:10.1073/pnas.97.8.4321)

Wikler, A. 1973 Dynamics of drug dependence, implication of a conditioning theory for research and treatment. *Arch. Gen. Psychiatry* **28**, 611–16.

Wilson, C. J. & Kawaguchi, Y. 1996 The origins of two-state spontaneous membrane potential fluctuations of neo-striatal spiny neurons. *J. Neurosci.* **16**, 2397–410.

Wyvell, C. L. & Berridge, K. C. 2000 Intra-accumbens amphetamine increases the conditioned incentive salience of sucrose reward: enhancement of reward "wanting" without enhanced "liking" or response reinforcement. *J. Neurosci.* **20**, 8122–30.

Xi, Z. X., Baker, D. A., Shen, H., Carson, D. S. & Kalivas, P. W. 2002 Group II metabotropic glutamate receptors modulate extracellular glutamate in the nucleus accumbens. *J. Pharmacol. Exp. Ther.* **300**, 162–71. (doi:10.1124/jpet.300.1.162)

Zironi, I., Burattini, C., Aicardi, G. & Janak, P. H. 2006 Context is a trigger for relapse to alcohol. *Behav. Brain Res.* **167**, 150–5. (doi:10.1016/j.bbr.2005.09.007)

Part 4

Causes and Consequences of Addiction

Transcriptional mechanisms of addiction: Role of ΔFosB

*Eric J. Nestler**

Regulation of gene expression is considered a plausible mechanism of drug addiction, given the stability of behavioural abnormalities that define an addicted state. Among many transcription factors known to influence the addiction process, one of the best characterized is ΔFosB, which is induced in the brain's reward regions by chronic exposure to virtually all drugs of abuse and mediates sensitized responses to drug exposure. Since ΔFosB is a highly stable protein, it represents a mechanism by which drugs produce lasting changes in gene expression long after cessation of drug use. Studies are underway to explore the detailed molecular mechanisms by which ΔFosB regulates target genes and produces its behavioural effects. We are approaching this question by use of DNA expression arrays coupled with the analysis of chromatin remodelling—changes in the post-translational modifications of histones at drug-regulated gene promoters—to identify genes that are regulated by drugs of abuse via induction of ΔFosB and to gain insight into the detailed molecular mechanisms involved. Our findings establish chromatin remodelling as an important regulatory mechanism underlying drug-induced behavioural plasticity, and promise to reveal fundamentally new insight into how ΔFosB contributes to addiction by regulating the expression of specific target genes in brain reward pathways.

Key Words: Chromatin remodelling; epigenetics; nucleus accumbens; orbitofrontal cortex; ventral tegmental area.

14.1 Introduction

The study of transcriptional mechanisms of addiction is based on the hypothesis that regulation of gene expression is one important mechanism by which chronic exposure to a drug of abuse causes long-lasting changes in the brain that underlie the behavioural abnormalities that define a state of addiction (Nestler 2001). A corollary of this hypothesis is that drug-induced changes in dopaminergic and glutamatergic transmission and in the morphology of certain neuronal cell types in the brain, which have been correlated with an addicted state, are mediated in part via changes in gene expression.

Work over the past 15 years has provided increasing evidence for a role of gene expression in drug addiction, as several transcription factors—proteins that bind to specific responses elements in the promoter regions of target genes and regulate those genes' expression—have been implicated in drug action. Prominent examples include ΔFosB (a Fos family protein), CREB (cAMP response element binding protein), ICER (inducible cAMP early repressor), ATFs (activating transcription factors), EGRs (early growth response proteins), NAC1 (nucleus accumbens 1), NFκB (nuclear factor κB), and glucocorticoid receptor (O'Donovan et al. 1999; Mackler et al. 2000; Ang et al. 2001; Carlezon et al. 2005; Deroche-Gamonet et al. 2003; Green et al. 2006, 2008). This review focuses on ΔFosB, which appears to play a

* eric.nestler@mssm.edu

unique role in the addiction process, as a way to illustrate the types of experimental approaches that have been used to investigate transcriptional mechanisms of addiction.

14.2 Induction of ΔFosB in nucleus accumbens by drugs of abuse

ΔFosB is encoded by the *fosB* gene (Fig. 14.1) and shares homology with other Fos family transcription factors, which include c-Fos, FosB, Fra1, and Fra2 (Morgan & Curran 1995). These Fos family proteins heterodimerize with Jun family proteins (c-Jun, JunB, or JunD) to form active AP-1 (activator protein-1) transcription factors that bind to AP-1 sites (consensus sequence: TGAC/GTCA) present in the promoters of certain genes to regulate their transcription. These Fos family proteins are induced rapidly and transiently in specific brain regions after acute administration of many drugs of abuse (Fig. 14.2) (Graybiel et al. 1990; Young et al. 1991; Hope et al. 1992). These responses are seen most prominently in nucleus accumbens and dorsal striatum, which are important mediators of the rewarding and locomotor actions of the drugs. All of these Fos family proteins, however, are highly unstable and return to basal levels within hours of drug administration.

Very different responses are seen after chronic administration of drugs of abuse (Fig. 14.2). Biochemically modified isoforms of ΔFosB (M_r 35–37 kD) accumulate within the same brain regions after repeated drug exposure, whereas all other Fos family members show tolerance (i.e. reduced induction compared with initial drug exposures) (Chen et al. 1995, 1997; Hiroi et al. 1997). Such accumulation of ΔFosB has been observed for virtually all drugs of abuse (Table 14.1) (Hope et al. 1994; Nye et al. 1995; Moratalla et al. 1996; Nye & Nestler 1996; Pich et al. 1997; Muller & Unterwald, 2005; McDaid et al. 2006b), although different drugs differ somewhat in the relative degree of induction seen in nucleus accumbens

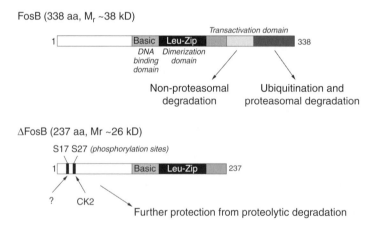

Fig. 14.1 Biochemical basis of ΔFosB's unique stability. ΔFosB and FosB are encoded by the *fosB* gene. ΔFosB is generated by alternative splicing and lacks the C-terminal 101 amino acids present in FosB. Two mechanisms are known that account for ΔFosB's stability. First, ΔFosB lacks two degron domains present in the C-terminus of full length FosB (and found in all other Fos family proteins as well). One of these degron domains targets FosB for ubiquitylation and degradation in the proteasome. The other degron domain targets FosB degradation by a ubiquitin- and proteasome-independent mechanism. Second, ΔFosB is phosphorylated by casein kinase 2 (CK2) and probably by other protein kinases at its N-terminus, which further stabilizes the protein.

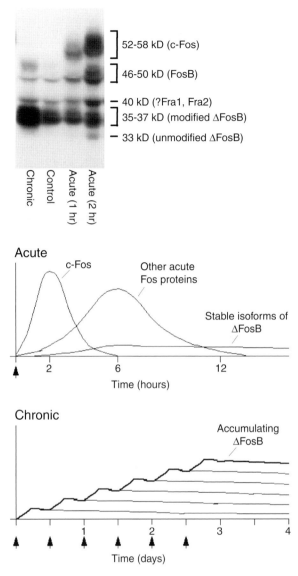

Fig. 14.2 Scheme showing the gradual accumulation of ΔFosB versus the rapid and transient induction of other Fos family proteins in response to drugs of abuse. *Top:* The autoradiogram illustrates the differential induction of Fos family proteins in the nucleus accumbens by acute stimulation (1–2 h after a single cocaine exposure) versus chronic stimulation (1 day after repeated cocaine exposure). *Bottom:* Upper graph shows several waves of Fos family proteins (comprised of c-Fos, FosB, ΔFosB [33 kD isoform], Fra1, Fra2) are induced in nucleus accumbens and dorsal striatal neurons by acute administration of a drug of abuse. Also induced are biochemically modified isoforms of ΔFosB (35–37 kD); they are induced at low levels by acute drug administration, but persist in brain for long periods due to their stability. The lower graph shows that with repeated (e.g. twice daily) drug administration, each acute stimulus induces a low level of the stable ΔFosB isoforms. This is indicated by the lower set of overlapping lines, which indicate ΔFosB induced by each acute stimulus. The result is a gradual increase in the total levels of ΔFosB with repeated stimuli during a course of chronic treatment. This is indicated by the increasing stepped line in the graph.

Table 14.1 Drugs of abuse known to induce ΔFosB in nucleus accumbens after chronic administration.

Opiates[1]
Cocaine[1]
Amphetamine
Methamphetamine
Nicotine[1]
Ethanol[1]
Phencyclidine
Cannabinoids

[1]Induction reported for self-administered drug in addition to investigator-administered drug. Drug induction of ΔFosB has been demonstrated in both rats and mice, except as follows: mouse only, cannabinoids; rat only, methamphetamine, phencyclidine.

core vs. shell and dorsal striatum (Perrotti et al. 2008). At least for some drugs of abuse, induction of ΔFosB appears selective for the dynorphin-containing subset of medium spiny neurons located in these brain regions (Nye et al. 1995; Moratalla et al. 1996; Muller & Unterwald, 2005; Lee et al. 2006), although more work is needed to establish this with certainty. The 35–37 kD isoforms of ΔFosB dimerize predominantly with JunD to form an active and long-lasting AP-1 complex within these brain regions (Chen et al. 1997; Hiroi et al. 1998). Drug induction of ΔFosB in the nucleus accumbens seems to be a response to the pharmacological properties of the drug per se and not related to volitional drug intake, since animals that self-administer cocaine or receive yoked drug injections show equivalent induction of this transcription factor in this brain region (Perrotti et al. 2008).

The 35–37 kD ΔFosB isoforms accumulate with chronic drug exposure due to their extraordinarily long half-lives (Chen et al. 1997; Alibhai et al. 2007). In contrast, there is no evidence that the splicing of ΔFosB or the stability of its mRNA is regulated by drug administration. As a result of its stability, therefore, the ΔFosB protein persists in neurons for at least several weeks after cessation of drug exposure. We now know that this stability is due to two factors (Fig. 14.1): (1) the absence in ΔFosB of two degron domains, which are present at the C-terminus of full length FosB and all other Fos family proteins and target those proteins to rapid degradation and (2) the phosphorylation of ΔFosB at its N-terminus by casein kinase 2 and perhaps other protein kinases (Ulery et al. 2006; Carle et al. 2007). The phosphorylation of ΔFosB also enhances its transcriptional properties (Ulery and Nestler, 2007). The stability of the ΔFosB isoforms provides a novel molecular mechanism by which drug-induced changes in gene expression can persist despite relatively long periods of drug withdrawal. We have, therefore, proposed that ΔFosB functions as a sustained 'molecular switch' that helps initiate and then maintain an addicted state (Nestler et al. 2001; McClung et al. 2004).

14.3 Role of ΔFosB in nucleus accumbens in regulating behavioural responses to drugs of abuse

Insight into the role of ΔFosB in drug addiction has come largely from the study of bitransgenic mice in which ΔFosB can be induced selectively within the nucleus accumbens and dorsal striatum of adult animals (Kelz et al. 1999). Importantly, these mice over express

ΔFosB selectively in the dynorphin-containing medium spiny neurons, where the drugs are believed to induce the protein. The behavioural phenotype of the ΔFosB-over expressing mice, which in certain ways resembles animals after chronic drug exposure, is summarized in Table 14.2. The mice show augmented locomotor responses to cocaine after acute and chronic administration (Kelz et al. 1999). They also show enhanced sensitivity to the rewarding effects of cocaine and of morphine in place conditioning assays (Kelz et al. 1999; Zachariou et al. 2006) and self-administer lower doses of cocaine than littermates that do not over express ΔFosB (Colby et al. 2003). ΔFosB over expression in nucleus accumbens also exaggerates the development of opiate physical dependence and promotes opiate analgesic tolerance (Zachariou et al. 2006). In contrast, ΔFosB expressing mice are normal in several other behavioural domains, including spatial learning as assessed in the Morris water maze (Kelz et al. 1999).

Specific targeting of ΔFosB over expression to the nucleus accumbens, by use of viral-mediated gene transfer, has yielded equivalent data (Zachariou et al. 2006), which indicates that this particular brain region can account for the phenotype observed in the bitransgenic mice, where ΔFosB is also expressed in dorsal striatum and to a lesser extent in certain other brain regions. Moreover, targeting the enkepahlin-containing medium spiny neurons in nucleus accumbens and dorsal striatum in different lines of bitransgenic mice fail to show most of these behavioural phenotypes, which specifically implicates dynorphin+ nucleus accumbens neurons in these phenomena. In contrast to over expression of ΔFosB, over expression of a mutant Jun protein (ΔcJun or ΔJunD)—which functions as a dominant negative antagonist of AP-1 mediated transcription—by use of bitransgenic mice or viral-mediated gene transfer produces the opposite behavioural effects (Peakman et al. 2003; Zachariou et al. 2006). These data indicate that induction of ΔFosB in dynorphin-containing medium spiny neurons of the nucleus accumbens increases an animal's sensitivity to cocaine and other drugs of abuse, and may represent a mechanism for relatively prolonged sensitization to the drugs.

Table 14.2 Behavioral phenotype upon ΔFosB induction in dynorphin+ neurons of nucleus accumbens and dorsal striatum[1]

Stimulus	Phenotype
Cocaine	Increased locomotor responses to acute administration
	Increased locomotor sensitization to repeated administration
	Increased conditioned place preference at lower doses
	Increased acquisition of cocaine self-administration at lower doses
	Increased incentive motivation in progressive ratio procedure
Morphine	Increased conditioned place preference at lower drug doses
	Increased development of physical dependence and withdrawal
	Decreased initial analgesic responses, enhanced tolerance
Alcohol	Increased anxiolytic responses
Wheel running	Increased wheel running
Sucrose	Increased incentive for sucrose in progressive ratio procedure
High fat	Increased anxiety-like responses upon withdrawal of high fat diet
Sex	Increased sexual behavior

[1]The phenotypes described in this table are established upon inducible overexpression of ΔFosB in inducible, bitransgenic mice where ΔFosB expression is targeted to dynorphin+ neurons of the nucleus accumbens and dorsal striatum; several fold lower levels of ΔFosB are seen in hippocampus and frontal cortex. In many cases, the phenotype has been directly linked to ΔFosB expression in nucleus accumbens *per se* by use of viral-mediated gene transfer.

The effects of ΔFosB may extend well beyond a regulation of drug sensitivity *per se* to more complex behaviours related to the addiction process. Mice overexpressing ΔFosB work harder to self-administer cocaine in progressive ratio self-administration assays, suggesting that ΔFosB may sensitize animals to the incentive motivational properties of cocaine and thereby lead to a propensity for relapse after drug withdrawal (Colby et al. 2003). ΔFosB overexpressing mice also show enhanced anxiolytic effects of alcohol (Picetti et al. 2001), a phenotype that has been associated with increased alcohol intake in humans. Together, these early findings suggest that ΔFosB, in addition to increasing sensitivity to drugs of abuse, produces qualitative changes in behaviour that promote drug-seeking behaviour, and support the view, stated above, that ΔFosB functions as a sustained molecular switch for the addicted state. An important question under current investigation is whether ΔFosB accumulation during drug exposure promotes drug-seeking behaviour after extended withdrawal periods, even after ΔFosB levels have normalized (see below).

14.4 Induction of ΔFosB in nucleus accumbens by natural rewards

The nucleus accumbens is believed to function under normal conditions by regulating responses to natural rewards, such as food, drink, sex, and social interactions. As a result, there is considerable interest in a possible role of this brain region in so-called natural addictions (e.g. pathological over-eating, gambling, exercise, etc.). Animal models of such conditions are limited; nevertheless, we and others have found that high levels of consumption of several types of natural rewards leads to the accumulation of the stable 35–37 kD isoforms of ΔFosB in nucleus accumbens. This has been seen after high levels of wheel running (Werme et al. 2002) as well as after chronic consumption of sucrose, high fat food, or sex (Teegarden & Bale 2007; Wallace et al. 2008). In some cases, this induction is selective for the dynorphin+ subset of medium spiny neurons (Werme et al. 2002). Studies of inducible, bitransgenic mice and of viral-mediated gene transfer have demonstrated that overexpression of ΔFosB in nucleus accumbens increases the drive and consumption for these natural rewards (Table 14.2) (Werme et al. 2002; Olausson et al. 2006; Wallace et al. 2008). In addition, a recent report has shown that ΔFosB expression increases anxiety-like responses seen upon withdrawal of a high fat diet (Teegarden et al., in press). Together, these findings suggest that ΔFosB in this brain region not only sensitizes animals for drug rewards, but for natural rewards as well, and may contribute to states of natural addiction by enhancing motivation for the rewards and by contributing to withdrawal symptoms when the rewards are withheld.

14.5 Induction of ΔFosB in nucleus accumbens by chronic stress

Given the substantial evidence that ΔFosB is induced in nucleus accumbens by chronic exposure to drug and natural rewards, it was interesting to observe that ΔFosB is also highly induced in this brain region after several forms of chronic stress, including restraint stress, chronic unpredictable stress, and social defeat (Perrotti et al. 2004; Vialou et al. 2007). Unlike drugs and natural rewards, however, this induction is seen more broadly in this brain region in that it is observed prominently in both dynorphin+ and enkephalin+ subsets of medium spiny neurons. Early evidence suggests that this induction of ΔFosB may represent a positive, coping response that helps an individual adapt to the stress. This hypothesis is supported by preliminary findings that overexpression of ΔFosB in nucleus accumbens, by use of inducible, bitransgenic mice or viral-mediated gene transfer, exerts antidepressant-like responses in several behavioural assays including social defeat, while ΔcJun expression causes prodepression-like effects (Vialou et al. 2007). Moreover, chronic administration of standard antidepressant medications exerts an effect similar to stress and induces ΔFosB in this brain region. While further work is needed to validate these findings, such a role would be consistent with the observations that ΔFosB increases the sensitivity of the brain's reward circuitry and may thereby help animals cope under periods of stress. Interestingly, this hypothesized antidepressant-like role for ΔFosB in nucleus accumbens is similar to that shown recently for periaqueductal gray where the transcription factor is also induced by chronic stress (Berton et al. 2007).

14.6 Target genes for ΔFosB in nucleus accumbens

Since ΔFosB is a transcription factor, it presumably produces this interesting behavioural phenotype in nucleus accumbens by enhancing or repressing expression of other genes. As shown in Fig. 14.1, ΔFosB is a truncated product of the *fosB* gene that lacks most of the C-terminal transactivation domain present in full-length FosB but retains the dimerization and DNA binding domains. ΔFosB is able to bind to Jun family members with the heterodimers than binding to AP-1 sites in DNA. Some *in vitro* studies suggest that because ΔFosB lacks much of its transactivation domain, it functions as a negative regulator of AP-1 activity, while several others show that ΔFosB can activate transcription at AP-1 sites (Nakabeppu & Nathans 1991; Dobrazanski et al. 1991; Yen et al. 1991; Chen et al. 2007).

Using our inducible, bitransgenic mice that overexpress ΔFosB or its dominant negative ΔcJun and analyzing gene expression on Affymetrix chips, we demonstrated that—in the nucleus accumbens *in vivo*—ΔFosB functions primarily as a transcriptional activator, while it does serve as a repressor for a smaller subset of genes (McClung & Nestler 2003). Interestingly, this differential activity of ΔFosB is a function of the duration and degree of ΔFosB expression, with short-term, lower levels leading to more gene repression and long-term, higher levels leading to more gene activation. This is consistent with the finding that short-term and long-term ΔFosB expression leads to opposite effects on behaviour: short-term ΔFosB expression, like the expression of ΔcJun, reduces cocaine preference, while longer-term ΔFosB expression increases cocaine preference (McClung & Nestler 2003). The mechanism responsible for this shift is currently under investigation; one novel possibility, which remains speculative, is that ΔFosB, at higher levels, may form homodimers that activate AP-1 transcription (Jorissen et al. 2007).

Several target genes of ΔFosB have been established using a candidate gene approach (Table 14.3). One candidate gene is GluR2, an AMPA glutamate receptor subunit (Kelz et al. 1999). ΔFosB overexpression in inducible bitransgenic mice selectively increases GluR2 expression in nucleus accumbens, with no effect seen on several other AMPA glutamate receptor subunits analyzed, while ΔcJun expression blocks the ability of cocaine to up-regulate GluR2 (Peakman et al. 2003). AP-1 complexes comprising ΔFosB (and most likely JunD) bind a consensus AP-1 site present in the GluR2 promoter. Furthermore, GluR2 overexpression via viral-mediated gene transfer increases the rewarding effects of cocaine, much like prolonged ΔFosB overexpression (Kelz et al. 1999). Since GluR2-containing AMPA channels have a lower overall conductance compared to AMPA channels that do not contain this subunit, the cocaine- and ΔFosB-mediated up-regulation of GluR2 in nucleus accumbens could account, at least in part, for the reduced glutamatergic responses seen in these neurons after chronic drug exposure (Kauer & Malenka 2007).

Table 14.3 Examples of validated targets for ΔFosB in nucleus accumbens[1]

Target	Brain region
↑ GluR2	Decreased sensitivitiy to glutamate
↓ Dynorphin[2]	Downregulation of κ opioid feedback loop
↑ Cdk5	Expansion of dendritic processes
↑ NF-κB	Expansion of dendritic processes; regulation of cell survival pathways
↓ c-Fos	Molecular switch from short-lived Fos family proteins induced acutely to ΔFosB induced chronically

[1]Although ΔFosB regulates the expression of numerous genes in brain (e.g. McClung & Nestler 2003), the table lists only those genes that meet at least three of the following criteria: (1) increased (↑) or decreased (↓) expression upon ΔFosB overexpression; (2) reciprocal or equivalent regulation by ΔcJun, a dominant negative inhibitor of AP-1-mediated transcription; (3) ΔFosB-containing AP-1 complexes bind to AP-1 sites in the promoter region of the gene; and (4) ΔFosB causes a similar effect on gene promoter activity *in vitro* as seen *in vivo*.

[2]Despite evidence that ΔFosB represses the dynorphin gene in drug abuse models (Zachariou et al. 2006), there is other evidence that it may activate the gene under different circumstances (see Cenci 2002).

Another candidate target gene of ΔFosB in nucleus accumbens is the opioid peptide, dynorphin. Recall that ΔFosB appears to be induced by drugs of abuse specifically in dynorphin-producing cells in this brain region. Drugs of abuse have complex effects on dynorphin expression, with increases or decreases seen depending on the treatment conditions used. The dynorphin gene contains AP-1-like sites, which can bind ΔFosB-containing AP-1 complexes. Moreover, we have shown that induction of ΔFosB represses dynorphin gene expression in nucleus accumbens (Zachariou et al. 2006). Dynorphin is thought to activate κ opioid receptors on VTA dopamine neurons and inhibit dopaminergic transmission and thereby down-regulate reward mechanisms (Shippenberg & Rea 1997). Hence, ΔFosB repression of dynorphin expression could contribute to the enhancement of reward mechanisms mediated by this transcription factor. There is now direct evidence supporting the involvement of dynorphin gene repression in ΔFosB's behavioural phenotype (Zachariou et al. 2006).

Recent evidence has shown that ΔFosB also represses the *c-fos* gene that helps create the molecular switch—from induction of several short-lived Fos family proteins after acute drug exposure to the predominant accumulation of ΔFosB after chronic drug exposure—cited earlier (Renthal et al. 2008). The mechanism responsible for ΔFosB repression of *c-fos* expression is complex and is covered below.

The second approach used to identify target genes of ΔFosB has measured the gene expression changes that occur upon the inducible overexpression of ΔFosB (or ΔcJun) in nucleus accumbens using DNA expression arrays, as described earlier. This approach has lead to the identification of many genes that are up- or down-regulated by ΔFosB expression in this brain region (Chen et al. 2000, 2003; Ang et al. 2001; McClung & Nestler 2003). Two genes that appear to be induced through ΔFosB's actions as a transcriptional activator are cyclin-dependent kinase-5 (Cdk5) and its cofactor P35 (Bibb et al. 2001; McClung & Nestler 2003). Cdk5 is also induced by chronic cocaine in the nucleus accumbens, an effect blocked upon ΔcJun expression, and ΔFosB binds to and activates the Cdk5 gene through an AP-1 site in its promoter (Chen et al. 2000; Peakman et al. 2003). Cdk5 is an important target of ΔFosB since its expression has been directly linked to changes in the phosphorylation state of numerous synaptic proteins including glutamate receptor subunits (Bibb et al. 2001), as well as increases in dendritic spine density (Norrholm et al. 2003; Lee et al. 2006), in the nucleus accumbens that are associated with chronic cocaine administration (Robinson & Kolb 2004). Recently, regulation of Cdk5 activity in nucleus accumbens has been directly linked to alterations in the behavioural effects of cocaine (Taylor et al. 2007).

Another ΔFosB target identified by use of microarrays is NFκB. This transcription factor is induced in nucleus accumbens by ΔFosB overexpression and by chronic cocaine, an effect blocked by ΔcJun expression (Ang et al. 2001; Peakman et al. 2003). Recent evidence suggests that induction of NFκB may also contribute to cocaine's ability to induce dendritic spines in nucleus accumbens neurons (Russo et al. 2007). As well, NFκB has been implicated in some of the neurotoxic effects of methamphetamine in striatal regions (Asanuma & Cadet 1998). The observation that NFκB is a target gene for ΔFosB emphasizes the complexity of the mechanisms by which ΔFosB mediates the effects of cocaine on gene expression. Thus, in addition to genes regulated by ΔFosB directly via AP-1 sites on the gene promoters, ΔFosB would be expected to regulate many additional genes via altered expression of NFκB and presumably other transcriptional regulatory proteins.

The DNA expression arrays provide a rich list of many additional genes that may be targeted—directly or indirectly—by ΔFosB. Among these genes are additional neurotransmitter receptors, proteins involved in pre- and post-synaptic function, many types of ion channels, and intracellular signalling proteins, as well as proteins that regulate the neuronal cytoskeleton and cell growth (McClung & Nestler 2003). Further work is needed to confirm each of these numerous proteins as *bona fide* targets of cocaine acting through ΔFosB and to establish the precise role that each protein plays in mediating the complex neural and behavioural aspects of cocaine action. Ultimately, of course, it will be crucial to move beyond the analysis of individual target genes to the regulation of groups of genes whose coordinated regulation is likely required to mediate the addicted state.

14.7 Induction of ΔFosB in other brain regions

The discussion up to now has focused solely on nucleus accumbens. While this is a key brain reward region and important for the addicting actions of cocaine and other drugs of abuse, many other brain regions are also crucial in the development and maintenance of a state of addiction. An important question, then, is whether ΔFosB acting in other brain regions beyond the nucleus accumbens may also influence drug addiction. Indeed, there is now increasing evidence that stimulant and opiate drugs of abuse induce ΔFosB in several brain regions implicated in diverse aspects of addiction (Nye et al. 1995; Perrotti et al. 2005, 2008; McDaid et al. 2006a, 2006b; Liu et al. 2007).

A recent study systematically compared ΔFosB induction in numerous brain regions across four different drugs of abuse: cocaine, morphine, cannabinoids, and ethanol (Perrotti et al. 2008; Table 14.4). All four drugs induce the transcription factor to varying degrees in nucleus accumbens and dorsal striatum as well as in prefrontal cortex, amygdala, hippocampus, bed nucleus of the stria terminalis, and interstitial nucleus of the posterior limb of the anterior commissure. Cocaine and ethanol alone induce ΔFosB in lateral septum, all of the drugs, except for cannabinoids, induce ΔFosB in the periaqueductal grey, and cocaine is unique in inducing ΔFosB in GABAergic cells in the posterior ventral tegmental area (Perrotti et al. 2005, 2008). In addition, morphine has been shown to induce ΔFosB in ventral pallidum (McDaid et al. 2006a). In each of these regions, it is the 35–37 kD isoforms of ΔFosB that accumulate with chronic drug exposure and persist for relatively long periods during withdrawal.

Table 14.4 Comparison of brain regions that show ΔFosB induction after chronic exposure to representative drugs of abuse[1]

	Cocaine	Morphine	Ethanol	Cannabinoids	
Nucleus accumbens					
Core	+	+	+	+	
Shell	+	+	+	+	
Dorsal striatum	+	+	+	+	
Ventral pallidum[2]	nd	+	nd	nd	
Prefrontal cortex[3]	+	+	+	+	
Lateral septum	+	−	+	−	
Medial septum	−	−	−	−	
BNST		+	+	+	+
IPAC		+	+	+	+
Hippocampus					
Dentate gyrus	+	+	−	+	
CA1	+	+	+	+	
CA3	+	+	+	+	
Amygdala					
Basolateral	+	+	+	+	
Central	+	+	+	+	
Medial	+	+	+	+	
Periaqueductal gray	+	+	+	−	
Ventral tegmental area	+	−	−	−	
Substantia nigra	−	−	−	−	

[1]The table does not show the relative levels of ΔFosB induction by the various drugs. See Perrotti et al. 2008 for this information.

[2]The effect of cocaine, ethanol, and cannabinoids on ΔFosB induction in ventral pallidum has not yet been studied, but such induction has been observed in response to methamphetamine (McDaid et al. 2006b).

[3]ΔFosB induction is seen in several subregions of prefrontal cortex, including infralimbic (medial prefrontal) and orbitofrontal cortex.

BNST, bed nucleus of the stria terminalis; IPAC, interstitial nucleus of the posterior limb of the anterior commisure; PAG, periaqueductal gray; VTA, ventral tegmental area; SN, substantia nigra.

A major goal for future research is to carry out studies, analogous to those described above for nucleus accumbens, to delineate the neural and behavioural phenotype mediated by ΔFosB for each of these brain regions. This represents an enormous undertaking, yet it is crucial for understanding the global influence of ΔFosB on the addiction process.

We have recently taken a significant step in this regard by using viral-mediated gene transfer to characterize the actions of ΔFosB in a particular subregion of prefrontal cortex, namely, orbitofrontal cortex. This region has been strongly implicated in addiction, in particular, in contributing to the impulsivity and compulsivity that characterizes an addicted state (Kalivas & Volkow 2005). Interestingly, unlike the nucleus accumbens where self-administered and yoked cocaine induce comparable levels of ΔFosB as noted earlier, we observed that cocaine self-administration causes a several-fold greater induction of ΔFosB in orbitofrontal cortex, suggesting that this response may be related to volitional aspects of drug administration (Winstanley et al. 2007). We then used rodent tests of attention and decision-making (e.g. 5 choice serial reaction time and delay discounting tests) to determine whether ΔFosB within the orbitofrontal cortex contributes to drug-induced alterations in cognition. We found that chronic cocaine treatment produces tolerance to the cognitive impairments caused by acute cocaine. Viral-mediated overexpression of ΔFosB within this region mimicked the effects of chronic cocaine, while overexpression of the dominant negative antagonist, ΔJunD, prevents this behavioural adaptation (Winstanley et al. 2007). In addition, ΔFosB overexpression in this region mimics the increase in impulsive behaviour exhibited by animals withdrawing from chronic cocaine self-administration (Winstanley et al., 2009). DNA expression microarray analyses identified several potential molecular mechanisms underlying these behavioural changes, including a cocaine- and ΔFosB-mediated increase in transcription of the metabotropic glutamate receptor mGluR5 and $GABA_A$ receptor as well as substance P (Winstanley et al. 2007). The influence of these and many other putative ΔFosB targets requires further investigation.

These findings indicate that ΔFosB helps mediate tolerance to the cognitive-disrupting effects of cocaine. Users who experience tolerance to the deleterious effects of cocaine are more likely to become cocaine-dependent, whereas those who find the drug more disruptive at work or school are less likely to become addicted (Shaffer & Eber 2002). Tolerance to the cognitive disruption caused by acute cocaine in cocaine-experienced individuals may therefore facilitate the maintenance of addiction. Increased impulsive behaviour, seen during withdrawal from cocaine self-administration, also appears to be mediated at least in part via ΔFosB in the orbitofrontal cortex. In these ways, ΔFosB induction in this prefrontal cortical region may promote an addicted state, similar to its actions in the nucleus accumbens, where ΔFosB promotes addiction by enhancing the rewarding and incentive motivational effects of the drug.

14.8 Epigenetic mechanisms of ΔFosB action

Until recently, all studies of transcriptional regulation in brain have relied on measurements of steady-state mRNA levels. For example, the search for ΔFosB target genes has involved identifying mRNA's up- or down-regulated upon ΔFosB or ΔcJun overexpression, as stated earlier. This level of analysis has been very useful in identifying putative targets for ΔFosB; however, it is inherently limited in providing insight into the underlying mechanisms involved. Rather, all studies of mechanisms have relied on *in vitro* measures such as ΔFosB binding to a gene's promoter sequences in gel shift assays or ΔFosB regulation of a gene's promoter activity in cell culture. This is unsatisfying because mechanisms of transcription regulation show dramatic variations from cell type to cell type, leaving it virtually completely unknown how a drug of abuse, or ΔFosB, regulate their specific genes in the brain *in vivo*.

Studies of epigenetic mechanisms make it possible, for the first time, to push the envelope one step further and directly examine transcriptional regulation in the brains of behaving animals (Tsankova et al. 2007). Historically, the term epigenetics describes mechanisms by which cellular traits can be inherited without a change in DNA sequence. We use the term more broadly to encompass 'the structural adaptation of chromosomal regions so as to register, signal, or perpetuate altered activity states' (Bird 2007). Thus, we now know that the activity of genes is controlled by the covalent modification (e.g. acetylation, methylation) of histones in the genes' vicinity and the recruitment of diverse types of coactivators or corepressors of transcription. Chromatin immunoprecipitation (ChIP) assays make it is possible to take advantage of this growing knowledge of chromatin biology to determine the activation state of a gene in a particular brain region of an animal treated with a drug of abuse (Renthal and Nestler 2008).

Examples of how studies of chromatin regulation can help us understand the detailed molecular mechanisms of action of cocaine and ΔFosB are given in Fig. 14.3. As stated above, ΔFosB can function as either a transcriptional activator or repressor depending on the target gene involved. To gain insight into these actions, we analyzed the chromatin state of two representative gene targets for ΔFosB, *cdk5* that is induced by ΔFosB and *c-fos* that is repressed, in nucleus accumbens. Chromatin immunoprecipitation studies demonstrated that cocaine activates the *cdk5* gene in this brain region through the following cascade: ΔFosB binds to the *cdk5* gene and then recruits histone acetyltransferases (which acetylate nearby histones) and SWI-SNF factors; both actions promote gene transcription (Kumar et al. 2005; Levine et al. 2005). Chronic cocaine further augments histone acetylation through the phosphorylation and inhibition of histone deacetylases (which normally deactylate and repress genes) (Renthal et al. 2007). In contrast, cocaine represses the *c-fos* gene: when ΔFosB binds to this gene, it recruits histone deacetylases and histone methyltransferases (which methylate nearby histones) and thereby inhibits c-Fos transcription (Fig. 14.3) (Renthal et al. 2008). A central question is what determines whether ΔFosB activates or represses a gene when it binds to that gene's promoter.

Activation of the *cdk*5 gene by ΔFosB

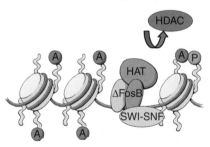

Repression of the *c-fos* gene by ΔFosB

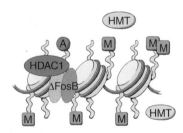

Fig. 14.3 Epigenetic mechanisms of ΔFosB action. The figure illustrates the very different consequences when ΔFosB binds to a gene that it activates (e.g. *cdk5*) versus represses (e.g. *c-fos*). At the *cdk5* promoter [*Top*], ΔFosB recruits histone acetyltransferases (HAT) and SWI-SNF factors, which promote gene activation. There is also evidence for exclusion of histone deacetylases (HDAC) (see text). In contrast, at the *c-fos* promoter [*Bottom*], ΔFosB recruits HDACs as well as histone methytransferases (HMT), which repress gene expression. A, P, and M depict histone acetylation, phosphorylation, and methylation, respectively.

These early studies of epigenetic mechanisms of drug addiction are exciting because they promise to reveal fundamentally new information concerning the molecular mechanisms by which drugs of abuse regulate gene expression in nucleus accumbens and other brain regions. Combining DNA expression arrays with so-called ChIP on chip assays (where alterations in chromatin structure or transcription factor binding can be analyzed genome-wide) will lead to the identification of drug and ΔFosB target genes with much greater levels of confidence and completeness (Kumar et al. 2007). In addition, epigenetic mechanisms are particularly attractive candidates to mediate the very long-lived phenomena central to a state of addiction. In this way, drug- and ΔFosB-induced changes in histone modifications and related epigenetic alterations provide potential mechanisms by which transcriptional changes can persist long after drug exposure ceases and perhaps even after ΔFosB degrades to normal levels.

14.9 Conclusions

The pattern of induction of ΔFosB in nucleus accumbens by chronic exposure to natural rewards, stress, or drugs of abuse raises an interesting hypothesis concerning the protein's normal functioning in this brain region. As depicted in Fig. 14.2, there is an appreciable level of ΔFosB in nucleus accumbens under normal conditions. This is unique to striatal regions, as ΔFosB is virtually undetectable elsewhere throughout brain at baseline. We hypothesize that levels of ΔFosB in nucleus accumbens represent a readout of an individual's exposure to emotional stimuli, both positive and negative, integrated over relatively long periods of time, given the temporal properties of the protein. The partial differences in the cellular specificity of ΔFosB induction by rewarding vs. aversive stimuli are poorly understood, and further work is needed to elucidate the functional consequences of these distinctions. We hypothesize further that as higher levels of emotional stimulation induce more ΔFosB in nucleus accumbens neurons, the neurons' functioning is altered so that they become more sensitive to rewarding stimuli. In this way, induction of ΔFosB would promote reward-related (i.e. emotional) memory through afferent projects of the nucleus accumbens. Under normal circumstances, induction of moderate levels of ΔFosB by rewarding or aversive stimuli would be adaptive by enhancing an animal's adjustments to environmental challenges. However, the excessive induction of ΔFosB seen under pathological conditions (e.g. chronic exposure to a drug of abuse) would lead to excessive sensitization of the nucleus accumbens circuitry and ultimately contribute to pathological behaviours (e.g. compulsive drug seeking and taking) associated with drug addiction. ΔFosB induction in other brain regions would presumably contribute to distinct aspects of an addicted state, as suggested by recent findings of ΔFosB action in orbitofrontal cortex.

If this hypothesis is correct, it raises the interesting possibility that levels of ΔFosB in nucleus accumbens or perhaps other brain regions could be used as a biomarker to assess the state of activation of an individual's reward circuitry, as well as the degree to which an individual is 'addicted', both during the development of an addiction and its gradual waning during extended withdrawal or treatment. The use of ΔFosB as a marker of a state of addiction has been demonstrated in animal models. Adolescent animals show much greater induction of ΔFosB compared to older animals, consistent with their greater vulnerability for addiction (Ehrlich et al. 2002). As well, attenuation of the rewarding effects of nicotine with a $GABA_B$ receptor positive allosteric modulator is associated with the blockade of nicotine induction of ΔFosB in nucleus accumbens (Mombereau et al. 2007). Although highly speculative, it is conceivable that a small molecule PET ligand, with high affinity for ΔFosB, could be used to help diagnosis addictive disorders as well as monitor progress during treatment.

Finally, ΔFosB itself, or any of the numerous genes it regulates—identified through DNA expression arrays or ChIP on chip assays—represent potential targets for the development of fundamentally novel treatments for drug addiction. We believe it is imperative to look beyond traditional drug targets (e.g. neurotransmitter receptors and transporters) for potential treatment agents for addiction. The genome-wide transcriptional maps capable with today's advanced technologies provide a promising source of such novel targets in our efforts to better treat and ultimately cure addictive disorders.

References

Alibhai, I. N., Green, T. A., Potashkin, J. A. & Nestler, E. J. 2007 Regulation of *fosB* and *ΔfosB* mRNA expression: in vivo and in vitro studies. *Brain Res* **1143**, 22–33.

Ang, E., Chen, J. S., Zagouras, P. et al. 2001 Induction of NFκB in nucleus accumbens by chronic cocaine administration. *J Neurochem* **79**, 221–24.

Asanuma, M. & Cadet, J. L. 1998 Methamphetamine-induced increase in striatal NF-kappaB DNA-binding activity is attenuated in superoxide dismutase transgenic mice. *Mol Brain Res* **60**, 305–9.

Berton, O., Covington, H. E., Ebner, K. et al. 2007 Induction of ΔFosB in the periaqueductal gray by stress promotes active coping responses. *Neuron* **55**, 289–300.

Bibb, J. A., Chen, J. S., Taylor, J. R. et al. 2001 Effects of chronic exposure to cocaine are regulated by the neuronal protein Cdk5. *Nature* **410**, 376–80.

Bird, A. 2007 Perceptions of epigenetics. *Nature* **447**, 396–8.

Carle, T. L., Ohnishi, Y. N., Ohnishi, Y. H. et al. 2007 Absence of conserved C-terminal degron domain contributes to ΔFosB's unique stability. *Eur J Neurosci* **25**, 3009–19.

Carlezon, W. A., Jr., Duman, R. S., & Nestler, E. J. 2005. The many faces of CREB. *Trends Neurosci* **28**, 436–45.

Cenci, M. A. 2002 Transcription factors involved in the pathogenesis of L-DOPA-induced dyskinesia in a rat model of Parkinson's disease. *Amino Acids* **23**, 105–9.

Chen, J. S., Kelz, M. B., Hope, B. T., Nakabeppu, Y., & Nestler, E. J. 1997 Chronic FRAs: Stable variants of ΔFosB induced in brain by chronic treatments. *J Neurosci* **17**, 4933–41.

Chen, J., Kelz, M. B., Hope, B. T., Nakabeppu, Y. & Nestler, E. J. 1997 Chronic FRAs: Stable variants of ΔFosB induced in brain by chronic treatments. *J Neurosci* **17**, 4933–41.

Chen, J. S., Nye, H. E., Kelz, M. B. et al. 1995 Regulation of ΔFosB and FosB-like proteins by electroconvulsive seizure (ECS) and cocaine treatments. *Mol Pharmacol* **48**, 880–9.

Chen, J. S., Zhang, Y. J., Kelz, M. B. et al. 2000 Induction of cyclin-dependent kinase 5 in hippocampus by chronic electroconvulsive seizures: role of ΔFosB. *J Neurosci* **20**, 8965–71.

Chen, J., Newton, S. S., Zeng, L. et al. 2003 Downregulation of the CCAAT-enhancer binding protein beta in DeltaFosB transgenic mice and by electroconvulsive seizures. *Neuropsychopharmacology* **29**, 23–31.

Colby, C. R., Whisler, K., Steffen, C., Nestler, E. J. & Self, D. W. 2003 ΔFosB enhances incentive for cocaine. *J Neurosci* **23**, 2488–93.

Deroche-Gamonet, V., Sillaber, I., Aouizerate, B. et al. 2003 The glucocorticoid receptor as a potential target to reduce cocaine abuse. *J Neurosci* **23**, 4785–90.

Dobrazanski, P., Noguchi, T., Kovary, K., Rizzo, C. A., Lazo, P. S. & Bravo, R. 1991 Both products of the fosB gene, FosB and its short form, FosB/SF, are transcriptional activators in fibroblasts. *Mol Cell Biol* **11**, 5470–8.

Ehrlich, M. E., Sommer, J., Canas, E. & Unterwald, E. M. 2002 Periadolescent mice show enhanced DeltaFosB upregulation in response to cocaine and amphetamine. *J Neurosci* **22**, 9155–9.

Graybiel, A. M., Moratalla, R. & Robertson, H. A. 1990 Amphetamine and cocaine induce drug-specific activation of the c-fos gene in striosome-matrix compartments and limbic subdivisions of the striatum. *Proc Natl Acad Sci USA* **87**, 6912–16.

Green, T. A., Alibhai, I. N., Hommel, J. D., et al. 2006. Induction of ICER expression in nucleus accumbens by stress or amphetamine increases behavioral responses to emotional stimuli. *J Neurosci* **26**, 8235–42

Green, T. A., Alibhai, I. N., Unterberg, S., et al. 2008. Induction of activating transcription factors ATF2, ATF3, and ATF4 in the nucleus accumbens and their regulation of emotional behavior. *J Neurosci* **28**, 2025–32.

Hiroi, N., Brown, J., Haile, C., Ye, H., Greenberg, M. E. & Nestler, E. J. 1997 FosB mutant mice: loss of chronic cocaine induction of Fos-related proteins and heightened sensitivity to cocaine's psychomotor and rewarding effects. *Proc Natl Acad Sci USA* **94**, 10397–402.

Hiroi, N., Brown, J., Ye, H. et al. 1998 Essential role of the fosB gene in molecular, cellular, and behavioral actions of electroconvulsive seizures. *J Neurosci* **18**, 6952–62.

Hope, B., Kosofsky, B., Hyman, S. E. & Nestler, E. J. 1992 Regulation of IEG expression and AP-1 binding by chronic cocaine in the rat nucleus accumbens. *Proc Natl Acad Sci USA* **89**, 5764–8.

Hope, B. T., Nye, H. E., Kelz, M. B. et al. 1994 Induction of a long-lasting AP-1 complex composed of altered Fos-like proteins in brain by chronic cocaine and other chronic treatments. *Neuron* **13**, 1235–44.

Jorissen, H., Ulery, P., Henry, L., Gourneni, S., Nestler, E. J. & Rudenko, G. 2007 Dimerization and DNA-binding properties of the transcription factor deltaFosB. *Biochemistry* **46**, 8360–72.

Kalivas, P. W. & Volkow, N. D. 2005 The neural basis of addiction: a pathology of motivation and choice. *Am J Psychiatry* **162**, 1403–13.

Kauer, J. A. & Malenka, R. C. 2007 Synaptic plasticity and addiction. *Nature Rev Neurosci* **8**, 844–58.

Kelz, M. B., Chen, J. S., Carlezon, W. A. et al. 1999 Expression of the transcription factor ΔFosB in the brain controls sensitivity to cocaine. *Nature* **401**, 272–6.

Kumar, A., Choi, K.-H., Renthal, W. et al. (2005) Chromatin remodeling is a key mechanism underlying cocaine-induced plasticity in striatum. *Neuron* **48**, 303–14.

Kumar, A., Sikder, D., Renthal, W. et al. (2007) Genome-wide epigenetic changes underlying chronic cocaine-induced neuroadaptations in the mouse nucleus accumbens. *Soc Neurosci Abs* 767.5.

Lee, K. W., Kim, Y., Kim, A. M., Helmin, K., Nairn, A. C. & Greengard, P. 2006 Cocaine-induced dendritic spine formation in D1 and D2 dopamine receptor-containing medium spiny neurons in nucleus accumbens. *Proc Natl Acad Sci USA* **103**, 3399–404.

Levine, A., Guan, Z., Barco, A., Xu, S., Kandel, E. & Schwartz, J. 2005 CREB-binding protein controls response to cocaine by acetylating histones at the fosB promoter in the mouse striatum. *Proc Natl Acad Sci USA* **102**, 19186–91.

Mackler, S. A., Korutla, L., Cha, X. Y. et al. 2000 NAC-1 is a brain POZ/BTB protein that can prevent cocaine-induced sensitization in the rat. *J Neurosci* **20**, 6210–17.

Liu, H. F., Zhou, W. H., Zhu, H. Q., Lai, M. J. & Chen, W. S. 2007 Microinjection of M(5) muscarinic receptor antisense oligonucleotide into VTA inhibits FosB expression in the NAc and the hippocampus of heroin sensitized rats. *Neurosci Bull* **23**, 1–8.

McClung, C. A. & Nestler, E. J. 2003 Regulation of gene expression and cocaine reward by CREB and ΔFosB. *Nature Neurosci* **11**, 1208–15.

McClung, C. A., Ulery, P. G., Perrotti, L. I., Zachariou, V., Berton, O. & Nestler, E. J. 2004 ΔFosB: A molecular switch for long-term adaptation in the brain. *Mol Brain Res* **132**, 146–54.

McDaid, J., Dallimore, J. E., Mackie, A. R. & Napier, T. C. 2006a Changes in accumbal and pallidal pCREB and deltaFosB in morphine-sensitized rats: correlations with receptor-evoked electrophysiological measures in the ventral pallidum. *Neuropsychopharmacology* **31**, 1212–26.

McDaid, J., Graham, M. P. & Napier, T. C. 2006b Methamphetamine-induced sensitization differentially alters pCREB and Delta-FosB throughout the limbic circuit of the mammalian brain. *Mol Pharmacol* **70**, 2064–74.

Mombereau, C., Lhuillier, L., Kaupmann, K. & Cryan J. F. 2007 GABAB receptor-positive modulation-induced blockade of the rewarding properties of nicotine is associated with a reduction in nucleus accumbens DeltaFosB accumulation. J Pharmacol Exp Ther 321, 172–7.

Moratalla, R., Elibol, R., Vallejo, M. & Graybiel, A. M. 1996 Network-level changes in expression of inducible Fos-Jun proteins in the striatum during chronic cocaine treatment and withdrawal. *Neuron* **17**, 147–56.

Morgan, J. I. & Curran, T. 1995 Immediate-early genes: ten years on. *Trends Neurosci* **18**, 66–7.

Muller, D. L. & Unterwald, E. M. 2005 D1 dopamine receptors modulate deltaFosB induction in rat striatum after intermittent morphine administration. *J Pharmacol Exp Ther* **314**, 148–55.

Nakabeppu, Y. & Nathans, D. 1991 A naturally occurring truncated form of FosB that inhibits Fos/Jun transcriptional activity. *Cell* **64**, 751–9.

Nestler, E. J. 2001 Molecular basis of long-term plasticity underlying addiction. *Nature Rev Neurosci* **2**, 119–28.

Norrholm, S. D., Bibb, J. A., Nestler, E. J., Ouimet, C. C., Taylor, J. R., & Greengard, P. 2003 Cocaine-induced proliferation of dendritic spines in nucleus accumbens is dependent on the activity of the neuronal kinase Cdk5. *Neuroscience* **116**, 19–22.

Nye, H., Hope, B. T., Kelz, M., Iadarola, M. & Nestler, E. J. 1995 Pharmacological studies of the regulation by cocaine of chronic Fra (Fos-related antigen) induction in the striatum and nucleus accumbens. *J Pharmacol Exp Ther* **275**, 1671–80.

Nye, H. E. & Nestler, E. J. 1996 Induction of chronic Fras (Fos-related antigens) in rat brain by chronic morphine administration. *Mol Pharmacol* **49**, 636–45.

O'Donovan, K. J., Tourtellotte, W. G., Millbrandt, J. & Baraban, J. M. 1999 The EGR family of transcription-regulatory factors: progress at the interface of molecular and systems neuroscience. *Trends Neurosci* **22**, 167–73.

Olausson, P., Jentsch, J. D., Tronson, N., Neve, R., Nestler, E. J. & Taylor, J. R. 2006 ΔFosB in the nucleus accumbens regulates food-reinforced instrumental behavior and motivation. *J Neurosci* **26**, 9196–204.

Peakman, M. C., Colby, C., Perrotti, L. I. et al. 2003 Inducible, brain region specific expression of a dominant negative mutant of c-Jun in transgenic mice decreases sensitivity to cocaine. *Brain Res* **970**, 73–86.

Perrotti, L. I., Bolaños, C. A., Choi, K.-H. et al. 2005 ΔFosB accumulates in a GABAergic cell population in the posterior tail of the ventral tegmental area after psychostimulant treatment. *Eur J Neurosci* **21**, 2817–24.

Perrotti, L. I., Hadeishi, Y., Ulery, P. et al. 2004 Induction of ΔFosB in reward-related brain regions after chronic stress. *J Neurosci* **24**, 10594–602.

Perrotti, L. I., Weaver, R. R., Robison, B. et al. 2008 Distinct patterns of ΔFosB induction in brain by drugs of abuse. *Synapse* **62**, 358–369.

Picetti, R., Toulemonde, F., Nestler, E. J., Roberts, A. J. & Koob, G. F. 2001 Ethanol effects in ΔFosB transgenic mice. *Soc Neurosci Abs* 745.16

Pich, E. M., Pagliusi, S. R., Tessari, M., Talabot-Ayer, D., hooft van Huijsduijnen, R. & Chiamulera, C. 1997 Common neural substrates for the addictive properties of nicotine and cocaine. *Science* **275**, 83–86.

Renthal, W., Carle, T. L., Maze, I. et al. 2008 ΔFosB mediates epigenetic desensitization of the *c-fos* gene after chronic amphetamine. *J Neurosci* **28**, 7344–9.

Renthal, W. & Nestler, E. J. 2008 Epigenetic mechanisms of drug addiction. *Trends Mol Med* **14**, 341–50.

Renthal, W., Maze, I., Krishnan, V. et al. 2007 Histone deacetylase 5 epigenetically controls behavioral adaptations to chronic emotional stimuli. *Neuron* **56**, 517–29.

&Robinson, T. E. & Kolb, B. 2004 Structural plasticity associated with exposure to drugs of abuse. *Neuropharmacology* **47**, S33–46.

Russo, S. J., Renthal, W., Kumar, A. et al. 2007 NFκB signaling regulates cocaine-induced behavioral and cellular plasticity. *Soc Neurosci Abs* 611.5.

Shaffer, H. J. & Eber, G. B. 2002 Temporal progression of cocaine dependence symptoms in the US National Comorbidity Survey. *Addiction* **97**, 543–54.

Shippenberg, T. S. & Rea, W. 1997 Sensitization to the behavioral effects of cocaine: modulation by dynorphin and kappa-opioid receptor agonists. *Pharmacol Biochem Behav* **57**, 449–55

Taylor, J. R., Lynch, W. J., Sanchez, H., Olausson, P., Nestler, E. J. & Bibb, J. A. 2007 Inhibition of Cdk5 in the nucleus accumbens enhances the locomotor activating & incentive motivational effects of cocaine. *Proc Natl Acad Sci USA* **104**, 4147–52.

Teegarden, S. L. & Bale, T. L. 2007 Decreases in dietary preference produce increased emotionality and risk for dietary relapse. *Biol Psychiatry* **61**, 1021–9.

Teegarden, S. L., Nestler, E. J. & Bale, T. L. 2008 ΔFosB-mediated alterations in dopamine signaling are normalized by a palatable high fat diet. *Biol Psychiatry* **64**, 941–50.

Tsankova, N., Renthal, W., Kumar, A. & Nestler, E. J. 2007 Epigenetic regulation in psychiatric disorders. *Nature Rev Neurosci* **8**, 355–67.

Ulery, P. G., Rudenko, G. & Nestler, E. J. 2006 Regulation of ΔFosB stability by phosphorylation. *J Neurosci* **26**, 5131–42.

Ulery, P. G. & Nestler, E. J. 2007 Regulation of ΔFosB transcriptional activity by ser27 phosphorylation. *Eur J Neurosci* **25**, 224–30.

Vialou, V. F., Steiner, M. A., Krishnan, V., Berton, O. & Nestler, E. J. 2007 Role of deltaFosB in the nucleus accumbens in chronic social defeat. *Soc Neurosci Abs* 98.3.

Wallace, D., Vialou, V., Rios, L. et al. 2008 The influence of ΔFosB in the nucleus accumbens on natural reward-related behavior. *J Neurosci* **28**, 10272–7.

Werme, M., Messer, C., Olson, L. et al. 2002 ΔFosB regulates wheel running. *J Neurosci* **22**, 8133–8.

Winstanley, C. A., Bachtell, R. K., Theobald, D. E. H. et al. 2009 Increased impulsivity during withdrawal from cocaine self-administration: Role for ΔFosB in the orbitofrontal cortex. *Cerebral Cortex* **19**, 435–44.

Winstanley, C. A., LaPlant, Q., Theobald, D. E. H. et al. 2007 ΔFosB induction in orbitofrontal cortex mediates tolerance to cocaine-induced cognitive dysfunction. *J Neurosci* **27**, 10497–507.

Yen, J., Wisdom, R. M., Tratner, I. & Verma, I. M. 1991 An alternative spliced form of FosB is a negative regulator of transcriptional activation and transformation by Fos proteins. *Proc Natl Acad Sci USA* **88**, 5077–81.

Young, S. T., Porrino, L. J. & Iadarola, M. J. 1991 Cocaine induces striatal c-fos-immunoreactive proteins via dopaminergic D1 receptors. *Proc Natl Acad Sci USA* **88**, 1291–5.

Zachariou, V., Bolanos, C. A., Selley, D. E. et al. 2006 An essential role for ΔFosB in the nucleus accumbens in morphine action. *Nature Neurosci* **9**, 205–11.

15

Parallel studies of neural and cognitive impairment in humans and monkeys

Linda J. Porrino,* Colleen A. Hanlon, Kathryn E. Gill, and Thomas J.R. Beveridge

Cocaine users display profound impairments in executive function. Of all the components of executive function, inhibition, or the ability to withhold responding, has been studied most extensively and may be most impaired. Consistent with these deficits, evidence from imaging studies points to dysregulation in medial and ventromedial prefrontal cortex, areas activated during performance of inhibition tasks. Other aspects of executive function including updating, shifting, and decision-making are also deficient in cocaine users, and these deficits are paralleled by abnormalities in patterns of prefrontal cortical activation. The extent to which cocaine plays a role in these effects, however, is not certain and cannot be determined solely on the basis of human studies. Investigations using a non-human primate model of increasing durations of cocaine exposure revealed that initially the effects of cocaine were restricted to ventromedial and orbital prefrontal cortex, but as exposure was extended, the intensity and spatial extent of the effects on functional activity also expanded rostrally and laterally. Given the spatial overlap in prefrontal pathology between human and monkey studies, these longitudinal mapping studies in non-human primates provide a unique window of understanding into the dynamic neural changes that are occurring early in human cocaine abuse.

Key Words: Cocaine; executive function; imaging; non-human primate; prefrontal cortex; functional activity.

There is considerable consensus that cocaine users suffer from significant neuropsychological impairments (Bolla et al. 1998; Cadet & Bolla 1996; Garavan & Hester 2007). Deficits in cognitive function can hinder the ability of substance abusers to benefit from treatment, especially those based on cognitive therapies, as well as impede the decision to enter treatment. Neuropsychological impairments may also impact the course of substance abuse by interfering with decisions about experimentation and continued drug seeking (Rogers & Robbins 2001).

Characterizing the nature and underlying causes of these deficits, however, has proven to be less than straightforward. There is little standardization of the batteries of neuropsychological and/or individual cognitive tests administered to substance abusers. Additionally, there are considerable differences across studies in the characteristics of the stimulant abusers included in terms of the duration and pattern of use, number of abstinence episodes, and the degree of drug use other than stimulants. This is compounded further by similar discrepancies in control populations as well as difficulties in matching user populations to controls on characteristics such as age, IQ, education, and socioeconomic status. Finally, the potential influence of pre-morbid psychiatric conditions on the cognitive performance of chronic cocaine users remains a significant confound that cannot be easily ruled out. Here we present a brief, non-comprehensive review of the profile of neuropsychological deficits associated with chronic cocaine abuse and the disruptions in functional brain activity associated with

* lporrino@wfubmc.edu

these deficits. This is followed by a comparison of these findings to those in a non-human primate model of cocaine self-administration.

15.1 Cognitive deficits exhibited by cocaine users

Cognitive impairments exhibited by chronic cocaine users are often related to problems in executive function. This is generally thought of as a group of processes involved in the learning, control, and monitoring of complex goal-directed behaviour (Garavan & Hester 2007; Stuss & Knight 2002; Teuber 1972). Executive functioning can be differentiated into three components: (1) updating, or the ability to monitor and update incoming information relevant to the task at hand, while discarding old information, (2) inhibition, or the ability to inhibit pre-potent, automatic, or impulsive responses, and (3) shifting, or the ability to shift mental sets back and forth between multiple tasks and operations (Miyake et al. 2000). Additionally, the process of decision-making has sometimes been identified as a separate component within the organization of executive function (Verdejo-Garcia & Perez-Garcia 2007), although decision-making tasks frequently combine some or all of the aforementioned elements. There is a growing body of literature describing the neuropsychological impairments of cocaine users on these four components of executive function, often relating the deficits to dysfunction in areas of the prefrontal cortex.

15.1.1 Updating

The executive function component of updating is typically measured by tasks that rely heavily on working memory, fluency, and analytic reasoning (c.f. Miyake et al. 2000; Verdejo-Garcia & Perez-Garcia 2007). More difficult tasks that tax working memory, such as the 2- and 3-back conditions on a standard n-back task, regularly elicit poor performance by substance abusers (Tomasi et al. 2007; Verdejo-Garcia et al. 2006), while less challenging tasks, such as sustained attention tasks, rarely yield differences between groups (Goldstein et al. 2007).

Hester & Garavan (2004) altered a classic Go/NoGo response inhibition task by embedding a working memory component into the presentation of the task. Increasing working memory load by increasing the number of letters to be remembered, from one to three to five in this case, significantly reduced the number of correct inhibitions in both cocaine users and healthy subjects. Controls, however, performed significantly better than cocaine users at all load levels and that advantage was amplified as working memory load increased (Hester & Garavan 2004). Recently, our group has used another measure of working memory function, the Delayed Match to Sample task (Fig. 15.1a), to examine the updating component of executive function in current cocaine users. Preliminary data indicate that cocaine users are not significantly impaired compared to age-matched controls at shorter delays, but perform more poorly than controls at longer delays (Hanlon et al., unpublished observations). These results are consistent with other findings that suggest significant impairments in working memory function, particularly as the load is increased.

These deficits in memory function of cocaine users appear to persist even during prolonged periods of abstinence (Di Sclafani et al. 2002; Verdejo-Garcia et al. 2006). At six weeks of abstinence, for example, crack-cocaine users performed more poorly than controls on attention tasks, memory tasks, reaction time tasks, and an analytic reasoning task. These results are striking in that the deficits in performance continue to be significant even after six

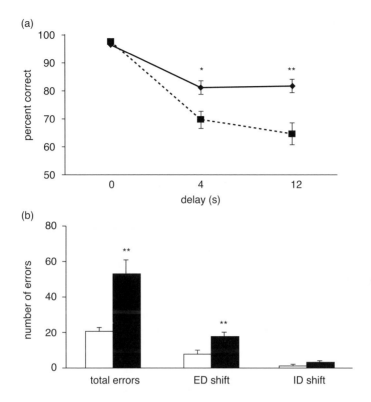

Fig. 15.1 Impaired performance on two tests of executive function by cocaine users ($n = 37$) and healthy controls ($n = 57$). (a) Percent correct on the Delayed Match to Sample task (working memory) at three delay intervals for cocaine users (dashed) and controls (solid). (b) Total errors on the Intra- and Extra-Dimensional Set Shift task (attentional set-shifting) in cocaine users (black) and controls (white). $*p < 0.05$, $**p < 0.005$, and t-test for independent groups.

months of abstinence in those subjects that did not relapse before the second test session (Di Sclafani et al. 2002; Verdejo-Garcia et al. 2006). This lack of recovery could imply that any neuroadaptations consequent to heavy cocaine use produce permanent behavioural and cognitive deficits. An alternate interpretation, however, might suggest that such deficits are symptomatic of differences in performance that pre-date any drug use. The absence of correlations between duration of use and degree of impairment might be considered support for the latter interpretation (but see conclusions).

15.1.2 Shifting

Cocaine users also display significant impairments in the shifting component of executive function. Here, tasks of probabilistic response reversal have been used to examine behavioural adaptation to changing reward contingencies (cf. Cools et al. 2002; Hornak et al. 2004). Chronic cocaine users have problems altering behaviour on such tasks after a change in the reward contingencies and tend to perseverate on previously rewarded responses (Ersche et al. 2008; Fillmore & Rush 2006). Other investigators have found that cocaine-dependent individuals perform more poorly than controls on tasks requiring switching within and between the modalities of verbal and visuospatial attention (Kubler et al. 2005). Recent data from our group indicate that cocaine users make significantly more errors on the Intra/Extra Dimensional Set Shifting task (Cambridge Cognition Ltd., Cambridge, UK) than healthy control participants (Fig. 15.1b). Users make the most errors on the extra-dimensional shift stage of the task (Hanlon et al., unpublished observations), which requires shifts not only of dimension of the current stimulus set, but across stimulus sets as well.

However, a number of studies have reported that there are, at most, only marginal differences in perseverative responding between cocaine users and healthy controls on the Wisconsin Card Sorting Task, another measure of set shifting behaviour (Bechara et al. 2000; Verdejo-Garcia et al. 2006). Yet, Bolla et al. (1999) did find significant negative correlations among the total dose of cocaine and the duration of use with the three outcome measures of the Wisconsin Card Sort task: categories completed, number of correct responses, and number of perseverations. As with the updating component of executive function, it is difficult to rule out the impact of antecedent differences in ability due to IQ or education or general life experience. Furthermore, the inconsistencies across reports may be due to differences in the characteristics of the cocaine user population, or to differences in the neural processes that are tapped into by Wisconsin Card Sorting and other set-shifting tasks.

15.1.3 Inhibition

This aspect of executive function is of particular interest since poor inhibitory control or an inability to gate inappropriate responses to external influences may increase the likelihood of risky behaviours such as drug seeking. One frequently used task to measure inhibitory control is the Go/NoGo task, in which subjects must respond to some stimuli while with-holding responses to others. One such study by Kaufman et al. (2003) observed that cocaine users made significantly more errors of commission on this task than healthy controls. Furthermore, other reports have shown that cocaine users not only exhibit impaired inhibi-tory control, but are also less aware of their errors than healthy controls. Thus they exhibit significantly more difficulty in adjusting their performance appropriately immediately after failing to inhibit a response (Hester et al. 2007).

Other groups, however, have reported that these deficits may be due to factors other than poor inhibition, such as a disruption of sensory information processing. In a Go/NoGo task of visual similarity, Go trials were defined as two identical images, easy NoGo trials were two obviously dissimilar images, and hard NoGo trials were two very similar images. Cocaine users were more impaired than controls on the most difficult NoGo trials only, leading to the conclusion that the response inhibition deficits were more likely to be caused by attentional processing deficits rather than an inability to inhibit responding (Lane et al. 2007).

The 'stop signal' paradigm is based on a cognitive model of control, which asserts that the ability to inhibit a response is determined by the outcome of competing activating and inhibitory processes elicited by cues to perform or withhold a response (Logan 1994; Logan et al. 1984). The task provides a measure of the time required by an individual to inhibit a pre-potent motor response (Chamberlain et al. 2006; Fillmore & Rush 2002). When tested on this task, cocaine users required more time to make inhibitory responses and had a significantly lower probability of inhibiting their responses than controls (Fillmore & Rush 2002). These data are more consistent with the concept that cocaine users have deficiencies in inhibitory control rather than in sensory processing. Compromised inhibitory control is the one aspect of deficient executive functioning about which there is the greatest degree of consensus. However, the question of whether this is due to cocaine exposure or to other factors remains unanswered. Indeed, pre-existing deficits in inhibitory control would be expected to increase the likelihood of drug experimentation and other risky behaviours.

15.1.4 Decision-making

Although not typically considered an element of executive function, decision-making tasks frequently combine multiple executive function processes. Poor performance on the Iowa Gambling Task (Bechara et al. 1994) or tasks such as the Cambridge Gambling Task (Rogers et al. 1999) could result from impairments of inhibitory control, set-shifting, and/or updating. Cocaine users perform very poorly on the Iowa Gambling Task relative to control partici- pants (Bechara et al. 2000; Stout et al. 2004; Verdejo-Garcia et al. 2007). Although controls tend to learn to make more advantageous choices over the course of the task, cocaine users continue to make choices that provide immediate gains, regardless of the losses accrued over time. Their poor performance on such tasks suggests that users are unable to process future negative consequences in the presence of an opportunity for immediate gratification. Again, such deficits might lead to increased likelihood of drug experimentation and vulnerability for addiction.

Neuropsychological dysfunction in cocaine abusers, then, is severe and widespread, spanning multiple components of executive function. These cognitive deficits may contrib- ute to onset of use, transition from recreational use to dependence, and the continuance of drug-seeking behaviours. They also may interfere with treatment programs that rely heavily on cognitive therapies for successful abstinence. Whether these deficits are the result of cocaine use, however, remains an unanswered question when so many other factors can impact cogni- tive function. Efforts to understand further the executive functioning deficits of cocaine users have led to examinations of brain function during performance of many cognitive tasks using neuroimaging methods.

15.2 Neuroanatomical substrates of cognitive deficits exhibited by cocaine users

Much of our understanding of the neurobiological consequences of chronic drug use in humans has come from imaging studies using positron emission tomography (PET) and functional magnetic resonance imaging (fMRI) to measure cerebral metabolism, blood flow, or blood volume. One consistent finding of these studies of chronic cocaine users is that of 'hypofrontality' or decreased function of the prefrontal cortex of cocaine abusers when compared to non-drug using controls. Numerous reports have demonstrated that cocaine users have lower rates of glucose utilization as measured with fluorodeoxyglucose and PET (Goldstein et al. 2004; Goldstein & Volkow 2002; Volkow et al. 1991, 1992, 2005). These depressed rates of functional activity have been reported to persist for up to 3 months of abstinence (Volkow et al. 1993), a finding that has been recently confirmed in our laboratory (Hanlon et al. 2006). In addition, disruptions in cerebral perfusion have also been consis- tently observed in prefrontal brain regions (Adinoff et al. 2003; Holman et al. 1991; Tucker et al. 2004; Tumeh et al. 1990; Weber et al. 1993). The majority of these studies, however, were conducted at rest when subjects were lying quietly in the scanner.

But then, what is the consequence of this 'hypofrontality' on executive function of cocaine users? Prefrontal cortex integrity is essential for executive function as demonstrated by investigations in both healthy adults and populations of patients with pathologies specific to the frontal cortex (Koechlin & Hyafil 2007; Robbins 2007; Salmon & Collette 2005). A number of recent neuroimaging studies of cocaine abusers have specifically addressed the role of prefrontal cortical dysfunction on the components of executive function: response inhibition, updating, set-shifting, and decision-making.

Perhaps the most well-studied component of executive function in cocaine users is response inhibition (Bolla et al. 2003; Goldstein et al. 2001; Hester & Garavan 2004; Kaufman et al. 2003). In healthy controls, performance on tasks such as the Go/NoGo task that require the inhibition of a pre-potent response is accompanied by activation in the anterior cingulate (Bush et al. 2000; Hester & Garavan 2004; Kaufman et al. 2003), dorsolateral prefrontal (Blasi et al. 2006; Garavan et al. 1999), inferior frontal (Aron et al. 2003), and orbitofrontal cortices (Horn et al. 2003). Cocaine users, however, have consistently lower levels of activity in the anterior cingulate and medial prefrontal cortex while performing such tasks (Kaufman et al. 2003). On other tasks requiring inhibitory control such as the Stroop task, cocaine users perform more poorly and exhibit decreased cerebral glucose metabolism in the orbitofrontal cortex as compared to controls (Goldstein et al. 2001). Furthermore, baseline levels of glucose metabolism in the orbitofrontal cortex were positively correlated with task performance (Goldstein et al. 2001), thus baseline function could predict task accuracy. This positive correlation between orbitofrontal function and Stroop performance may provide some functional basis for the recent observation that better performance on this task predicts greater treatment compliance (Streeter et al. 2008).

The updating component of executive function is frequently investigated with paradigms that challenge working memory. A key variable in working memory tasks is the degree of cognitive demand or load. Higher loads are associated with longer durations of time that items need to remain in memory, as well as greater amounts of information that must be held in memory. In non-drug using individuals, higher working memory demands are associated with greater elevations in activity in the prefrontal and the anterior cingulate cortex (Barch et al 1998, Smith & Jonides 1999). Given that chronic cocaine users have impaired working memory performance (Dackis & O'Brien 2001; Goldstein et al. 2007; Kubler et al. 2003; O'Malley & Gawin 1990; Tomasi et al. 2007), investigations of the brain substrates of increasing cognitive load could provide insights into the function of the prefrontal cortex after cocaine abuse. A recent study by Hester and Garavan (2004) investigated the effects of varying working memory load on response inhibition performance in cocaine users. Relative to controls, the cocaine users had significantly lower activity in right prefrontal and the left anterior cingulate cortex when working memory demands were increased. This is consistent with results from our laboratory demonstrating that, as working memory demands increase, the deficits in dorsolateral prefrontal cortex activity in cocaine users relative to controls are amplified (Fig. 15.2). A similar study by Tomasi and colleagues (2007) that varied working memory load revealed that cocaine abstainers performed more poorly than controls with increasing load. Abstinent cocaine users had significantly lower activity in the dorsolateral prefrontal cortex compared to controls, a difference that was amplified with increasing memory load. Thus, these studies suggest that as working memory performance diminishes in cocaine users as a function of cognitive load, activity in the dorsolateral prefrontal cortex also decreases.

Performance of set-shifting tasks in healthy control populations is generally accompanied by increased functional activity within the anterior cingulate, orbitofrontal, and dorsolateral prefrontal cortices (Cools et al. 2004; Dias et al. 1996; Fellows & Farah 2003; Wager et al. 2005). Cocaine users, in contrast, exhibit *reduced* activity in both the anterior cingulate and medial prefrontal regions (Bolla et al. 2004; Kubler et al. 2005). Activity in the dorsolateral aspects of the prefrontal cortex, however, has not generally been found to differ

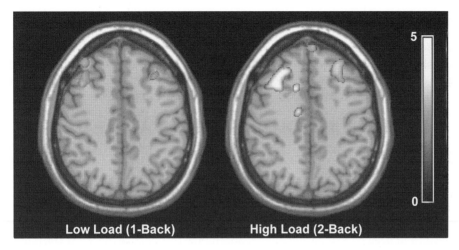

Fig. 15.2 (See also Plate 7) BOLD signal in the superior frontal gyrus is greater in non-drug using controls than cocaine users during performance of a standard verbal working memory task. This difference is amplified in conditions of higher cognitive demand (high load, right image). The color bar indicates *z* scores from the group-level analysis (Hanlon et al., unpublished observations).

significantly from that of controls (Kubler et al. 2005). The selective impairment of medial and ventral prefrontal regions of cocaine users suggests that, depending upon the processes tested, functional deficits associated with cocaine abuse may have a specific, rather than global, distribution within the prefrontal cortex.

Performance on the Iowa Gambling Task by healthy controls is associated with activity in the anterior cingulate cortex as well as dorsolateral prefrontal areas (Adinoff et al. 2003; Bechara et al. 2000, 2001; Bolla et al. 2003). Cocaine users have reduced functional activation relative to control participants in both the dorsolateral prefrontal cortex and rostral anterior cingulate, as well as greater activation in orbital prefrontal areas during gambling task performance (Bolla et al. 2003). Users with the lowest resting cerebral blood flow levels in the dorsolateral prefrontal cortex and anterior cingulate had the poorest task performance (Adinoff et al. 2003). The presence of these dorsolateral prefrontal functional abnormalities in cocaine users when performing the gambling task is in contrast to results from set-shifting studies, where there was little evidence for dorsolateral prefrontal disruption.

In summary, although cocaine users appear to have impaired processing throughout much of the prefrontal cortex, the most consistent deficits in functional activity are within ventromedial orbital and anterior cingulate cortex, regardless of the task, although there are also deficiencies in the dorsolateral prefrontal cortex, particularly in the more rostral portions of this region. Whether the deficits in these portions of the prefrontal cortex are the result of specific structural adaptations that accompany cocaine exposure or the result of disrupted connectivity with areas that have incurred damage remains an open question.

15.3 Addressing the confounds of human studies

Many of these investigations into the cognitive and neurobiological consequences of cocaine use often imply or assume that cocaine exposure is the cause of these deficits. However, the influence of factors such as concomitant psychiatric illness, lifestyle differences, and the use of multiple licit and illicit substances can be significant confounds in the interpretation of these data. Perhaps most difficult is assessing whether any of these impairments actually occur as a result of drug exposure itself or pre-date any drug experiences.

Because of these and many other problems, it is virtually impossible to isolate and address the issue of the consequences of chronic cocaine exposure in human populations. This is a critical question for treatment and prevention. An alternate approach to pursuing questions about the long-term effects of chronic exposure to drugs is the use of animal models in which carefully controlled experiments can be conducted. Animal models allow systematic evaluation of dose, session length, duration of experience, total lifetime intake, duration of abstinence, etc. Importantly, animal models allow us to assess the role of the drug itself on structure and function by directly examining the temporal course of drug exposure and the accompanying neuroadaptations. Using a non-human primate model of cocaine self-administration, our laboratory has investigated the long-term effects of chronic drug exposure.

Non-human primates have been used in intravenous self-administration studies for close to 60 years and have proved a valid and reliable model of human drug abuse (Griffiths et al. 1980; Johanson & Fischman 1989; Mello & Negus 1996; Thompson & Schuster 1964). Monkeys share cytoarchitectural, neurochemical, and ultrastructural similarities with humans, particularly with respect to the prefrontal cortex (Carmichael & Price 1994, 1996; Hardman et al. 2002; Porrino & Lyons 2000). Given that connectivity patterns of the prefrontal cortex are highly homologous to those of humans (Ongur et al. 2003) and monkeys can perform higher order cognitive tasks, non-human primates may provide insights into the psychiatric and cognitive deficits observed in human drug users.

Our current model of cocaine exposure makes use of rhesus monkeys initially trained to respond for food reinforcement. Once stable baselines are established, some animals remain on the food reinforcement schedule (controls), whereas others go on to self-administer cocaine on a similar schedule. Animals self-administer high doses of cocaine (9.0 mg/kg) daily for increasing durations, which are chosen to model different stages of the addiction process. With this model, we have been able to document significant dysregulation in neurotransmitter systems including increases in the density of norepinephrine (Beveridge et al. 2005) and dopamine transporters (Letchworth et al. 2001), increases in dopamine D_1 receptors (Nader et al. 2002), as well as decreases in the concentration of dopamine D_2 receptors (Nader et al. 2002). Thus, these studies have clearly shown that chronic exposure to cocaine in and of itself can produce substantial neuroadaptations in both brain structure and function over the temporal course of drug exposure.

15.4 Metabolic mapping of the functional consequences of chronic cocaine exposure in the prefrontal cortex of non-human primates

Important questions, then, are how functional activity within the prefrontal cortex has changed over the course of cocaine exposure, and how such changes might account for the cognitive impairments associated with cocaine use in human substance-abusing populations. To address this question, we have used the 2-[^{14}C]deoxyglucose method (2DG) to map the changes in cerebral metabolism after increasing durations of cocaine exposure. By assessing these changes in metabolism following the final infusion of cocaine at the end of a self-administration session, we are effectively measuring the response of the brain to a cocaine challenge in animals with different drug histories. Using this approach, we have been able to characterize alterations in the pattern and intensity of the changes in functional activity in the prefrontal cortex after increasing durations of cocaine self-administration experience: (1) initial exposure, designed to model the initial phases of drug exposure, when cocaine use is still considered casual or recreational (5 days of cocaine self-administration); (2) chronic exposure, designed to model the effects of repeated cocaine self-administration (3.3 months of self-administration); and (3) prolonged exposure, designed to more closely model investigations of human addicts in which the minimum inclusion criterion is typically at least one year of heavy use, and actual duration of use is frequently much longer (1.2 years of cocaine self-administration). We have recently undertaken a detailed re-analysis of the effects of cocaine on functional activity in the prefrontal cortex in order to map more carefully the topography of the initial effects and any potential shifts in this topography with continued exposure.

In the initial stages of drug exposure, cocaine produced a highly restricted pattern of changes in functional activity throughout the brain. Within the prefrontal cortex, significant decreases in cerebral metabolism were focused along the more caudal sectors of the medial wall in the gyrus rectus (area 14), cingulate areas 24 and 25, and caudal portions of area 32 (Fig. 15.3 (initial middle and caudal)). These regions have been shown to be involved in visceromotor functioning, providing cortical influence over autonomic and endocrine function (Price 1999). Decreases were also found in anterior insula cortex (area Ia), an area believed to be responsible for associations between taste and smell, specifically linking olfactory and

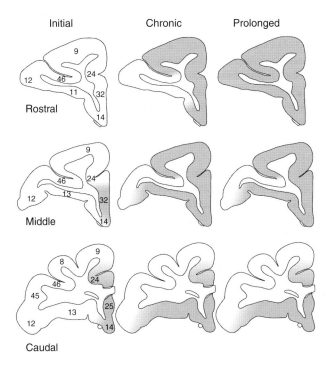

Fig. 15.3 Time course of effects on local cerebral glucose metabolism in prefrontal cortex of non-human primate brain at three levels (rostral, middle and caudal). Schematic diagram illustrating the spatial extent of the effects of increasing durations of cocaine self-administration histories on functional activity (initial, 5 days; chronic, 3.3 months; prolonged, 1.2 years). Areas shaded in grey represent regions exhibiting significant decreases in functional activity. Numbers represent Brodmann's areas.

gustatory cues to reward (Rolls 1996). These decreases were accompanied by increases in dorsomedial and dorsolateral portions of the prefrontal cortex (areas 45, 46, and 9). In primates as in humans, these regions are essential for working memory function (Baddeley 1986; Fuster 1997). These effects may result from a continuing representation of the drug-associated environment that persists beyond the end of the session. This continued activation at a time when access to cocaine has ceased may constitute the basis for the formation of memories for cues that can elicit cravings, even in abstinence. Thus, it appears that even in the initial stages of drug experience, cocaine may influence higher-order processing of converging sensory and visceral information, as well as the formation of associations between various stimuli with the presence of reward.

After chronic self-administration, however, adaptations to repeated cocaine exposure became evident. In these studies, monkeys had total intakes of at least 900 mg/kg of cocaine over more than a 3-month period. In contrast to the rather restricted pattern of changes in cerebral metabolism in the initial stages of exposure, the pattern after repeated exposure shifted to encompass larger expanses of the prefrontal cortex. In addition, the changes were greater in magnitude compared to earlier stages of cocaine experience. Although there was considerable overlap when comparing the initial and chronic stages along the medial wall of the prefrontal cortex (areas 14, 24, 25, and 32), the decreases extended rostrally into more anterior portions of the cingulate cortex (Fig. 15.3 (chronic rostral)). Furthermore, functional activity was altered in areas not seen previously, such as the orbitofrontal cortex (area 13), as well as caudal portions of area 12 (Fig. 15.3 (chronic middle and caudal)). These are areas that are critical for the processing of reward value and salience (Schultz et al. 2000; Tremblay & Schultz 2000). One other important difference at this time point was the absence of increases in cerebral metabolism. In fact, metabolism was decreased in portions of the dorsal prefrontal regions, suggesting that significant adaptations may be occurring within the dorsolateral prefrontal cortex as a result of the more chronic drug exposure.

Studies of the changes in functional activity associated with cocaine self-administration have recently been extended to include prolonged periods of cocaine exposure. The goal of these studies was to include durations of exposure more consistent with investigations of human addicts where subjects report extended periods of heavy use. In these studies, animals self-administered high doses of cocaine for a minimum of 300 sessions receiving on average of 2,700 mg/kg cocaine total intake. Although this data is still preliminary, glucose metabolism in the prolonged cocaine exposure group was significantly decreased in the medial and orbital regions of the prefrontal cortex, in a very similar pattern to that observed following chronic cocaine exposure (Fig. 15.3 (prolonged middle and caudal)). The overlap in terms of spatial extent between the two groups was striking. The only difference was an extension of functional changes into more rostral ventromedial and orbital cortex (areas 10, 11, and 12 (Fig. 15.3 (prolonged rostral)). Furthermore, there was very little change in the magnitude of the effects despite the much longer cocaine history.

15.5 Conclusions

Cocaine abusers have significant cognitive impairments that encompass all aspects of executive function. These deficits in cognitive performance are coincident with differences in functional activation observed throughout the prefrontal cortex of cocaine users when compared to healthy controls. It is difficult, however, to attribute these impairments directly to the consequences of chronic cocaine exposure on the basis of these data alone. Cognitive impairments can also be derived from concomitant psychiatric conditions, differences in lifestyle or educational experiences, as well as the use of other licit and illicit substances. Furthermore, it is not possible to rule out antecedent differences in function that may have impacted performance above and beyond the influence of cocaine itself. However, the shift in the functional consequences of cocaine use over time within the prefrontal cortex in the non-human primate model of drug exposure described here strongly supports the idea that cocaine is an important contributor to the significant impairments of cognitive performance experienced by drug users.

Our non-human primate studies have shown that the effects of cocaine are initially highly restricted to portions of the ventromedial prefrontal cortex, but with increasing experience and escalated intakes the effects rapidly spread rostrally and laterally to encompass the orbital and dorsolateral cortex. The increasing magnitude and the shift in topography of the alterations in functional activation in the prefrontal cortex after greater cocaine exposure parallel the association between cognitive decline and cocaine exposure reported in some studies in human users (Bolla et al. 2003, 1999; Colzato et al. 2007). Recently, Colzato et al. (2007) demonstrated a significant correlation between the magnitude of deficits in the performance of a stop-signal task and total lifetime cocaine intake. This study is of particular interest because these users were considered recreational. Their lifetime intakes were well within the range of those of the monkeys in the chronic stages of experience in our studies. Examining recreational users is distinct from most studies of cocaine users where the durations of use are often much longer. These studies, then, miss this dynamic period that we have identified as the time of most rapid adaptation.

After over a year of prolonged use, despite the fact that the duration of exposure to cocaine has been increased more than threefold, the alterations in functional activity do not continue to intensify or expand at the same rate as they had between the initial and chronic stages of drug exposure. Although the effects of chronic cocaine exposure undoubtedly continue to accumulate, they appear to do so at a much slower rate. This suggests that there may be a plateau in the rate of adaptations after a rapid acceleration early in the course of drug experience. Indeed, this may help to explain the frequent absence of positive correlations between duration of use and the degree of cognitive impairment in many studies, where the minimum reported drug use is often longer than one year and intakes are beyond those included even in these non-human primate studies.

One interesting aspect of the progression that has been identified is the growing involvement of frontopolar cortex (BA10) in the consequences of cocaine self-administration. Of all the areas of the orbitofrontal cortex, this region has undergone the greatest expansion in humans when compared to monkeys (Ongur et al. 2003). Both neuroimaging studies and lesion data have shown that this region of the prefrontal cortex is involved in prospective or intentional thinking and memory. Patients with lesions tend to have great difficulty remembering and developing intentions to act (Burgess et al. 2007). Other studies have pointed to this area as critical for exploratory decisions (Daw et al. 2006) where there is uncertainty about the outcomes of the selections. A recent paper has hypothesized that the frontopolar regions of cortex enable the considerations of multiple stimulus sets simultaneously, or so-called multi-tasking behaviour (Koechlin & Hyafil 2007). The common element in all of these functions is the ability to think about future events and anticipate consequences. It is easy to speculate how disruption of information processing in this brain region could impact decisions about drug use and impair treatment. The inability of substance abusers to consider potential future negative consequences is a hallmark characteristic of this disorder.

Although the imaging modalities and experimental designs vary, there is remarkable consistency in the spatial distribution of prefrontal cortical functional deficits in both the human and monkey literature. The anterior cingulate cortex, the medial prefrontal cortex, orbital frontal cortex, and to a lesser degree, the dorsolateral prefrontal cortex all appear to be affected after chronic cocaine use. In addition to the other limitations of human research, however, it is extremely difficult to assess the temporal progression of functional brain changes in human users. Instead, most imaging studies are performed on individuals that have been using cocaine for several years, a time point similar to that of our group of monkeys with the most cocaine experience. At this time point, we found that most of the prefrontal cortical brain changes had stabilized. The dynamic periods of functional alterations to chronic cocaine use are likely occurring early in use and before the typical user is enrolled in human imaging investigations. Given the spatial overlap in prefrontal pathology between human and monkey studies, these longitudinal mapping studies in non-human primates provide a unique window of understanding into the dynamic neural changes that occur early in human cocaine abuse, and may provide insights into the initial stages of the addiction process in humans.

Acknowledgements

This work was supported by NIH Grants DA09085, DA06634, and DA020074.

References

Adinoff, B., Devous, M. D., Sr., Cooper, D. B. et al. 2003 Resting regional cerebral blood flow and gambling task performance in cocaine-dependent subjects and healthy comparison subjects. *Am J Psychiatry* **160**, 1892–4.

Aron, A. R., Fletcher, P. C., Bullmore, E. T., Sahakian, B. J. & Robbins, T. W. 2003 Stop-signal inhibition disrupted by damage to right inferior frontal gyrus in humans. *Nat Neurosci* **6**, 115–16.

Baddeley, A. 1986 *Working Memory.* Oxford: Clarendon.

Barch, D. M., Braver, T. S., Nystrom, L. E., Forman, S. D., Noll, D. C. & Cohen, J. D.. 1998. Dissociating working memory from task difficulty in human prefrontal cortex *Neuropsychologia* **10,** 1373–80.

Bechara, A., Damasio, A. R., Damasio, H. & Anderson, S. W. 1994 Insensitivity to future consequences following damage to human prefrontal cortex. *Cognition* **50**, 7–15.

Bechara, A., Damasio, H. & Damasio, A. R. 2000 Emotion, decision making and the orbitofrontal cortex. *Cereb Cortex* **10**, 295–307.

Bechara, A., Dolan, S., Denburg, N., Hindes, A., Anderson, S. W. & Nathan, P. E. 2001 Decision-making deficits, linked to a dysfunctional ventromedial prefrontal cortex, revealed in alcohol and stimulant abusers. *Neuropsychologia* **39**, 376–89.

Beveridge, T. J., Smith, H. R., Nader, M. A. & Porrino, L. J. 2005 Effects of chronic cocaine self-administration on norepinephrine transporters in the nonhuman primate brain. *Psychopharmacology (Berl)* **180**, 781–8.

Blasi, G., Goldberg, T. E., Weickert, T. et al. 2006 Brain regions underlying response inhibition and interference monitoring and suppression. *Eur J Neurosci* **23**, 1658–64.

Bolla, K., Ernst, M., Kiehl, K. et al. 2004 Prefrontal cortical dysfunction in abstinent cocaine abusers. *J Neuropsychiatry Clin Neurosci* **16**, 456–64.

Bolla, K. I., Cadet, J. L. & London, E. D. 1998 The neuropsychiatry of chronic cocaine abuse. *J Neuropsychiatry Clin Neurosci* **10**, 280–9.

Bolla, K. I., Eldreth, D. A., London, E. D. et al. 2003 Orbitofrontal cortex dysfunction in abstinent cocaine abusers performing a decision-making task. *Neuroimage* **19**, 1085–94.

Bolla, K. I., Rothman, R. & Cadet, J. L. 1999 Dose-related neurobehavioral effects of chronic cocaine use. *J Neuropsychiatry Clin Neurosci* **11**, 361–9.

Burgess, P. W., Gilbert, S. J. & Dumontheil, I. 2007 Function and localization within rostral prefrontal cortex (area 10). *Philos Trans R Soc Lond B Biol Sci* **362**, 887–99.

Bush, G., Luu, P. & Posner, M. I. 2000 Cognitive and emotional influences in anterior cingulate cortex. *Trends Cogn Sci* **4**, 215–22.

Cadet, J. L. & Bolla, K. I. 1996 Chronic cocaine use as a neuropsychiatric syndrome: a model for debate. *Synapse* **22**, 28–34.

Carmichael, S. T. & Price, J. L. 1994 Architectonic subdivision of the orbital and medial prefrontal cortex in the macaque monkey. *J Comp Neurol* **346**, 366–402.

Carmichael, S. T. & Price, J. L. 1996 Connectional networks within the orbital and medial prefrontal cortex of macaque monkeys. *J Comp Neurol* **371**, 179–207.

Chamberlain, S. R., Muller, U., Blackwell, A. D., Clark, L., Robbins, T. W. & Sahakian, B. J. 2006 Neurochemical modulation of response inhibition and probabilistic learning in humans. *Science* **311**, 861–3.

Colzato, L. S., van den Wildenberg, W. P. & Hommel, B. 2007 Impaired inhibitory control in recreational cocaine users. *PLoS ONE* **2**, e1143.

Cools, R., Clark, L., Owen, A. M. & Robbins, T. W. 2002 Defining the neural mechanisms of probabilistic reversal learning using event-related functional magnetic resonance imaging. *J Neurosci* **22**, 4563–7.

Cools, R., Clark, L. & Robbins, T. W. 2004 Differential responses in human striatum and prefrontal cortex to changes in object and rule relevance. *J Neurosci* **24**, 1129–35.

Dackis, C. A. & O'Brien, C. P. 2001 Cocaine dependence: a disease of the brain's reward centers. *J Subst Abuse Treat* **21**, 111–17.

Daw, N. D., O'Doherty, J. P., Dayan, P., Seymour, B. & Dolan, R. J. 2006 Cortical substrates for exploratory decisions in humans. *Nature* **441**, 876–9.

Di Sclafani, V., Tolou-Shams, M., Price, L. J. & Fein, G. 2002 Neuropsychological performance of individuals dependent on crack-cocaine, or crack-cocaine and alcohol, at 6 weeks and 6 months of abstinence. *Drug Alcohol Depend* **66**, 161–71.

Dias, R., Robbins, T. W. & Roberts, A. C. 1996 Dissociation in prefrontal cortex of affective and attentional shifts. *Nature* **380**, 69–72.

Ersche, K. D., Roiser, J. P., Robbins, T. W. & Sahakian, B. J. 2008 Chronic cocaine but not chronic amphetamine use is associated with perseverative responding in humans. *Psychopharmacology (Berl)* **197**, 421–31.

Fellows, L. K. & Farah, M. J. 2003 Ventromedial frontal cortex mediates affective shifting in humans: evidence from a reversal learning paradigm. *Brain* **126**, 1830–7.

Fillmore, M. T. & Rush, C. R. 2002 Impaired inhibitory control of behavior in chronic cocaine users. *Drug Alcohol Depend* **66**, 265–73.

Fillmore, M. T. & Rush, C. R. 2006 Polydrug abusers display impaired discrimination-reversal learning in a model of behavioural control. *J Psychopharmacol* **20**, 24–32.

Fuster, J. 1997 *The prefrontal cortex. Anatomy, physiology and neuropsychology of the frontal lobe.* New York: Raven.

Garavan, H. & Hester, R. 2007 The role of cognitive control in cocaine dependence. *Neuropsychol Rev* **17**, 337–45.

Garavan, H., Ross, T. J. & Stein, E. A. 1999 Right hemispheric dominance of inhibitory control: an event-related functional MRI study. *Proc Natl Acad Sci U S A* **96**, 8301–6.

Goldstein, R. Z., Leskovjan, A. C., Hoff, A. L. et al. 2004 Severity of neuropsychological impairment in cocaine and alcohol addiction: association with metabolism in the prefrontal cortex. *Neuropsychologia* **42**, 1447–58.

Goldstein, R. Z., Tomasi, D., Alia-Klein, N., Zhang, L., Telang, F. & Volkow, N. D. 2007 The effect of practice on a sustained attention task in cocaine abusers. *Neuroimage* **35**, 194–206.

Goldstein, R. Z. & Volkow, N. D. 2002 Drug addiction and its underlying neurobiological basis: neuroimaging evidence for the involvement of the frontal cortex. *Am J Psychiatry* **159**, 1642–52.

Goldstein, R. Z., Volkow, N. D., Wang, G. J., Fowler, J. S. & Rajaram, S. 2001 Addiction changes orbitofrontal gyrus function: involvement in response inhibition. *Neuroreport* **12**, 2595–9.

Griffiths, R. R., Bigelow, G. E. & Henningfield, J. E. 1980 *Similarities in Animals and Huuman Drug-Taking Behavior. Advances in Substance Abuse.* Greenwich, CT: JAI Press.

Hanlon, C. A., Weisser, V. D., Livengood, L. B., Miller, M., Flowers, D. L. & Porrino, L. J. 2006 The effects of protracted cocaine abstinence on depression, cognitive planning and brain metabolism. In *College of Problems on Drug Dependence Annual Meeting.* Scottsdale: Arizona.

Hardman, C. D., Henderson, J. M., Finkelstein, D. I., Horne, M. K., Paxinos, G. & Halliday, G. M. 2002 Comparison of the basal ganglia in rats, marmosets, macaques, baboons, and humans: volume and neuronal number for the output, internal relay, and striatal modulating nuclei. *J Comp Neurol* **445**, 238–55.

Hester, R. & Garavan, H. 2004 Executive dysfunction in cocaine addiction: evidence for discordant frontal, cingulate, and cerebellar activity. *J Neurosci* **24**, 11017–22.

Hester, R., Simoes-Franklin, C. & Garavan, H. 2007 Post-error behavior in active cocaine users: poor awareness of errors in the presence of intact performance adjustments. *Neuropsychopharmacology* **32**, 1974–84.

Holman, B. L., Carvalho, P. A., Mendelson, J. et al. 1991 Brain perfusion is abnormal in cocaine-dependent polydrug users: a study using technetium-99m-HMPAO and ASPECT. *J Nucl Med* **32**, 1206–10.

Horn, N. R., Dolan, M., Elliott, R., Deakin, J. F. & Woodruff, P. W. 2003 Response inhibition and impulsivity: an fMRI study. *Neuropsychologia* **41**, 1959–66.

Hornak, J., O'Doherty, J., Bramham, J. et al. 2004 Reward-related reversal learning after surgical excisions in orbito-frontal or dorsolateral prefrontal cortex in humans. *J Cogn Neurosci* **16**, 463–78.

Johanson, C. E. & Fischman, M. W. 1989 The pharmacology of cocaine related to its abuse. *Pharmacol Rev* **41**, 3–52.

Kaufman, J. N., Ross, T. J., Stein, E. A. & Garavan, H. 2003 Cingulate hypoactivity in cocaine users during a GO-NOGO task as revealed by event-related functional magnetic resonance imaging. *J Neurosci* **23**, 7839–43.

Koechlin, E. & Hyafil, A. 2007 Anterior prefrontal function and the limits of human decision-making. *Science* **318**, 594–8.

Kubler, A., Murphy, K. & Garavan, H. 2005 Cocaine dependence and attention switching within and between verbal and visuospatial working memory. *Eur J Neurosci* **21**, 1984–92.

Kubler, A., Murphy, K., Kaufman, J., Stein, E. A. & Garavan, H. 2003 Co-ordination within and between verbal and visuospatial working memory: network modulation and anterior frontal recruitment. *Neuroimage* **20**, 1298–308.

Lane, S. D., Moeller, F. G., Steinberg, J. L., Buzby, M. & Kosten, T. R. 2007 Performance of cocaine dependent individuals and controls on a response inhibition task with varying levels of difficulty. *Am J Drug Alcohol Abuse* **33**, 717–26.

Letchworth, S. R., Nader, M. A., Smith, H. R., Friedman, D. P. & Porrino, L. J. 2001 Progression of changes in dopamine transporter binding site density as a result of cocaine self-administration in rhesus monkeys. *J Neurosci* **21**, 2799–807.

Logan, G. D. 1994 On the ability to inhibit thought and action: a users' guide to the stop-signal paradigm. In *Inhibitory Processes in Attention, Memory, and Language.* San Diego: Academic Press.

Logan, G. D., Cowan, W. B. & Davis, K. A. 1984 On the ability to inhibit simple and choice reaction time responses: a model and a method. *J Exp Psychol Hum Percept Perform* **10**, 276–91.

Mello, N. K. & Negus, S. S. 1996 Preclinical evaluation of pharmacotherapies for treatment of cocaine and opioid abuse using drug self-administration procedures. *Neuropsychopharmacology* **14**, 375–424.

Miyake, A., Friedman, N. P., Emerson, M. J., Witzki, A. H., Howerter, A. & Wager, T. D. 2000 The unity and diversity of executive functions and their contributions to complex "Frontal Lobe" tasks: a latent variable analysis. *Cognit Psychol* **41**, 49–100.

Nader, M. A., Daunais, J. B., Moore, T. et al. 2002 Effects of cocaine self-administration on striatal dopamine systems in rhesus monkeys: initial and chronic exposure. *Neuropsychopharmacology* **27**, 35–46.

O'Malley, S. S. & Gawin, F. H. 1990 Abstinence symptomatology and neuropsychological impairment in chronic cocaine abusers. *NIDA Res Monogr* **101**, 179–90.

Ongur, D., Ferry, A. T. & Price, J. L. 2003 Architectonic subdivision of the human orbital and medial prefrontal cortex. *J Comp Neurol* **460**, 425–49.

Porrino, L. J. & Lyons, D. 2000 Orbital and medial prefrontal cortex and psychostimulant abuse: studies in animal models. *Cereb Cortex* **10**, 326–33.

Price, J. L. 1999 Prefrontal cortical networks related to visceral function and mood. *Ann NY Acad Sci* **877**, 383–96.

Robbins, T. W. 2007 Shifting and stopping: fronto-striatal substrates, neurochemical modulation and clinical implications. *Philos Trans R Soc Lond B Biol Sci* **362**, 917–32.

Rogers, R. D., Owen, A. M., Middleton, H. C. et al. 1999 Choosing between small, likely rewards and large, unlikely rewards activates inferior and orbital prefrontal cortex. *J Neurosci* **19**, 9029–38.

Rogers, R. D. & Robbins, T. W. 2001 Investigating the neurocognitive deficits associated with chronic drug misuse. *Curr Opin Neurobiol* **11**, 250–7.

Rolls, E. T. 1996 The orbitofrontal cortex. *Philos Trans R Soc Lond B Biol Sci* **351**, 1433–43; discussion 1443–4.

Salmon, E. & Collette, F. 2005 Functional imaging of executive functions. *Acta Neurol Belg* **105**, 187–96.

Schultz, W., Tremblay, L. & Hollerman, J. R. 2000 Reward processing in primate orbitofrontal cortex and basal ganglia. *Cereb Cortex* **10**, 272–84.

Smith, E. E. & Jonides, J. 1999 Storage and executive processes in the frontal lobes. *Science* **5408**, 1657–61. Review.

Stout, J. C., Busemeyer, J. R., Lin, A., Grant, S. J. & Bonson, K. R. 2004 Cognitive modeling analysis of decision-making processes in cocaine abusers. *Psychon Bull Rev* **11**, 742–7.

Streeter, C. C., Terhune, D. B., Whitfield, T. H. et al. 2008 Performance on the Stroop predicts treatment compliance in cocaine-dependent individuals. *Neuropsychopharmacology* **33**, 827–36.

Stuss, D. T. & Knight, R. T. 2002 *Principles of Frontal Lobe Functioning.* New York: Oxford University Press.

Teuber, H. L. 1972 Unity and diversity of frontal lobe functions. *Acta Neurobiol Exp (Wars)* **32**, 615–56.

Thompson, T. & Schuster, C. R. 1964 Morphine self-administration, food-reinforced, and avoidance behaviors in rhesus monkeys. *Psychopharmacologia* **5**, 87–94.

Tomasi, D., Goldstein, R. Z., Telang, F. et al. 2007 Widespread disruption in brain activation patterns to a working memory task during cocaine abstinence. *Brain Res* **1171**, 83–92.

Tremblay, L. & Schultz, W. 2000 Modifications of reward expectation-related neuronal activity during learning in primate orbitofrontal cortex. *J Neurophysiol* **83**, 1877–85.

Tucker, K. A., Potenza, M. N., Beauvais, J. E., Browndyke, J. N., Gottschalk, P. C. & Kosten, T. R. 2004 Perfusion abnormalities and decision making in cocaine dependence. *Biol Psychiatry* **56**, 527–30.

Tumeh, S. S., Nagel, J. S., English, R. J., Moore, M. & Holman, B. L. 1990 Cerebral abnormalities in cocaine abusers: demonstration by SPECT perfusion brain scintigraphy. Work in progress. *Radiology* **176**, 821–4.

Verdejo-Garcia, A., Bechara, A., Recknor, E. C. & Perez-Garcia, M. 2006 Executive dysfunction in substance dependent individuals during drug use and abstinence: an examination of the behavioral, cognitive and emotional correlates of addiction. *J Int Neuropsychol Soc* **12**, 405–15.

Verdejo-Garcia, A., Benbrook, A., Funderburk, F., David, P., Cadet, J. L. & Bolla, K. I. 2007 The differential relationship between cocaine use and marijuana use on decision-making performance over repeat testing with the Iowa Gambling Task. *Drug Alcohol Depend* **90**, 2–11.

Verdejo-Garcia, A. & Perez-Garcia, M. 2007 Profile of executive deficits in cocaine and heroin polysubstance users: common and differential effects on separate executive components. *Psychopharmacology (Berl)* **190**, 517–30.

Volkow, N. D., Fowler, J. S., Wang, G. J. et al. 1993 Decreased dopamine D2 receptor availability is associated with reduced frontal metabolism in cocaine abusers. *Synapse* **14**, 169–77.

Volkow, N. D., Fowler, J. S., Wolf, A. P. et al. 1991 Changes in brain glucose metabolism in cocaine dependence and withdrawal. *Am J Psychiatry* **148**, 621–6.

Volkow, N. D., Hitzemann, R., Wang, G. J. et al. 1992 Long-term frontal brain metabolic changes in cocaine abusers. *Synapse* **11**, 184–90.

Volkow, N. D., Wang, G. J., Ma, Y. et al. 2005 Activation of orbital and medial prefrontal cortex by methylphenidate in cocaine-addicted subjects but not in controls: relevance to addiction. *J Neurosci* **25**, 3932–9.

Wager, T. D., Jonides, J., Smith, E. E. & Nichols, T. E. 2005 Toward a taxonomy of attention shifting: individual differences in fMRI during multiple shift types. *Cogn Affect Behav Neurosci* **5**, 127–43.

Weber, D. A., Franceschi, D., Ivanovic, M. et al. 1993 SPECT and planar brain imaging in crack abuse: iodine-123-iodoamphetamine uptake and localization. *J Nucl Med* **34**, 899–907.

16

Acute effects of cocaine on the neurobiology of cognitive control

Hugh Garavan,* Jacqueline N. Kaufman, and Robert Hester

Compromised ability to exert control over drug urges and drug-seeking behaviour is a characteristic of addiction. One specific cognitive control function, impulse control, has been shown to be a risk factor for the development of substance problems and has been linked in animal models to increased drug administration and relapse. We present evidence of a direct effect of cocaine on the neurobiology underlying impulse control. In a laboratory test of motor response inhibition, an intravenous cocaine administration improved task performance in 13 cocaine users. This improvement was accompanied by increased activation in right dorsolateral and inferior frontal cortex, regions considered critical for this cognitive function. Similarly, for both inhibitory control and action monitoring processes, cocaine normalized activation levels in lateral and medial prefrontal regions previously reported to be hypoactive in users relative to drug-naive controls. The acute amelioration of neurocognitive dysfunction may reflect a chronic dysregulation of those brain regions and the cognitive processes they subserve. Furthermore, the effects of cocaine on midline function suggest a dopaminergically mediated intersection between cocaine's acute reinforcing effects and its effects on cognitive control.

Key Words: Cocaine; impulsivity; functional magnetic resonance imaging; addiction.

16.1 Introduction

There is a growing appreciation that the compulsive behaviour of drug-dependent individuals may result, in part, from compromise in the cognitive processes that control behaviour (Moeller et al. 2001; Lubman et al. 2004). For example, among the core behaviours associated with drug abuse are disinhibition and an apparent loss of self-control (Lyvers 2000). Diagnostic criteria for substance dependence emphasize behavioural patterns of diminished control and drug use exceeding intended levels, consistent with compromised monitoring and inhibition of potentially harmful behaviour. Compromised impulse control might be expected to have significant consequences for an individual as it is a fundamental control process. Impulse control follows a developmental trajectory demarcating important cognitive milestones early in life and its diminution has been proposed to underlie many aspects of cognitive decline in the elderly (Diamond 1990; Perry & Hodges 1999). It represents an important element of individual differences in personality (Patton et al. 1995) and its dysfunction is associated with many clinical conditions including attention-deficit hyperactivity disorder (ADHD) (Barkley 1997; Rapport et al. 2001), schizophrenia (Carter et al. 2001) and mania (McGrath et al. 1997; Clark et al. 2001). The many manifestations of impulse control hint at it being a multifaceted construct. Typical measures of impulsivity include

* hugh.garavan@tcd.ie

perseverative behaviours, inability to delay gratification, inability to suppress prepotent responses, lack of premeditation prior to action, insufficient sampling of relevant information prior to decision making, resistance to extinction and more. As a consequence, investigations into the role of impulse control in addiction need to be cognizant of which particular aspect of the construct they are addressing as it is not yet clear to what extent these deficits are related, share common cognitive or neurobiological mechanisms or might coalesce to form a broad impulsive phenotype (Grant 2004).

Despite these conceptual uncertainties, there is evidence of addiction-related impairment in many of these different aspects of impulsivity suggesting that common (disrupted) mechanisms may be at play. For example, cocaine users show higher delayed discounting rates (Coffey et al. 2003; Simon et al. 2007), are slower or poorer at motor inhibition (Fillmore et al. 2002; Hester & Garavan 2004; Colzato et al. 2007), make riskier decisions on various gambling tasks (Bartzokis et al. 2000; Monterosso et al. 2001; Bolla et al. 2003; Fishbein et al. 2005; Verdejo-Garcia et al. 2007) and amphetamine users sample less of the available information prior to making decisions (Clark et al. 2006). A growing literature suggests both anatomical changes and functional dysregulation in lateral, ventral, and medial prefrontal cortex in chronic cocaine users (Volkowetal. 1993; Franklin et al. 2002). Anterior cingulate cortex (ACC) hypoactivity for performance monitoring processes has been demonstrated in chronic cocaine users (not currently under the influence of cocaine) when compared with non-using control participants (Kaufman et al. 2003); a similar effect has also been reported for opiate-dependent individuals (Forman et al. 2004) and cannabis users (Eldreth et al. 2004). Poor motor response inhibition in cocaine users has been associated with reduced activity in dorsolateral prefrontal cortex, insula, and the ACC, and increased activity in the cerebellum (Kaufman et al. 2003; Hester & Garavan 2004; Li et al. 2007). Stroop task performance has been associated with changes in orbitofrontal cortex in cocaine users (Goldstein et al. 2001).

One approach to understanding cocaine-related impairments on these cognitive control processes and their underlying neurobiology is to study the acute effects of a cocaine administration. Cocaine's powerful reinforcing properties have been well documented both experimentally and anecdotally (Johanson & Fischman 1989; Kuhar et al. 1991; Ahmed & Koob 1998). While research has focused primarily on elucidating the neurobiological mechanisms of cocaine's effects on putative reward systems, less research has explored the functional neuroanatomical regions associated with the cognitive changes that accompany cocaine use. Inhibitory control and action monitoring during and immediately after the consumption of cocaine are of particular importance as cocaine's stimulatory effects paired with its short half-life produce a physiological urge to seek more cocaine shortly after initial consumption. This urge may be facilitated by compromise in those cognitive processes involved in controlling behaviour. The present study aims to investigate cocaine's effects by identifying the cortical regions and psychological functions affected by an acute cocaine administration. Using a motor response inhibition task in which both motor impulsivity and the brain's response to errors can be assayed allows us to determine whether cocaine directly affects these processes thought central to controlling behaviour. In addition, the acute effects of cocaine on both brain function and cognitive control may suggest likely candidates for long-term impairment. Frequent drug-induced activation of these regions may lead to them subsequently being functionally downregulated, with negative consequences for the cognitive functions they perform (Garavan & Stout 2005).

16.2 Material and methods

16.2.1 Participants

Thirteen otherwise healthy, right-handed, active cocaine users (two female; mean age of 37 years, range of 21–45 years) participated in this study after providing written informed consent according to the procedures approved by the Medical College of Wisconsin's Institutional Review Board. Details on the screening and pretesting medical procedures are provided in the electronic supplementary material. Urine samples returned positive screens for cocaine or its metabolites, indicating that participants had used cocaine within the previous 72 hours. All users were able to estimate their last use, which ranged from 11 to 80 hours (average 36 hours) before the scan session; no user displayed overt behavioural signs of cocaine intoxication. The average amount of money spent on the last use of cocaine was $84 (range: $10–$400). Years of cocaine use ranged from 5 to 20 (average 12 years), and educational level ranged from 8 to 14 years (mean 12 years). A secondary follow-up comparison was also conducted, which included the data from 14 drug-naive controls from a previous study (10 females; mean age 30 years; range 19–45 years; Kaufman et al. 2003). All non-drug users had negative urine tests for all drugs.

16.2.2 Task and procedure

Task stimuli consisted of a 1 Hz serial visual stream of alternating letters X and Y (Garavan et al. 2002; Kaufman et al. 2003). Participants were instructed to press a button for each stimulus (Go trials) while still on screen. No-Go trials in which the stimuli did not alternate required inhibition of the response (i.e. participants would respond to each stimulus except the fifth in the sequence. … XYXYYX….). No-Go trials represented 6% (80 No-Go trials) of the total number of trials over four runs with task difficulty tailored for each participant by manipulating stimulus presentation rates (details in the electronic supplementary material). Go/No-Go runs were alternated with a simple event-related visuomotor finger-tapping task to be used as a measure of the effects of cocaine on the shape and size of the haemodynamic response function (Murphy et al. 2006). Cocaine-using participants completed both drug imaging sessions on the same day (drug order was counterbalanced), separated by approximately 2 hours. Each session comprised four Go/No-Go task runs alternated with two finger-tapping runs (see timeline in Fig. 16.1).

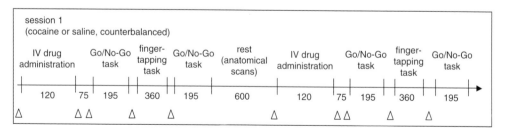

Fig. 16.1 Experimental design. The durations of the components are given in seconds and triangles represent the time points in which physiological measurements were made.

Cocaine-using participants were manually injected over 120 s through a catheter port with either cocaine at 40 mg/70 kg body weight, or normal saline; administration order in the two separate scanning sessions was counterbalanced across participants. Infusions occurred at rest points prior to task runs 1 and 3 of each session. The dose used was based on previous work in administering cocaine to users conducted at the Medical College of Wisconsin, and was of a reinforcing quality (producing a high and rush) comparable with the users' reported typical use. The rate of administration over 2 min was chosen from pilot data that demonstrated this rate to minimize the rush experience (important for keeping subjects 'on-task' and avoiding head movements during magnetic resonance imaging (MRI) acquisition) and to prolong the high period (to enable completion of the task during a drug-active window). Scanning of the Go/No-Go task was initiated approximately 75 s following completion of the injection (time required to obtain baseline physiological measures). The 3 min 15 s task run was followed by a 6 min event-related finger-tapping task. There then followed another 3 min 15 s task run and then a rest period during which the high-resolution anatomical images were collected. Vital statistics (blood pressure (BP) and heart rate (HR)) were measured between each run; the exact timings of these measurements varied between subjects due to small variations in data copying and scanner preparation time between runs. Approximately 40 min after the first injection, the second injection was administered and the three aforementioned functional runs were repeated. HR and BP were monitored for safety and to assess physiological responses to cocaine administration.

16.2.3 Image acquisition and analysis

High-resolution anatomical images and standard gradient-echo, echo-planar functional images were acquired (functional images were 7 mm contiguous sagittal slices: repeat time, 2000 ms; echo time, 40 ms; field of view 240 mm; 64 × 64 matrix; 3.75 × 3.75 mm in-plane resolution; see the electronic supplementary material). Imaging data were analysed using the AFNI software package (Cox 1996; http://afni.nimh.nih.gov/afni) and comparisons were carried out between the saline and cocaine conditions (full details in the electronic supplementary material). In brief, event-related changes in activation were calculated using deconvolution and curve-fitting techniques for successful inhibitions (STOPS) and commission errors (ERRORS) for each condition (cocaine and saline). Statistically significant activation maps were created for both STOPS and ERRORS for each condition based on the one-sample t-tests against the null hypothesis of no activation changes with thresholds ($p \leq 0.05$, corrected) determined through data simulation procedures (Garavan et al. 1999). Functionally defined region of interest maps were defined for each event type (STOPS and ERRORS) by combining the activated regions of both the intravenous (IV) cocaine and saline conditions as OR maps (e.g. for STOPS, a voxel was included in the region of interest if significant in either the cocaine or the saline condition) and between-condition comparisons were performed on the mean activations of the resulting functionally defined regions.

Additionally, data from healthy control participants were available from a previous study (Kaufman et al. 2003) in which drug-naive participants completed four runs of the same inhibitory control task using similar stimulus duration tailoring procedures as described above. In a secondary follow-up analysis, data from cocaine users following cocaine and saline injections were compared with these healthy controls using the regions identified in our original study. Although the procedures were not identical for the two studies (e.g. there were no IV lines for the controls) this follow-up analysis was deemed a worthwhile initial investigation of a cocaine administration's impact on those areas previously observed to be functionally hypoactive in users. Finally, details of the event-related finger-tapping control task analyses are reported in-depth elsewhere (Murphy et al. 2006).

16.3 Results

16.3.1 Physiological analyses

ANOVAs on each of the physiological measures revealed significant main effects for drug condition and time and significant interactions (all $p < 0.01$). Physiological measures showed the anticipated effects of cocaine infusion (Fig. 16.2) with beats per minute, systolic and diastolic BP rising from pre- to post-injection ($F_{9,4} = 50.0$, $p \leq 0.001$; $F_{9,4} = 19.18$, $p \leq 0.006$, and $F_{9,4} = 6.2$, $p \leq 0.05$, respectively). Whereas HR significantly differed between the

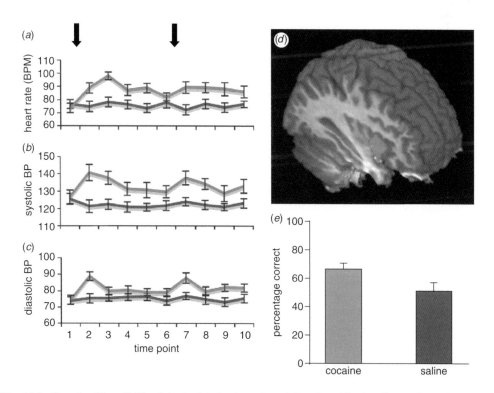

Fig. 16.2 (See also Plate 9) Physiological, behavioural, and functional brain effects of cocaine in performing an inhibitory control Go/No-Go task. Cocaine administration increased (*a*) HR, (*b*) systolic BP, and (*c*) diastolic BP and (*e*) improved the user's ability to inhibit a prepotent behaviour (all error bars are standard errors of the mean). Improved inhibitory control (successful inhibitions) was associated with increased activity in (*d*) right insula/inferior frontal gyrus (coronal section, y = 14) and right dorsolateral prefrontal cortex. Drug infusions occurred between time points 1 and 2 as well as between time points 6 and 7. The four runs of the Go/No-Go task commenced following time points 3, 5, 8, and 10. The event-related finger-tapping control task was performed following time points 4 and 9. Red, cocaine; blue, saline.

pre-injection time point 1 and each subsequent time point, systolic BP was significantly higher at time points 2, 3, and 7 compared with time point 1 ($p < 0.05$) and diastolic BP was significantly higher at all time points except time point 6. For saline administration, ANOVAs revealed no significant variance for HR, systolic, or diastolic BP over the course of the scan session (all $p > 0.25$).

16.3.2 Performance analyses

To examine behavioural effects of the drug manipulation, a 2 × 4 (drug condition × scan run) repeated-measures ANOVA assessed changes in performance (percentage of successful inhibitions for all No-Go trials) across each scan session's four runs in the users. Both main effects were significant (drug: $F_{1,12} = 11.7$, $p \leq 0.005$; scan run: $F_{3,10} = 4.8$, $p \leq 0.025$), as was the interaction ($F_{3,10} = 6.8$, $p \leq 0.009$). The main effects indicate that the percentage of successful inhibitions was higher in the cocaine condition (66.8 ± 4%) than in the saline condition (51.2 ± 6%) and that accuracy declined over the duration of each session. Performance was significantly better in the cocaine condition relative to the saline condition during runs 1 and 3 (run 1: $F_{1,12} = 23.8$, $p \leq 0.001$; run 3: $F_{1,12} = 5.5$, $p \leq 0.04$), but was not different from the saline condition for runs 2 and 4 (run 2: $F_{1,12} = 1.5$, $p \leq 0.24$; run 4: $F_{1,12} = 3.1$, $p \leq 0.10$), indicating that the performance was significantly better in the scan runs that immediately followed cocaine administration. A 2 × 4 (drug condition × scan run) repeated-measures ANOVA on omission errors across the four scan runs found a significant effect for drug ($F_{1,12} = 7.9$, $p \leq 0.02$), but not for run or the interaction (all $F < 1$); participants made significantly more omission errors in the saline condition (1.9 ± 5%) than in the cocaine condition (0.5 ± 0.2%). Finally, there was no difference in the Go response time between the conditions ($F < 1$) and there was no effect of the order of substance administration on any task performance measure (all $p > 0.10$). The absence of a condition effect on response time helps rule out the possibility that the improved inhibitory performance in the cocaine condition was secondary to more cautious, slower responding following cocaine.

Comparing performance with the control subjects from the previous investigation (Kaufman et al. 2003) revealed no significant difference between controls and users in the saline condition (51.2 versus 54.9%, respectively; $t = 0.52$, $p \leq 0.61$) and significantly better performance by users in the cocaine condition relative to controls (66.8 versus 54.9%, respectively; $t = 2.23$, $p \leq 0.03$).

16.3.3 Functional analyses

For successful inhibitions (STOPS) in the saline and cocaine conditions of the users, activation was primarily bilateral with large clusters evident in bilateral insula extending rostrally into the inferior frontal gyrus, as well as the medial frontal/superior frontal gyri. Smaller clusters were evident in the right middle frontal gyrus, left middle frontal gyrus, and in the cingulate gyrus anterior to the precentral gyrus (Table 16.1). Significant differences were observed for two regions, both of which produced higher blood–oxygen-level-dependent (BOLD) signal for the cocaine condition than the saline condition: the right insula/inferior frontal gyrus ($t_{(12)} = 2.89$, $p \leq 0.014$) and the right middle frontal gyrus ($t_{(12)} = 3.81$, $p \leq 0.003$; Fig. 16.2).

For commission errors (ERRORS), activation was bilateral and considerably more widespread, yet only five discrete regions showed significant differences between conditions, suggesting that differences observed were specific to both region and drug condition rather than

Table 16.1 Regions activated for failed inhibitions (ERRORS) and successful inhibitions (STOPS). (Asterisks identify brain regions in which comparisons revealed significant differences (with modified Bonferroni at $p < 0.05$) between activation in the cocaine and saline conditions.)

Structure	Brodmann area	Hemisphere	Volume (ml)	Centre-of-mass	(x, y, z)	
ERRORS						
Frontal lobe						
Middle frontal gyrus	46*	R	118	38	31	18
Medial frontal gyrus	6/24	R	111	20	1	51
	6/24/32	R	3993	1	−1	52
Post-central gyrus	3	L	407	−36	−25	47
			148	−22	−29	58
Pre-central gyrus	4	L	126	−48	−14	38
	3/4	R	116	47	−14	48
Cingulate gyrus	32	R	475	7	26	29
	29/30*	L	121	−16	−46	13
Parietal lobe						
Inferior parietal lobule	40*	L	156	−54	−43	25
	7	R	131	31	−51	52
Temporal lobe						
Parahippocampal gyrus	27	R	460	16	−362	2
	36	L	109	−22	−43	−5
Middle temporal gyrus	39	R	121	53	−54	10
	37	R	107	52	−619	9
Occipital lobe						
Lingual gyrus	19/30	L	183	−12	−46	−3
	18/30*	R	169	11	−556	6
	18*	L	157	−4	−67	−1
Declive	19	L	105	−20	−60	−12
Subcortical						
Putamen		R	3043	21	4	4
		L	1776	−24	−3	2
		L	111	20	1	51
Thalamus			2739	0	−198	8
Insula/claustrum	30	L	261	−30	16	2
STOPS						
Frontal lobe						
Middle frontal gyrus9	9*	R	192	36	40	35
	6	L	101	−20	57	57
Superior frontal gyrus	6	R	472	1	6	55
Cingulate gyrus	24/32	R	101	3	9	40
Subcortical						
Insula	*	R	1800	34	13	4
		L	1636	−30	11	3

a general effect of cocaine administration. In four of these five regions, users showed greater error-related activation following cocaine relative to the saline condition: right posterior cingulate/lingual gyrus ($t_{(12)} = 3.4$, $p \leq 0.005$); culmen of vermis/left lingual gyrus ($t_{(12)} = 3.7$, $p \leq 0.003$); left inferior parietal lobule ($t_{(12)} = 3.1$, $p \leq 0.01$); and right middle frontal gyrus ($t_{(12)} = 3.9$, $p \leq 0.002$). Conversely, participants were found to be hypoactive in the cocaine condition compared with the saline condition in the left posterior cingulate ($t_{(12)} = -6.4$, $p \leq 0.001$).

Comparisons of neural activation for cocaine users in both the cocaine and saline conditions with that of non-using controls from a previous investigation (Kaufman et al. 2003) were carried out using regions of interest identified from the original study, i.e. regions in which users were previously shown to be hypoactive relative to controls. Confirming this previous result, the activation levels were significantly reduced in users ($p \leq 0.05$, corrected) following the saline injection compared with non-using controls for STOPS; this hypoactivity was observed in right inferior parietal lobule, right insula into superior temporal gyrus and right middle frontal gyrus. Following IV cocaine, hypoactivity relative to controls persisted in just the right middle frontal gyrus. For ERRORS, similar to the original study, users in the saline condition demonstrated hypoactivity in an anterior cingulate cortex region; although less robust, this hypoactivity approached significance ($p \leq 0.056$). By contrast, cocaine users in the cocaine condition showed no significant differences in activation compared with controls, with the exception of the left thalamus that had significantly more activation ($p \leq 0.02$) in users for ERRORS.

Because the results comparing users and controls in the ACC, a region shown previously to be significantly hypoactive, were only marginally significant, we examined this region further. The functionally defined region of interest (ROI) that we used was not only largely right hemispheric but also incorporated the interhemispheric space and some left ACC. To limit activation measures to the parenchyma, we masked the functional ROI with an anatomically defined map of the ACC, thereby only including the right hemisphere in the ROI. The resulting right hemisphere ACC ROI showed a significant difference between control participant data and the IV saline condition in users ($p \leq 0.05$), which disappeared following the IV cocaine administration (controls versus IV cocaine in users: $p \leq 0.66$).

Given cocaine's potent vasoactive effect, it was important to determine that any observed BOLD effects were due to changes in the neural level rather than being due to changes in vascular functioning or neuronal-vascular coupling. While a vascular basis for the observed effects is unlikely, given the regional specificity of the cortical effects, this was confirmed with the finger-tapping control data that showed no differences in the haemodynamic response in either amplitude (area under the curve) or shape (individual parameters of a gamma-variate model: $y = k\ t^r e^{-t/b}$) that was fit voxelwise to the haemodynamic response between the IV cocaine and saline conditions. Additional data also confirm no differences in event-related haemodynamic properties between the users and the cocaine-naive controls (Murphy et al. 2006).

16.4 Discussion

The present study has addressed the effects of an IV cocaine administration on neurocognitive function in cocaine-dependent individuals. The results demonstrate that a cocaine-induced improvement in inhibitory control was accompanied by increased activation in two frontal areas, right dorsolateral prefrontal cortex and right insula extending into right inferior frontal gyrus. The importance of these regions for inhibitory control, and particularly the more ventral region, has been demonstrated by functional imaging, human lesion studies and, more recently, by transcranial magnetic stimulation (Aron et al. 2004; Buchsbaum et al. 2005; Chambers et al. 2006, 2007; Garavan et al. 2006). That improved performance should be associated with increased activity in these regions adds further support to their central role in inhibitory control. Similarly, the cocaine administration was observed to increase activation levels in frontal and parietal areas that responded to performance errors.

Previously, we have shown that the subjective awareness of errors in one's performance is associated with increased frontoparietal activity (Hester et al. 2005) and that cocaine users have poorer awareness of their errors (Hester et al. 2007). Thus, an increase in error-related activity may be functionally significant insofar as error-related activation levels tend to be greater in better, more attentive performers (Hester et al. 2004) and when errors are made more salient through within-subject manipulations (Taylor et al. 2006).

The availability of data from a previous control participant study allowed us to observe that an acute cocaine administration rendered activation levels in users largely indistinguishable with that of controls, seemingly 'normalizing' the cortical hypoactivity associated with chronic drug abuse. This normalization of function was observed in midline cingulate areas previously shown to be hypoactive for errors in cocaine users (Kaufman et al. 2003) and in right hemisphere parietal and insular regions. By contrast, the right dorsolateral prefrontal cortex region active for STOPS remained hypoactive relative to controls in both the IV cocaine and saline conditions, despite this region increasing in activity in the users following cocaine relative to the saline condition. Although the comparison between users and previously tested controls was imperfect experimentally and should be interpreted with some caution, it is also important to note that stable group differences between users and controls such as sex or education levels cannot account for the different patterns of results observed when comparing controls first to users in the IV saline condition and then to users in the IV cocaine condition. Furthermore, although the user and control groups did differ in sex composition, we have previously shown that neither performance on the task nor error-related midline activity differs between males and females (Hester et al. 2004).

Much evidence exists for the capacity of stimulant drugs to enhance cognitive performance. This holds true not only for populations with known dysfunction in brain regions targeted by the mesolimbic dopamine system, such as ADHD (Vaidya et al. 1998; Aron et al. 2003; Bedard et al. 2003), but also for normal healthy control populations for whom no pre-existing cognitive deficits are identified (Sostek et al. 1980; Koelega 1993; Wiegmann et al. 1996). As stimulant medications are used in these populations to enhance cognitive performance, it is possible that one aspect of the reinforcing nature of chronic cocaine use is the drug's capacity to improve cognitive function through its action on cortical structures involved in cognitive control. A related possibility is that the cocaine administration alleviated a withdrawal or craving state in the users. While this or other motivational differences may have existed between the cocaine and saline conditions, it is important to note that a similar effect, an increase in electrophysiological error-related signal following D-amphetamine (de Bruijn et al. 2003), has been observed in drug-naive controls for whom withdrawal would not have applied. Furthermore, we found no relationships between the time since the users' last use, which may indirectly index their craving or withdrawal levels, and their performance or activation levels on the task or, most critically, on the change in activation between the IV cocaine and saline conditions.

The phasic modulation of activity levels in specific cortical regions is consistent with cocaine having either a direct or indirect long-term detrimental effect on those same cortical structures. For example, if drug use produces a phasic increase in activity in a brain region and the brain's homeostatic response is to down-regulate receptors in that region (Volkow et al. 2002) then, relative to a control condition, one may identify regions of possible down-regulation by their increased phasic activity following a drug administration. Tonic down-regulation of medial or lateral prefrontal regions may result from repeated exposure to a drug-induced hyperdopaminergic state, which has been suggested to account for decreased dopamine receptor levels in users, and consequently, decreased metabolism in response to stimuli other than the drug itself (Volkow et al. 1999). In this regard, the cognitive tests can serve as functional probes of cocaine's effects. The cognitive tests can also identify the profile of deficits, linked to specific brain structures, likely to accompany drug abuse. Although there is much evidence of impaired cognitive abilities in cocaine users (Fillmore & Rush 2002; Goldstein et al. 2004), the relationship between these behavioural impairments and their underlying neurobiology is not yet very well understood. In this regard, the present results nicely complement previous investigations that have demonstrated diminished inhibitory control in cocaine users (Fillmore & Rush 2002; Colzato et al. 2007). Identifying the neurocognitive profile of this group should inform therapeutic interventions and may also provide an assay of the efficacy of these interventions.

In the human model, it is unclear whether observed deficits reflect a consequence of drug abuse or a pre-existing difference. Neurofunctional deficits such as those observed may render an individual susceptible to the development of addiction (i.e. the transition from recreational to uncontrolled use; Tarter et al. 2003; Dalley et al. 2007; Verdejo-Garcia et al. 2008) and may be related to the psychiatric comorbidities observed in drug-dependent users, or such deficits may result from the effects that prolonged cocaine use may have on the brain or a combination of both these factors. These uncertainties notwithstanding, the present results demonstrate that an acute cocaine administration affects the functioning of brain areas critical for cognitive control, thereby showing a direct relationship between cocaine and impulse control, as mediated by right prefrontal cortex, and performance monitoring as mediated by the ACC. Curiously, the results run counter to a hypothesis that acute cocaine would disrupt these control processes. Instead, the observation of improved performance and increased activation levels are consistent with similar ameliorative effects on inhibitory control that have been observed with methylphenidate in patients with ADHD (Scheres et al. 2003). By contrast, alcohol has been shown to impair error monitoring (Ridderinkhof et al. 2002), but this effect was observed in non-alcoholics and is thus in keeping with the neurofunctional effects of drugs of abuse being determined by a history of use and its associated brain changes (discussed further below). That said, as noted above, D-amphetamine increased an electrophysiological marker of error monitoring (but not performance) in drug-naive controls (de Bruijn et al. 2003); D-amphetamine improved information processing but had no effect on inhibitory control in drug-naive controls (Fillmore et al. 2005a,b), while D-amphetamine and cocaine administrations have also been observed to impair inhibitory control in users (Fillmore et al. 2002, 2003).

One important consideration in attempting to reconcile these findings is the role of dose on the observed patterns of cortical activation and behavioural performance. While the beneficial effects of stimulant medications such as methylphenidate to enhance cognitive performance in both children and adults have been demonstrated (Chelonis et al. 2002; Aron et al. 2003; Bedard et al. 2003, 2004), these benefits appear to vary by dose, with more unfavourable behaviours appearing at higher doses (Stein et al. 2003). Similar inverted U-shaped function curves for behaviour are observed in studies of chronic cocaine users (Johnson et al. 1998). A relevant series of studies by Fillmore and colleagues have demonstrated the importance of drug dose insofar as inhibitory control performance on a Go/No-Go task was found to be disimproved following oral cocaine administration in the 50–150 mg dose range (Fillmore et al. 2002), but improved following administration in the 100–300 mg dose range (Fillmore et al. 2005a,b; but see also Fillmore et al. (2006), in which performance was shown to increase with dose but with different dose-response effects on two different tests of motor response inhibition). Although full dose-response studies are difficult for both methodological and safety reasons, the present results, having established a drug-related enhancement effect, may warrant further study of dose-related effects in future neuroimaging studies.

A further consideration when interpreting a drug's beneficial or deleterious effects on cognitive performance is the drug use history of one's participants. The present study did not include a drug-naive control group. Even if one might surmount the significant ethical and safety issues involved in administering cocaine to drug-naive controls, it is likely the case that the response of controls, given, for example, their baseline levels of dopaminergic activity, might be quite different from those of experienced cocaine users. Individual variation of this kind can be observed in drug-naive controls who, based on working memory capacity measures thought to reflect tonic dopaminergic activity, can show widely divergent performance and brain activation responses following a dopaminergic challenge (Gibbs & D'Esposito 2005). Fillmore and colleagues note that earlier findings of improved inhibitory control following D-amphetamine in drug-naive controls (de Wit et al. 2000) were limited to those subjects who displayed poor inhibitory abilities (Fillmore et al. 2005a,b). These observations suggest that the effects of a drug administration will be modulated by where the recipient falls on that drug's dose-response function curve.

The present results showing ACC hypoactivity relative to controls to be present following saline but not cocaine, coupled with the similar effects of D-amphetamine (de Bruijn et al. 2003) and the evidence that ACC dysfunction in cocaine users may be related to D_2 receptor availability (Volkow et al. 1993), suggest that the neurotransmitter dopamine may be implicated in performance monitoring functions. This conclusion is supported by recent functional MRI and electrophysiological evidence linking the brain's error response to genetic markers of dopamine function (Frank et al. 2007; Klein et al. 2007; Krämer et al. 2007). Additionally, patients with Parkinson's disease show reduced ACC responses to errors that are partly moderated by dopaminergic medication (Frank et al. 2004). It has been proposed that the midline error-related signal is driven by the same mesocorticolimbic dopamine system that generates ventral striatal responses related to expected and unexpected rewards and losses (Holroyd & Coles 2002). Thus, the present results lead to a hypothesized intersection between cocaine's dopaminergically mediated reinforcing effects and a cognitive dysregulation, with dopamine function in the ACC hypothesized to be on the cognitive–affective interface. Disruption to the ACC may be of particular relevance for understanding the behaviour of cocaine users given that the performance monitoring functions of this region includes the assessment of risky behaviour and decision making (Magno et al. 2006; Bjork et al. 2007). Deficits in those cognitive processes central to the endogenous control of behaviour may render the behaviour of the drug-dependent individual inordinately influenced by habitual behavioural patterns or by environmental stimuli such as drug-related cues.

This work was supported by USPHS grant DA1 4100 and General Clinical Research Center grant M01 RR00058. We gratefully acknowledge the assistance of Veronica Dixon, Kevin Murphy, Stacy Claesges, Linda Piacentine, Robert Risinger, Tom Ross and Elliot Stein.

References

Ahmed, S. H. & Koob, G. F. 1998 Transition from moderate to excessive drug intake: change in hedonic set point. *Science* **282**, 298–300. (doi:10.1126/science.282.5387.298)

Aron, A. R., Dowson, J. H., Sahakian, B. J. & Robbins, T. W. 2003 Methylphenidate improves response inhibition in adults with attention-deficit/hyperactivity disorder. *Biol. Psychiatry* **54**, 1465–68. (doi:10.1016/S0006-3223(03) 00609-7)

Aron, A. R., Robbins, T. W. & Poldrack, R. A. 2004 Inhibition and the right inferior frontal cortex. *Trends Cogn. Sci.* **8**, 170–7. (doi:10.1016/j.tics.2004.02.010)

Barkley, R. A. 1997 Behavioral inhibition, sustained attention, and executive functions: constructing a unifying theory of ADHD. *Psychol. Bull.* **121**, 65–94. (doi:10. 1037/0033-2909.121.1.65)

Bartzokis, G., Lu, P. H., Beckson, M., Rapoport, R., Grant, S., Wiseman, E. J. & London, E. D. 2000 Abstinence from cocaine reduces high-risk responses on a gambling task. *Neuropsychopharmacology* **22**, 102–3. (doi:10.1016/ S0893-133X(99)00077-9)

Bedard, A.-C., Ickowicz, A., Logan, G. D., Hogg-Johnson, S., Schachar, R. & Tannock, R. 2003 Selective inhibition in children with attention-deficit hyperactivity disorder off and on stimulant medication. *J. Abnorm. Child Psychol.* **31**, 315–27. (doi:10.1023/A:1023285614844)

Bedard, A. C., Martinussen, R., Ickowicz, A. & Tannock, R. 2004 Methylphenidate improves visual-spatial memory in children with attention-deficit/hyperactivity disorder. *J. Am. Acad. Child Adolesc. Psychiatry* **43**, 260–8. (doi: 10.1097/00004583-200403000-00006)

Bjork, J. M., Smith, A. R., Danube, C. L. & Hommer, D. W. 2007 Developmental differences in posterior mesofrontal cortex recruitment by risky rewards. *J. Neurosci.* **27**, 4839–44. (doi:10.1523/JNEUROSCI.5469-06.2007)

Bolla, K. I. et al. 2003 Orbitofrontal cortex dysfunction in abstinent cocaine abusers performing a decision-making task. *Neuroimage* **19**, 1085–94. (doi: 10.1016/S1053-8119(03)00113-7)

Buchsbaum, B. R., Greer, S., Chang, W. L. & Berman, K. F.2005 Meta-analysis of neuroimaging studies of the Wisconsin Card-Sorting task and component processes. *Hum. Brain Mapp.* **25**, 35–45. (doi:10.1002/hbm.20128)

Carter, C. S., MacDonald III, A. W., Ross, L. L. & Stenger, V. A. 2001 Anterior cingulate cortex activity and impaired self-monitoring of performance in patients with schizophrenia: an event-related fMRI study. *Am. J. Psychiatry* **158**, 1423–8. (doi:10.1176/appi.ajp.158.9.1423)

Chambers, C. D., Bellgrove, M. A., Stokes, M. G., Henderson, T. R., Garavan, H., Robertson, I. H. & Mattingley, J. B. 2006 Executive 'brake failure' following deactivation of human frontal lobe. *J. Cogn. Neurosci.* **18**, 444–55.

Chambers, C. D., Bellgrove, M. A., Gould, I. C., English, T., Garavan, H., McNaught, E., Kamke, M. & Mattingley, J. B. 2007 Dissociable mechanisms of cognitive control in human prefrontal cortex. *J. Neurophysiol.* **98**, 3638–47. (doi:10.1152/jn.00685.2007)

Chelonis, J. J., Edwards, M. C., Schulz, E. G., Baldwin, R., Blake, D. J., Wenger, A. & Paule, M. G. 2002 Stimulant medication improves recognition memory in children diagnosed with attention-deficit/hyperactivity disorder. *Exp. Clin. Psychopharmacol.* **10**, 400–7. (doi: 10.1037/1064-1297. 10.4.400)

Clark, L., Iversen, S. D. & Goodwin, G. M. 2001 A neuropsychological investigation of prefrontal cortex involvement in acute mania. *Am. J. Psychiatry* **158**, 1605–11. (doi:10.1176/appi.ajp. 158.10.1605)

Clark, L., Robbins, T. W., Ersche, K. D. & Sahakian, B. J. 2006 Reflection impulsivity in current and former substance users. *Biol. Psychiatry* **60**, 515–22. (doi: 10. 1016/j.biopsych.2005.11.007)

Coffey, S. F., Gudleski, G. D., Saladin, M. E. & Brady, K. T. 2003 Impulsivity and rapid discounting of delayed hypothetical rewards in cocaine-dependent individuals. *Exp. Clin. Psychopharmacol.* **11**, 18–25. (doi:10.1037/1064-1297.11.1.18)

Colzato, L. S., van den Wildenberg, W. P. & Hommel, B. 2007 Impaired inhibitory control in recreational cocaine users. *PLoS ONE2*, e1143. (doi:10.1371/journal.pone.0001143)

Cox, R. W 1996 AFNI: Software for analysis and visualization of functional magnetic resonance neuro-images. *Comput. Biomed. Res.* **29**, 162–73. (doi:10. 1006/cbmr.1996.0014)

Dalley, J. W. et al. 2007 Nucleus accumbens D2/3 receptors predict trait impulsivity and cocaine reinforcement. *Science* **315**, 1267–70. (doi:10.1126/science.1137073)

de Bruijn, E. R., Hulstijn, W., Meulenbroek, R. G. & van Galen, G. P. 2003 Action monitoring in motor control: ERPs following selection and execution errors in a force production task. *Psychophysiology* **40**, 786–95. (doi:10. 1111/1469-8986.00079)

de Wit, H., Crean, J. & Richards, J. B. 2000 Effects of d-amphetamine and ethanol on a measure of behavioral inhibition in humans. *Behav. Neurosci.* **114**, 830–7. (doi:10.1037/0735-7044.114.4.830)

Diamond, A. 1990 Developmental time course in human infants and infant monkeys, and the neural bases of, inhibitory control in reaching. *Ann. N. Y. Acad. Sci.* **608**, 637–69. (doi:10.1111/j.1749-6632.1990.tb48913.x)

Eldreth, D. A., Matochik, J. A., Cadet, J. L. & Bolla, K. I. 2004 Abnormal brain activity in prefrontal brain regions in abstinent marijuana users. *NeuroImage* **23**, 914–20. (doi: 10.1016/j.neuroimage. 2004.07.032)

Fillmore, M. T. & Rush, C. R. 2002 Impaired inhibitory control of behavior in chronic cocaine users. *Drug Alcohol Depend.* **66**, 265–73. (doi:10.1016/S0376-8716(01) 00206-X)

Fillmore, M. T., Rush, C. R. & Hays, L. 2002 Acute effects of oral cocaine on inhibitory control of behavior in humans. *Drug Alcohol Depend.* **67**, 157–67. (doi:10.1016/S0376-8716(02)00062-5)

Fillmore, M. T., Rush, C. R. & Marczinski, C. A. 2003 Effects of d-amphetamine on behavioral control in stimulant abusers: the role of prepotent response tendencies. *Drug Alcohol Depend.* **71**, 143–52. (doi:10. 1016/S0376-8716(03)00089-9)

Fillmore, M. T., Kelly, T. H. & Martin, C. A. 2005a Effects of d-amphetamine in human models of information processing and inhibitory control. *Drug Alcohol Depend.* **77**, 151–9. (doi:10.1016/j. drugalcdep.2004.07.013)

Fillmore, M. T., Rush, C. R. & Hays, L. 2005b Cocaine improves inhibitory control in a human model of response conflict. *Exp. Clin. Psychopharmacol.* **3**, 327–35.

Fillmore, M. T., Rush, C. R. & Hays, L. 2006 Acute effects of cocaine in two models of inhibitory control: implications of non-linear dose effects. *Addiction* **101**, 1323–32. (doi:10.1111/j.1360-0443. 2006.01522.x)

Fishbein, D. H. et al. 2005 Risky decision making and the anterior cingulate cortex in abstinent drug abusers and nonusers. *Cogn. Brain Res.* **23**, 119–36. (doi:10.1016/ j.cogbrainres.2004.12.010)

Forman, S. D. et al. 2004 Opiate addicts lack error-dependent activation of rostral anterior cingulate. *Biol. Psychiatry* **55**, 531–7. (doi:10.1016/j.biopsych.2003.09.011)

Frank, M. J., Seeberger, L. C. & O'Reilly, R. C. 2004 By carrot or by stick: cognitive reinforcement learning in parkinsonism. *Science* **306**, 1940–3. (doi:10.1126/ science.1102941)

Frank, M. J., D'Lauro, C. & Curran, T. 2007 Cross-task individual differences in error processing: neural, electro-physiological, and genetic components. *Cogn. Affect. Behav. Neurosci.* **7**, 297–308.

Franklin, T. R., Acton, P. D., Maldjian, J. A., Gray, J. D., Croft, J. R., Dackis, C. A., O'Brian, C. P. & Childress, A. R. 2002 Decreased gray matter concentration in the insular, orbitofrontal, cingulate, and temporal cortices of cocaine patients. *Biol. Psychiatry* 51, 134–42. (doi: 10. 1016/S0006-3223(01)01269-0)

Garavan, H. & Stout, J. C. 2005 Neurocognitive insights into substance abuse. *Trends Cogn. Sci.* 9, 195-201. (doi:10. 1016/j.tics. 2005.02.008)

Garavan, H., Ross, T. J. & Stein, E. A. 1999 Right hemispheric dominance of inhibitory control: an event-related functional MRI study. *Proc. Natl Acad. Sci. USA* **96**, 8301–6. (doi:10.1073/ pnas.96.14.8301)

Garavan, H., Ross, T. J., Murphy, K., Roche, R. A. P. & Stein, E. A. 2002 Dissociable executive functions in the dynamic control of behavior: inhibition, error detection and correction. *NeuroImage* 17, 1820–9. (doi:10.1006/ nimg.2002.1326)

Garavan, H., Hester, R., Murphy, K., Fassbender, C. & Kelly, C. 2006 Individual differences in the neuroanatomy of inhibitory control. *Brain Res.* **1105**, 130–42. (doi:10. 1016/j.brainres.2006.03.029)

Gibbs, S. E. & D'Esposito, M. 2005 Individual capacity differences predict working memory performance and prefrontal activity following dopamine receptor stimulation. *Cogn. Affect. Behav. Neurosci.* **5**, 212–21.

Goldstein, R. Z., Volkow, N. D., Wang, G. J., Fowler, J. S. & Rajaram, S. 2001 Addiction changes orbitofrontal gyrus function: involvement in response inhibition. *Neuro-Report* **12**, 2595–9. (doi:10.1097/00001756-2001080 80-00060)

Goldstein, R. Z., Leskovjan, A. C., Hoff, A. L., Hitzemann, R., Bashan, F., Khalsa, S. S., Wang, G. J., Fowler, J. S. & Volkow, N. D. 2004 Severity of neuropsychological impairment in cocaine and alcohol addiction: association with metabolism in the prefrontal cortex. *Neuropsychologia* 42, 1447–1458. (doi:10.1016/j.neuropsychologia.2004. 04.002)

Grant, S. 2004 Let's not be impulsive: comments on Lubman et al. (2004). *Addiction* **99**, 1504–1505. (doi:10.1111/ j.1360-0443.2004.00895.x)

Hester, R. & Garavan, H. 2004 Executive dysfunction in cocaine addiction: evidence for discordant frontal, cingulate and cerebellar activity. *J. Neurosci.* **24**, 11017–22. (doi:10.1523/JNEUROSCI.3321-04.2004)

Hester, R., Fassbender, C. & Garavan, H. 2004 Individual differences in error processing: a review and meta-analysis of three event-related fMRI studies using the GO/NOGO task. *Cereb. Cortex* 14, 986-994. (doi:10.1093/cercor/ bhh059)

Hester, R., Shpaner, M., Molholm, S., Foxe, J. J. & Garavan, H. 2005 Neural correlates of error detection with and without awareness. *NeuroImage* 27, 602–8. (doi:10. 1016/j.neuroimage.2005.04.035)

Hester, R., Simões-Franklin, C. & Garavan, H. 2007 Post-error behaviour in active cocaine users: poor awareness of errors in the presence of intact performance adjustments. *Neuropsychopharmacology* **32**, 1974–84. (doi:10.1038/ sj.npp.1301326)

Holroyd, C. B. & Coles, M. G. 2002 The neural basis of human error processing: reinforcement learning, dopamine, and the error-related negativity. *Psychol. Rev.* **109**, 679–709. (doi:10.1037/0033-295X.109.4.679)

Johanson, C. E. & Fischman, M. W 1989 The pharmacology of cocaine related to its abuse. *Pharmacol. Rev.* 41, 3–52.

Johnson, B., Overton, D., Wells, L., Kenny, P., Abramson, D., Dhother, S., Chen, Y. R. & Bordnick, P. 1998 Effects of acute intravenous cocaine on cardiovascular function, human learning, and performance in cocaine addicts. *Psychiatry Res.* **77**, 35–42. (doi:10.1016/S0165-1781(97) 00127-3)

Kaufman, J. N., Ross, T. J., Stein, E. A. & Garavan, H. 2003 Cingulate hypoactivity in cocaine users during a GO/NOGO task as revealed by event-related functional magnetic resonance imaging. *J. Neurosci.* **23**, 7839–43.

Klein, T. A., Neumann, J., Reuter, M., Hennig, J., Yves von Cramon, D. & Ullsperger, M. 2007 Genetically determined differences in learning from errors. *Science* **318**, 1642–5. (doi:10.1126/ science.1145044)

Koelega, H. S. 1993 Stimulant drugs and vigilance performance: a review. *Psychopharmacology* **111**, 1–16. (doi: 10.1007/BF02257400)

Krämer, U. M. et al. 2007 The impact of catechol-*O*-methyltransferase and dopamine D_4 receptor genotypes on neurophysiological markers of performance monitoring. *J. Neurosci.* **19**, 14190–8. (doi: 10.1523/ JNEUROSCI.4229-07.2007)

Kuhar, M. J., Ritz, M. C. & Boja, J. W 1991 The dopamine hypothesis of the reinforcing properties of cocaine. *Trends Neurosci.* **14**, 299–302. (doi:10.1016/0166-2236(91)90 141-G)

Li, C.-S. R., Huang, C., Yan, P., Bhagwagar, Z., Milivojevic, V. & Sinha, R. 2007 Neural correlates of impulse control during stop signal inhibition in cocaine-dependent men. *Neuropsychopharmacology* **33**, 1798–806. (doi:10.1038/ sj.npp.1301568)

Lubman, D. I., Yucel, M. & Pantelis, C. 2004 Addiction, a condition of compulsive behaviour? Neuroimaging and neuropsychological evidence of inhibitory dysregulation. *Addiction* **99**, 1491–502. (doi:10.1111/j.1360-0443. 2004.00808.x)

Lyvers, M. 2000 "Loss of control" in alcoholism and drug addiction: a neuroscientific interpretation. *Exp. Clin. Psychopharmacol.* **8**, 225–49. (doi: 10.1037/1064-1297. 8.2.225)

Magno, E., Foxe, J. J., Molholm, S., Robertson, I. & Garavan, H. 2006 The anterior cingulate and error avoidance. *J. Neurosci.* **26**, 4769–73. (doi:10.1523/ JNEUROSCI.0369-06.2006)

McGrath, J., Scheldt, S., Welham, J. & Clair, A. 1997 Performance on tests sensitive to impaired executive ability in schizophrenia, mania and well controls: acute and subacute phases. *Schizophr. Res.* **26**, 127–37. (doi:10. 1016/S0920-9964(97)00070-4)

Moeller, G. F., Barratt, E. S., Dougherty, D. M., Schmitz, J. M. & Swann, A. C. 2001 Psychiatric aspects of impulsivity. *Am. J. Psychiatry* **158**, 1783–93. (doi:10. 1176/appi.ajp.158.11.1783)

Monterosso, J., Ehrman, R., Napier, K L., O'Brien, C. P. & Childress, A. R. 2001 Three decision-making tasks in cocaine-dependent patients: do they measure the same construct? *Addiction* 96, 1825–37. (doi:10.1046/j.1360-0443.2001.9612182512.x)

Murphy, K., Dixon, V., LaGrave, K., Kaufman, J., Risinger, R., Bloom, A. & Garavan, H. 2006 A validation of event-related fMRI comparisons between drug groups and controls. *Am. J. Psychiatry* **163**, 1245-1251. (doi: 10. 1176/appi.ajp.163.7.1245)

Patton, J., Standford, M. & Barratt, E. 1995 The factor structure of the Barratt impulsiveness scale. *J. Clin. Psychol.* **51**, 768–75. (doi:10.1002/1097-4679(199511) 51:6<768::AID-JCLP2270510607>3.0.CO;2-1)

Perry, R. J. & Hodges, J. R. 1999 Attention and executive deficits in Alzheimer's disease: a critical review. *Brain* **122**, 383–404. (doi: 10.1093/brain/122.3.383)

Rapport, L. J., Van Voorhis, A., Tzelepis, A. & Friedman, S. R. 2001 Executive functioning in adult attention-deficit hyperactivity disorder. *Clin. Neuropsychol.* **15**, 479–91.

Ridderinkhof, K. R., de Vlugt, Y., Bramlage, A., Spaan, M., Elton, M., Snel, J. & Band, G. P. 2002 Alcohol consumption impairs detection of performance errors in mediofrontal cortex. *Science* **298**, 2209–11. (doi: 10. 1126/science. 1076929)

Scheres, A., Oosterlaan, J., Swanson, J., Morein-Zamir, S., Meiran, N., Schut, H., Vlasveld, L. & Sergeant, J. A. 2003 The effect of methylphenidate on three forms of response inhibition in boys with AD/HD. *J. Abnorm. Child Psychol.* **31**, 105–20. (doi:10.1023/A:1021729501230)

Simon, N. W., Mendez, I. A. & Setlow, B. 2007 Cocaine exposure causes long-term increases in impulsive choice. *Behav. Neurosci.* **121**, 543–9. (doi:10.1037/0735-7044. 121.3.543)

Sostek, A. J., Buchsbaum, M. S. & Rapoport, J. L. 1980 Effects of amphetamine on vigilance performance in normal and hyperactive children. *J. Abnorm. Child Psychol.* **8**, 491–500. (doi:10.1007/BF00916502)

Stein, M. A., Sarampote, C. S., Waldman, I. D., Robb, A. S., Conlon, C., Pearl, P. L., Black, D. O., Seymour, K. E. & Newcorn, J. H. 2003 A dose-response study of OROS methylphenidate in children with attention-deficit/hyper-activity disorder. *Pediatrics* **112**, 404–13. (doi:10.1542/peds.112.5.e404)

Tarter, R. E., Kirisci, L., Mezzich, A., Cornelius, J. R., Pajer, K., Vanyukov, M., Gardner, W., Blackson, T. & Clark, D. 2003 Neurobehavioral disinhibition in childhood predicts early age at onset of substance use disorder. *Am. J. Psychiatry* **160**, 1078–85. (doi:10.1176/appi.ajp. 160.6.1078)

Taylor, S. F., Martis, B., Fitzgerald, K. D., Welsh, R. C., Abelson, J. L., Liberzon, I., Himle, J. A. & Gehring, W. J. 2006 Medial frontal cortex activity and loss-related responses to errors. *J. Neurosci.* **26**, 4063–70. (doi:10. 1523/JNEUROSCI.4709-05.2006)

Vaidya, C. J., Austin, G., Kirkorian, G., Ridlehuber, H. W., Desmond, J. E., Glover, G. H. & Gabrieli, J. D. 1998 Selective effects of methylphenidate in attention deficit hyperactivity disorder: a functional magnetic resonance study. *Proc. Natl Acad. Sci. USA* **95**, 14 494–14 499. (doi:10.1073/pnas.95.24.14494)

Verdejo-Garcia, A. J., Perales, J. C. & Perez-Garcia, M. 2007 Cognitive impulsivity in cocaine and heroin polysubstance abusers. *Addict. Behav.* **32**, 950–66. (doi:10.1016/ j.addbeh.2006.06.032)

Verdejo-Garcia, A., Lawrence, A. J. & Clark, L. 2008 Impulsivity as a vulnerability marker for substance-use disorders: review of findings from high-risk research, problem gamblers and genetic association studies. *Neurosci. Biobehav. Rev* **32**, 777–810. (doi:10.1016/ j.neubiorev.2007.11.003)

Volkow, N. D., Fowler, J. S., Wang, G. J., Hitzemann, R., Logan, J., Schlyer, D. J., Dewey, S. L. & Wolf, A. P. 1993 Decreased dopamine D_2 receptor availability is associated with reduced frontal metabolism in cocaine abusers. *Synapse* **14**, 169–77. (doi:10.1002/syn.890140210)

Volkow, N. D., Fowler, J. S. & Wang, G. J. 1999 Imaging studies on the role of dopamine in cocaine reinforcement and addiction in humans. *J. Psychopharmacol.* **13**, 337–45.

Volkow, N. D., Fowler, J. S., Wang, G.-J. & Goldstein, R. Z. 2002 Role of dopamine, the frontal cortex and memory circuits in drug addiction: insight from imaging studies. *Neurobiol. Learn. Mem.* **78**, 610–24. (doi:10.1006/nlme. 2002.4099)

Wiegmann, D. A., Stanny, R. R., McKay, D. L., Neri, D. F. & McCardie, A. H. 1996 Methamphetamine effects on cognitive processing during extended wakefulness. *Int. J. Aviat. Psychol.* **6**, 379–97. (doi:10.1207/s 15327 108ijap0604_5)

17

Evidence-based treatments of addiction

*Charles P. O'Brien**

Both pharmacotherapy and behavioural treatment are required to relieve the symptoms of addictive disorders. This paper reviews the evidence for the benefits of pharmacotherapy and discusses mechanisms where possible. Animal models of addiction have led to some medications that are effective in reducing symptoms and improving function but they do not produce a cure. Addiction is a chronic disease that tends to recur when treatment is stopped; thus, long-term treatment is recommended.

Key Words: Addiction; relapse; withdrawal; endophenotype.

17.1 Introduction

Most theories of drug-addiction mechanisms have been based on animal models and, until recently, these theories have made the assumption that all subjects are alike in their responses to drugs (Deroche-Gamonet et al. 2004). In reality, human subjects are quite variable in how they respond to drugs. Moreover, data from the studies of non-human primates indicate that genetic variation is also important in other higher species. Drugs that demonstrate rewarding properties in animals also tend to be abused by humans, but only by a relatively small percentage of those humans exposed (Table 17.1). The most obvious effects of chronic drug use are tolerance and physiological dependence and these phenomena translate well from animals to humans. However, tolerance and its complement, physiological dependence, are normal reactions and do not imply addiction.

At the clinical level, the theoretical model of addiction is similar to that of an infectious disease such as tuberculosis. The development of addiction depends on the interaction of agent, host, and environment (Fig. 17.1). The progression from use to abuse to addiction is determined by this interaction. An understanding of addiction requires addressing all three of these classes of variables. Treatment and prevention efforts that fail to consider all three have not been successful. Therefore, it follows that pharmacological treatments must be imbedded in a comprehensive rehabilitation programme that addresses these variables to the extent possible. While first use is under cognitive control, albeit usually influenced by social pressures, the user with genetic vulnerability will progress to a stage of compulsive use. At this point, volitional control is greatly diminished. As an example, the reader need only think of friends and relatives who repeatedly relapse to compulsive cigarette smoking despite the knowledge of the hazards to their health and despite having expressed a conscious desire to abstain from smoking. At the neuronal level, this compulsive relapse suggests plasticity, a memory trace. No treatment has even been theorized, however, that could selectively 'erase' addiction memories while not impairing adaptive memories and new memory formation.

* obrien@mail.trc.upenn.edu

Table 17.1 In a relatively small percentage of those humans exposed, the risk of becoming addicted to nicotine was approximately double the risk of cocaine. (By other measures, cocaine has more powerful pharmacological effects than nicotine and this implies a role for host (genetics) and environmental factors. Source: Anthony et al. (1994).)

| | **Risk of addiction** | | |
	ever used (%)	**Dependence (Addiction) (%)**	**Risk (%)**
Tobacco	75.6	24.1	31.9
Cocaine	16.2	2.7	16.7
Heroin	1.5	0.4	23.1
Alcohol	91.5	14.1	15.4
Cannabis	46.3	4.2	9.1

The mechanisms involved in the production of euphoria vary according to the pharmacological category of the drug and have been discussed in earlier papers of this issue. All have in common the activation of brain reward pathways that have evolved to ensure survival, which largely explains the compelling nature of drug reward. The activation of the reward system produces reinforcement of drug acquisition behaviours and associations between environmental cues that signal the arrival of drug effects or drug withdrawal symptoms as drugs disappear from the body through metabolism. The environmental stimuli that become neurologically associated with drug effects are variable and may include persons, places and situations. Treatment approaches, therefore, have attempted to diminish the strength of these conditioned reflexes that lead to relapse and facilitate the development of new memories that produce natural rewards. In this paper, pharmacological approaches that reduce aversive effects of drug cessation, reduce drug reward or reduce drug desire or craving will be discussed. Behavioural approaches are also necessary in combination with medication, but will not be discussed here.

The modern definition of addiction emphasizes uncontrolled drug use rather than tolerance and physiological dependence as essential features of the disorder. It is generally recognized that addiction has strong hereditary influences and once established, it behaves as a chronic brain disorder with relapses and remissions over the long term (McLellan et al. 2000). The diagnostic criteria, which are signs of compulsive drug seeking, are the same for all drug categories (ethanol, opioids, stimulants, sedatives, nicotine, and cannabinoids), even though the mechanisms for activating the reward system are quite different.

With active drug use, euphoria alternates with craving to establish a cycle of addiction that becomes increasingly entrenched and uncontrollable, despite medical and psychosocial hazards. Craving (a strong desire for a drug) can be precipitated by environmental cues, stress

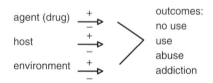

Fig. 17.1 Addiction: resultant of interacting variables. Each class of variables can increase or decrease the risk of addiction. For example, high drug availability and low price (agent) would increase the risk, but genetic factors (host) or opportunities for other pleasures in life (environment) could offset the increased risk. Treatment approaches must also address all of these variables.

or exposure to a small dose of the addictive agent (priming). Cue-induced craving has been associated with limbic system activation in a large number of human neuroimaging studies using positron emission tomography and functional magnetic resonance imaging (Childress et al. 1999), and this pernicious and persistent phenomenon might be reversed by agents that dampen limbic activation. Human neuroimaging studies also demonstrate reductions in frontal lobe metabolism with stimulant, opioid, and alcohol dependence, thus providing a possible explanation for deficiencies in behavioural inhibition among addicts (Franklin et al. 2002). Numerous animal studies indicate that chronic exposure to addictive agents disturbs reward function (Koob et al. 2004). These findings support a biological basis for addiction and are guiding neuronal strategies that target specific clinical components of addiction.

The clinical data fit best when addiction is considered to be a syndrome characterized by compulsive drug-seeking behaviour that impairs psychosocial functioning or health. Even after detoxification and long periods of abstinence, relapse frequently occurs despite sincere efforts to avoid further drug use. People or situations previously associated with drug use elicit involuntary reactions and may provoke relapse (Wikler 1973; O'Brien et al. 1975). The biological mechanisms for these reflex patterns are suggested by the data from animal models at the neurochemical and molecular levels, as discussed in this issue. At the clinical level, conditioned cues produce intense craving through involuntary limbic activation, leading to self-destructive drug use even after long periods of abstinence. In cocaine addicts, even a brief exposure (33 ms) to drug cues evokes limbic system activation (Childress et al. 2008). A key point for the clinician to realize is that the proneness to relapse is based on changes in brain function, which continue for months or years after the last use of the drug. Of course, these changes in brain function interact with environmental factors such as social stress and situational triggers.

If tolerance and withdrawal symptoms were the only elements of addictive illness, treatment would simply consist of detoxification, a process that allows the body to cleanse itself while receiving descending doses of a medication that reduces withdrawal symptoms (O'Brien 2006). If drug taking does not resume, homeostatic mechanisms will gradually readapt to the absence of the drug (LeBlanc et al. 1969) and tolerance will be diminished or lost. We now know that detoxification is, at best, a first step in treatment and that simply achieving a drug-free state is not the most significant accomplishment. The more difficult aspect is the prevention of relapse to drug-taking behaviour.

17.2 Detoxification

It is unfortunate that the majority of drug-dependent persons are merely treated with detoxification and little or no long-term follow-up care. This is not logical, but it is a fact of the current health-care system in the USA (McLellan et al. 2005). Detoxification is actually performed by the patient's own metabolic processes. Thus, it can be accomplished voluntarily (although not necessarily safely) through sheer will power by ceasing drug use or accomplished involuntarily when an addict is incarcerated or placed in a treatment programme where access to drugs is denied. The withdrawal syndrome from opiate addiction can be very uncomfortable, but it is not life-threatening unless the patient has pre-existing medical problems. The symptoms consist of sweating, muscle aches, cramps, nausea, diarrhoea, vomiting, lachrymation, rhinorrhoea, tremors, tachycardia and other signs of autonomic nervous system hyperactivity. The discomfort has been compared to a bad case of the flu. Several sorts of treatment of these symptoms are available. Withdrawal from sedatives, alcohol and stimulants will be considered below.

Replacing the drug of dependence or using another drug in the same pharmacological category in gradually decreasing doses is a direct way to block withdrawal symptoms. As in all forms of detoxification, transfer from a short-acting drug such as heroin to a longer acting drug such as methadone provides a smooth transition to the drug-free state. By appropriate dosing, detoxification can be achieved with minimal discomfort. A recent innovation for opiate dependence involves using the partial agonist buprenorphine as a transition to the drug-free state. The patient can be switched from dependence on heroin or methadone to buprenorphine, which is then stopped with few or no withdrawal symptoms.

The same principles apply in the detoxification from nicotine dependence using nicotine replacement and from sedative (ethanol) dependence using another sedative such as a benzodiazepine. Stimulant (cocaine and amphetamine) withdrawal does not usually require medication, but rapid return to drug use is frequent. A medication that reduces stimulant withdrawal symptoms such as modafinil (see §17.3.4) may reduce relapse.

In the treatment of patients dependent on alcohol or other sedatives, appropriate detoxification is critical because the sedative withdrawal syndrome is potentially life-threatening. Whereas the acute administration of alcohol and sedatives increases γ-aminobutyric acid (GABA) and decreases glutamate activation, the reverse occurs with chronic exposure, producing a GABA-deficiency state and glutamate hyperactivity that increases the risk of seizures during withdrawal (Dackis & O'Brien 2003). There is evidence that sensitization to alcohol withdrawal symptoms occurs, so repeated withdrawals become progressively more severe. The treatment of withdrawal symptoms with benzodiazepines may retard the sensitization process (Brown et al. 1988). Benzodiazepines effectively suppress the sedative withdrawal syndrome, and with proper attention to electrolytes and vitamins, the vast majority of patients can be safely eased into the alcohol-abstinent state in preparation for a long-term rehabilitation programme.

Symptoms of nicotine withdrawal can be diminished by nicotine replacement therapy through chewing gum, patch or nasal spray. Nicotine gum and nicotine patch do not achieve the peak plasma levels seen with cigarettes, and thus they do not produce the same magnitude of nicotine's pleasant effects. Comparisons with placebo treatment show large benefits for nicotine replacement at six weeks, but the advantage diminishes with time.

The withdrawal syndrome from stimulants such as cocaine and amphetamine consists of hypersomnia, hyperphagia, bradycardia, and a number of depressive symptoms that usually resolve over several days. Interestingly, cocaine withdrawal symptoms appear to be predictive of treatment outcome. Kampman et al. (2001) measured cocaine withdrawal symptoms in several trials using the Cocaine Selective Severity Assessment. They found that more withdrawal symptoms in subjects at the start of treatment accurately predicted poorer outcome following treatment. Given these findings, the pharmacological reversal of cocaine withdrawal symptoms with agents such as modafinil may improve clinical outcome (Dackis et al. 2005).

Heavy marijuana users also develop a physical dependence and may present for treatment when they are unable to stop daily use on their own (Haney et al. 2004). The symptoms consist of irritability, anxiety, marijuana craving, decreased quality and quantity of sleep and decreased food intake. Various medications have been used to alleviate these symptoms and some clinicians have reported success with dronabinol, the oral form of delta-9-tetrahydrocannabinol, but controlled clinical trials are lacking.

17.2.1 Detoxification by the suppression of autonomic hyperactivity

For opiate detoxification, methadone is not always available due to legal limitations and buprenorphine may be undesirable because it is a partial opiate agonist. Clonidine, an α_2-agonist, reverses opiate withdrawal by acting on autoreceptors producing presynaptic inhibition of locus coeruleus activity. This effectively reduces the large adrenergic component of opioid withdrawal (Gerra et al. 2001). Lofexidine, a similar medication, has been successfully used in the UK as an aid to opiate detoxification and is in clinical trials in the USA. Thus, clonidine and lofexidine have found a place in the clinic for treating the symptoms of opioid withdrawal. Very rapid detoxification under general anaesthesia has also been used, but there are no data to support an advantage over standard treatment.

17.3 Principles of relapse prevention

As a chronic disorder, addiction requires long-term treatment that should be measured in months and years. The strategies for preventing relapse have traditionally involved counselling or psychotherapy and, more recently, include pharmacotherapies that target clinical components of addictive illness. When psychiatric disorders co-occur with addiction, these disorders must be treated concomitantly and preferably by the same treatment team. This paper focuses on the medication for the primary addictive disorder, but counselling and medication of co-occurring disorders are equally important.

The treatment of addicted patients must always be individualized. This requires a complete evaluation so that coexisting medical, psychiatric and social problems can be addressed as needed. There are, however, common elements to treatment programmes. Treatments for addictive disorders may begin with detoxification, but the key to successful treatment is the long-term prevention of relapse by behavioural and pharmacological means. Usually, these approaches should be combined; insistence on behavioural treatment alone and without medication remains one of the chief weaknesses in many treatment programmes. The types of medication that have shown efficacy in combination with behavioural therapy in the prevention of relapse can be classified as agonists (including partial agonists), antagonists and anti-craving medications that work through a variety of mechanisms. Vaccines are an experimental approach that is currently being evaluated in clinical trials (Martell et al. 2005; Sofuoglu & Kosten 2006).

17.3.1 Agonists and partial agonists

The first use of an agonist for the treatment of addiction was reported in the 1960s by Vincent Dole and colleagues who demonstrated that daily methadone could transform the behaviour of opiate addicts, reducing craving and permitting the addict to engage in productive activities (Dole & Nyswander 1965).

Opiates (which are derivates of the opium poppy) and opioids (which may be peptides or synthetic compounds) activate opiate receptors that are located throughout the nervous system, as well as in the endocrine, cardiovascular, gastrointestinal and other systems of the body. The behavioural effects of opiates include intense euphoria and calming. The user becomes satisfied and relaxed, a state quite different from the euphoric excitement produced by stimulants. In the presence of pain, opiates, and opioids produce analgesia, so there is both relaxation and relief of severe pain.

While opioids produce prompt physiological dependence with repeated use, addiction seldom occurs in patients receiving opioids for the relief of severe pain (Adams et al. 2006). Of course, prescription opiates and opioids can be abused and it is the responsibility of the physician to provide humane pain relief to patients in need while exercising caution to reduce the likelihood that the prescribed medication will be obtained by deliberate abusers. The use of heroin or other opiates purchased on the street for the purpose of obtaining a 'high' has a significant risk of producing addiction.

Detoxification is not applicable to those opioid-dependent patients who prefer transition to maintenance using methadone or buprenorphine. Methadone has a slow onset by the oral route. It is a long-acting μ-opiate receptor agonist that largely prevents reward or euphoria if the patient 'slips' and takes a dose of an opiate. The mechanism for preventing euphoria is based on cross-tolerance in which tolerance (insensitivity) acquired by the use of one drug in a category conveys tolerance to all drugs in that category. Of course, the maintenance dose of methadone must be adjusted to the purity of heroin on the street. A dose of heroin significantly higher in opioid equivalents than the maintenance dose of methadone would override the cross-tolerance effect. Patients can be maintained for many years on a properly adjusted dose of methadone. Craving for opioids is diminished or absent, and patients are able to engage in constructive activities. Cognition and alertness are not impaired, and complex tasks including higher education can be accomplished (Kreek 1992). Currently, approximately 200 000 former opiate addicts are being maintained on methadone in the USA. Those with significant psychosocial problems require counselling or psychotherapy in addition to the medication.

As a partial agonist, buprenorphine produces limited opiate effects, and thus overdose is rare except when combined with benzodiazepines. Owing to its high affinity for the μ-receptor, buprenorphine effectively prevents access to the receptor by other opiates and opioids, thus reducing the likelihood that other opioids will be used. Patients treated with buprenorphine become physiologically dependent on it, as is the case with methadone, but if buprenorphine is stopped, withdrawal symptoms are quite mild. A limitation of buprenorphine is the ceiling on opiate agonist effects giving a maximal efficacy equivalent to approximately 40–50 mg of methadone. Addicts using large doses of street heroin may find that buprenorphine is not sufficiently potent to block withdrawal or drug craving.

Nicotine replacement has been listed in §17.2 as a treatment of nicotine withdrawal. The administration of nicotine as a patch, gum, or nasal spray can also be used as a maintenance treatment for extended periods as is the case with methadone. The levels obtained via a nicotine patch usually do not produce the pleasant responses achieved through smoking and there are usually no withdrawal symptoms on stopping the patch. Theoretically, smokers should be able to switch their nicotine dependence from administration via smoking to nicotine delivered by patch, chewing gum, or nasal spray. Although some smokers continue to chew nicotine gum for many months after giving up cigarettes, most discontinue nicotine replacement after a few weeks. The tendency to relapse may be strong, and thus it is important to teach patients behavioural techniques to resist the urge to smoke. An interesting approach that showed some efficacy in clinical trials is the combination of nicotine and mecamylamine, a nicotinic receptor antagonist, to prevent relapse to smoking. It was hypothesized that stimulation of receptors by both an agonist and an antagonist would be more effective, and the side effects of the two drugs would tend to cancel each other (Rose et al. 2001). The clinical data on this combination have been mixed, and more studies are needed.

Clinical serendipity played a role in the discovery of bupropion as an effective treatment of nicotine dependence (Ferry 1994). Originally used as an anti-depressant, bupropion was found to significantly improve abstinence rates in smokers whether or not they were depressed (Swan et al. 2003). The mechanism is unclear, but one effect of bupropion is the relief of negative affect in recently abstinent smokers (Lerman et al. 2002).

A recently introduced medication that applies the partial agonist principle in the treatment of tobacco use disorder is varenicline (Foulds 2006). This is an a4β2 nicotinic receptor partial agonist that has been reported to relieve cigarette craving and to result in a significantly higher rate of abstinence at 52 weeks (23%) than placebo (10.3%) or bupropion (14.6%) in company-sponsored double-blind trials (Jorenby et al. 2006).

Although agonist treatment is effective in opioid and nicotine addiction, agonists have not been found effective in patients addicted to stimulants. Experiments using methylphenidate or dextroamphetamine as agonists for cocaine and methamphetamine addiction have not been successful (Gorelick et al. 2004). Similarly, benzodiazepine treatment for alcohol or sedative dependence is ineffective. It is unclear why agonist treatment does not work in patients addicted to these substances.

17.3.2 Antagonist treatment

Advances in understanding how opioids interact with opiate receptors to produce their pharmacological effects led to the development of specific antagonists that have high affinity for these receptors, but do not activate the chain of cellular events producing opioid drug effects. Naltrexone is an antagonist that has great affinity for μ-opiate receptors and significant but less affinity for ∂- and kappa-opiate receptors. Unlike methadone, it has no agonist effects, so there are no opioid calming or other subjective effects. When first introduced, naltrexone was thought to be an ideal medication for heroin addiction because it occupied opiate receptors and blocked the effects of subsequent heroin injections. Experience has shown that most heroin addicts prefer methadone because it provides mild opioid-reinforcing effects that are absent in naltrexone. Thus, naltrexone has been used very little except for white-collar opiate addicts such as physicians, nurses and former addicts released from prison on probation (Cornish et al. 1997). The effects of blocking opiate receptors probably depend on the degree of tonic activation of the endogenous opioid system. Some normal volunteers given naltrexone experience nausea and dysphoria, while others experience no reaction. Although long-term blockade of opiate receptors might be expected to produce impairment of neuroendocrine function, remarkably few effects have been noted even in patients who have taken naltrexone daily for several years.

In 2006, a slow-release (depot) injectable preparation of naltrexone was given FDA approval and made available for prescription. Paradoxically, it was approved only for alcoholism because it was discovered in animal models that alcohol activated endogenous opioids (Altshuler et al. 1980). Subsequent work has clearly shown that endogenous opioids are involved in alcohol reinforcement. This was a discovery in an animal model that led directly to a completely novel treatment for alcoholism in humans. Such translational examples give hope that knowledge gained from basic research will eventually lead to new and better treatments. In 1983, clinical trials began and it was found that blocking opiate receptors with naltrexone significantly reduced relapse to clinically significant drinking (Volpicelli et al. 1990, 1992).

Of course, the depot form of naltrexone is also effective for the treatment of opioid addiction (Comer et al. 2006), and clinical trials are underway that will eventually lead to FDA approval for that indication in addition to alcoholism. Thus, opiate receptor antagonists have been found to be effective in the treatment of both opiate addiction (blocking external opiates) and alcoholism (blocking endogenous opioids). The availability of a depot form is expected to significantly improve the adherence to medication for this treatment method.

17.3.3 Genomic subcategories

The evidence for genetic influence on vulnerability to addiction is strong, but as with other complex psychiatric disorders, gene association studies based on diagnosis have not identified consistent susceptibility genes. Diagnosis in psychiatry still depends on behaviour rather than biomarkers. Recently, a sub-category of alcoholism based on a functional allele of the gene for the µ-opiate receptor has been studied as a candidate gene for an alcoholism endophenotype. The critical functional observation is an increased stimulation effect from alcohol in carriers of this gene. Recent reports of significantly improved treatment results in alcoholic patients selected on the basis of this genetic variant have raised the exciting prospect of alcoholism treatment guided by genomic testing (O'Brien 2008).

The variant is an A to G substitution at position 118 of exon 1 of the µ-opioid receptor gene and results in a receptor that has been reported to have greater affinity for β-endorphin (Bond et al. 1998). Individuals with this allele have been found to perceive greater stimulation from a given blood level of alcohol (Ray & Hutchison 2004) and the stimulation was found to be blocked by naltrexone pretreatment (Ray & Hutchison 2007). Reduced euphoria from alcohol was also reported in clinical trials of alcoholics randomized to naltrexone and in heavy-drinking volunteers with a family history of alcoholism given alcohol in the laboratory. A retrospective analysis of alcoholic patients in a naltrexone clinical trial found that those with the G allele did poorly when randomized to placebo, but had a significantly better outcome when randomized to naltrexone (Oslin et al. 2003). This finding was replicated in another clinical trial (Anton et al. 2008), but not in a small sample of U.S. Veterans Affairs alcoholics (Gelernter et al. 2007).

Taken together, the various lines of evidence suggest that alcohol activates the endogenous opioid system and this activation is exaggerated in carriers of this genetic variant. The proposed circuitry involves β-endorphin neurons that modulate ventral tegmental GABA neurons inhibiting dopamine (DA) neurons. Alcohol causes a release of β-endorphin or other endogenous opioids that inhibits GABA neurons, thus releasing DA neurons from inhibition and allowing dopaminergic stimulation. This mechanism is supported by microdialysis studies showing that the alcohol-induced DA increase is blocked by naltrexone (Gonzales & Weiss 1998).

17.3.4 Blockade of euphoria

There are different mechanisms whereby medications can block or diminish the euphoria produced by drugs of abuse. Antagonist treatment prevents the addictive agent from effective binding to brain receptors that mediate the euphoric response. This is best illustrated by naltrexone treatment in opiate dependence, since the mechanism of opiate euphoria results from the stimulation of µ-opiate receptors. The mechanism of stimulant euphoria is not well understood, so it has been more difficult to develop medications to block this essential clinical phenomenon. Nicotine replacement therapy for smokers can reduce the pleasure of smoking by a cross-tolerance mechanism similar to that of methadone for heroin euphoria.

Modafinil, a medication that retards sleep onset, has been shown to block cocaine-induced euphoria in three human laboratory studies of predominantly male subjects (Dackis et al. 2003; Malcolm et al. 2006; Hart et al. 2007). The mechanism of this blockade is unknown. Other medications block cocaine reward in animal studies (but not yet reliably demonstrated in humans) by increasing GABA-inhibitory effects on reward pathways such as ventral tegmental-ventral striatal DA pathways. These include medications such as topiramate (Kampman et al. 2004), vigabatrin (Brodie et al. 2005) and baclofen (Weerts et al. 2007). Animal models suggest that this GABA-enhancing mechanism may block the rewarding effects of alcohol as well as cocaine.

17.3.5 Medications that produce an aversive response

Until 1995, disulfiram was the only medication available to prevent relapse to uncontrolled drinking in detoxified alcoholics. This medication blocks the metabolism of alcohol, causing the accumulation of acetaldehyde, a noxious by-product. The resulting acetaldehyde reaction is so unpleasant that it effectively prevents patients from consuming any alcohol. Disulfiram has a place in the pharmacopoeia of medications for alcoholism but its usefulness is limited. Despite treatment contracts and even legal coercion, most alcoholics will not take disulfiram regularly and randomized clinical trials have not shown disulfiram to be efficacious (Fuller et al. 1986). Aversive conditioning has also been tried by timing an injection of emetine to produce vomiting while presenting the smell and taste of alcohol (Childress et al. 1985). A short-term success has been reported, but the technique has never become widespread.

17.3.6 Anti-craving medications

The pharmacological reversal of clinically significant neuroadaptations has long been employed with detoxification regimens, and the normalization of more persistent neuroadaptations might identify agents with anti-craving action (O'Brien 2005). In addition to chronic neuroadaptations in reward-related pathways, prefrontal cortical dysregulation has been demonstrated in stimulant, opioid and alcohol dependence (Dackis & O'Brien 2005), and is now viewed as a core component of addiction that contributes to poor impulse control, reduced motivation and denial in addicted individuals. Consequently, agents that enhance prefrontal cortical metabolism hold promise in the treatment of addiction.

Acamprosate, a medication that appears to decrease the desire for alcohol, was developed in Europe and has been available in the USA since 2004. Acamprosate appears to reduce the long-lasting neuronal hyperexcitability that follows chronic alcohol use (Kranzler & Gage 2008). The mechanisms are unclear but may include alterations in glutamate receptor gene expression. This medication suppresses the intake of alcohol in rats and, as with naltrexone, activity in the animal model predicts clinical efficacy. In double-blind studies, acamprosate has been shown to increase the likelihood of continuous abstinence in alcoholics and to shorten the period of drinking if the patient slips and consumes some alcohol.

The opiate receptor antagonist naltrexone has been reported in several clinical trials to reduce alcohol craving (O'Brien 2005) as well as alcohol reward. Human laboratory studies of alcohol priming in non-treatment-seeking alcoholics demonstrated a reduction in alcohol craving and alcohol drinking in spite of the alcohol priming drink in participants who were not seeking treatment (O'Malley et al. 2002).

Preclinical data have also shown an effect of alcohol on serotonergic systems. This has motivated trials using medications affecting that system. Ritanserin, a 5-hydroxytryptamine-2 (5-HT$_2$) receptor antagonist, was found to be no more effective than placebo in the treatment of alcoholism (Johnson et al. 1996). Ondansetron, a 5-HT$_3$ antagonist, was found to reduce drinking in early-onset alcoholics both alone (Johnson et al. 2000) and in combination with naltrexone (Ait-Daoud et al. 2001). Specific craving studies have not been addressed with the serotonergic medications.

17.4 Stimulant addiction

17.4.1 Cocaine sensitization

Sensitization is a progressive increase in the behavioural effects of a drug when a steady dose is repeatedly administered. This is a consistent finding in rodent studies, but it has not been clearly demonstrated in human cocaine addicts. Sensitization is typically measured by increased behavioural hyper-activity when the same dose is given daily to an animal. In human cocaine users, sensitization for euphoric effects of cocaine is not typically seen. On the contrary, some experienced users report that they require more cocaine over time to obtain euphoria, that is, drug tolerance. In the laboratory, tachyphylaxis (rapid tolerance) has been observed with reduced effects when the same dose was given repeatedly in one session. Since not all animals show behavioural sensitization to cocaine, and not all human cocaine users become addicted, it is possible that cocaine addicts whom we can observe in treatment are the minority of users who failed to sensitize.

Another possible explanation is that evidence of sensitization in human cocaine users may manifest as paranoid or psychotic symptoms. This idea is based on the fact that binge-limited paranoia begins after long-term cocaine use (mean interval 35 months) in vulnerable users (Satel & Edell 1991). Thus, a long-term exposure may be required to sensitize the patient to experience paranoia. The phenomenon of kindling has also been invoked to explain cocaine sensitization. Sub-convulsive doses of cocaine given repeatedly will eventually produce seizures in rats (Post et al. 1987). This observation has been compared to electrical kindling of seizures and may underlie the gradual development of paranoia.

Cocaine users experience intense craving when exposed to cocaine-related cues, which typically include the neighbourhood where they have used cocaine, the sight of cocaine, cocaine paraphernalia and cash (used to purchase cocaine). This response has been measured in the laboratory when abstinent cocaine users are shown video scenes associated with cocaine use (Ehrman et al. 1992). The conditioned response consists of physiological arousal and increased drug craving. Cue-induced craving leads directly to relapse in addicted patients, even after long periods of abstinence. Medications that block limbic activation in response to cocaine cues may prove effective against this relapse mechanism.

Numerous studies have been conducted on medications that might aid in the rehabilitation of cocaine addicts. A detailed review would not be useful since most are no longer used. Among those medications still under study in clinical trials as a treatment for stimulant addiction are modafinil (Dackis et al. 2005), disulfiram (Carroll et al. 2004) and topiramate (Kampman et al. 2006).

Buprenorphine, a partial opioid agonist, has been found to reduce cocaine self-administration in monkeys (Mello & Negus 2007), but studies in cocaine-dependent patients have yielded mixed results. A recent controlled study of buprenorphine in a population of combined opiate- and cocaine-dependent patients has shown a positive effect in reducing the use of both cocaine and opiates (Montoya et al. 2004). The results were consistent with the hypothesis that buprenorphine is effective for cocaine only in higher doses, 16 mg or greater.

Studies in animals have consistently shown that the enhancement of GABA activity reduces cocaine self-administration (Roberts et al. 1996). Preliminary results from clinical trials using baclofen, a $GABA_B$ agonist, and topiramate, which activates $GABA_A$ receptors, suggest that this approach may reduce cocaine use in human subjects as well (Shoptaw et al. 2003). Controlled clinical trials of treatment of cocaine and methamphetamine addicts using vigabatrin, an inhibitor of GABA transaminase, are just beginning (Brodie etal. 2005).

Another recent novel approach involves modafinil, a drug that produces alerting via a complex mechanism involving enhanced glutamate activity. As mentioned in §17.3.4, modafinil partially blocks cocaine-induced euphoria in the laboratory. In a randomized clinical trial, Dackis reported that modafinil-treated subjects significantly reduced their use of cocaine when compared with placebo-treated subjects (Dackis et al. 2005). Modafinil is currently under intense investigation as a potential first-line treatment for cocaine dependence.

17.4.2 Other stimulants

Amphetamine, dextroamphetamine, methamphetamine, phenmetrazine, methylphenidate and diethyl-propion all produce behavioural activation similar to that of cocaine. Amphetamines increase synaptic DA levels primarily by stimulating presynaptic DA release rather than by blockade of reuptake at the DA transporter, as is the case with cocaine. Intravenous or smoked methamphetamine is an important drug of abuse in the western half of the USA, and it produces an abuse/dependence syndrome similar to that of cocaine. Paranoid psychosis is more common with amphetamine abuse. In some geographical areas, methamphetamine abuse has reached epidemic proportions and there are intensive efforts to develop behavioural and medication treatments for this serious addiction (Rawson et al. 2000).

A different picture arises when oral stimulants are prescribed in a weight-reduction programme. These drugs do reduce appetite and weight on a short-term basis, but the effects diminish over time as tolerance develops. In rodents, there is a rebound of appetite and weight gain when amphetamine use is stopped. In obese humans, weight loss after amphetamine treatment is usually temporary. Anorectic medications, therefore, are not considered to be a treatment for obesity by themselves, but rather a short-term adjunct to behavioural treatment programmes. It is noteworthy that drug abuse manifested by drug-seeking behaviour occurs in only a small proportion of patients given stimulants to facilitate weight reduction.

17.4.3 Cannabinoids (marijuana)

Cannabinoids are the most widely abused illegal drugs. The frequency of addiction among marijuana users in the USA is approximately 9%. Tolerance to the effects of marijuana has been demonstrated in both humans and animals (Jones et al. 1981). Withdrawal symptoms and signs are not typically seen in clinical populations, but some patients report compulsive frequent marijuana use. In 2002, over 280 000 people entered treatment for cannabis dependence (NIDA 2007). There is no specific treatment for marijuana dependence at this time, but cannabinoid receptor antagonists are logical candidates for investigation. The withdrawal syndrome does not require medication unless persistent signs of depression are present. Prevention of relapse is accomplished by behavioural treatments such as those used in the treatment of alcoholism or cocaine addiction (Stephens et al. 2002). Medication such as the cannabinoid agonist dronabinol has been used clinically to treat withdrawal, but randomized trials are lacking. Cannabinoid receptor antagonists are available, but have not yet been tested in clinical trials for marijuana addiction.

17.4.4 Hallucinogenic drugs

Addiction in the usual sense does not occur with this category of drugs, so they will not be discussed in this paper. Their use carries significant risks and counselling is the only effective approach.

17.5 Therapeutics under development

17.5.1 The vaccine approach

Immunization against the effects of an abused drug was first tested using morphine. Monkeys were immunized with morphine-6-hemisuccinate-bovine serum albumin, and the resultant morphine antibodies were found to reduce self-administration of heroin but not cocaine (Killian et al. 1978). Recently, active immunization with a new, stable cocaine conjugate has been found to suppress cocaine, but not amphetamine-induced locomotor activity and stereotyped behaviour in rats (Rocio et al. 1995). Brain levels of cocaine were also lowered by the antibodies, and rats and mice were found to reduce intravenous cocaine self-administration after the passive transfer of cocaine antibodies (Kantak et al. 2000). A clinical trial involving 34 subjects showed that the vaccine caused few side effects and produced dose-related levels of antibodies (Martell et al. 2005). Recent studies have shown further improvement in the vaccine, but additional studies involving dose-response relationships to clinical response are necessary. In spite of cocaine antibodies, relapse may still be possible by using a high dose of the drug or by taking a different stimulant.

17.5.2 Current status of pharmacotherapy

Medications that target addiction phenomena, such as euphoria, withdrawal and craving, are being developed as adjunctive treatments that may significantly improve clinical outcome. In the case of alcoholism, a completely novel treatment that probably would not have been discovered in the clinic was developed from animal models. The development of new agents has been greatly facilitated by research, revealing the underlying neuronal mechanisms of these phenomena. Although the many types of drug use disorders have common aspects, there are also many differences that must be specifically addressed with different pharmacological strategies. In addition, all patients require a full evaluation and tailored treatment plans that take their unique set of problems into account. It is especially important to identify and stabilize co-occurring medical and psychiatric disorders in the addicted population. Currently, effective medications are available for some addictive disorders, and others will certainly be developed through continued research. When viewed in comparison with other chronic diseases, the current treatments for addiction are reasonably successful (O'Brien & McLellan 1996; McLellan et al. 2000). Long-term treatment is accompanied by improvements in physical status, as well as in mental, social, and occupational functions. Treatment is usually not curative. As is the case with other chronic diseases, when the treatment is ended, relapse eventually occurs in most cases.

References

Adams, E. H., Breiner, S., Cicero, T. J., Geller, A., Inciardi, J. A., Schnoll, S. H., Senay, E. C. & Woody, G. E. 2006 A comparison of the abuse liability of tramadol, NSAIDs, and hydrocodone in patients with chronic pain. *J. Pain Symptom Manage.* **31**, 465–76. (doi:10.1016/j.jpainsym-man.2005. 10.006)

Ait-Daoud, N., Johnson, B. A., Javors, M., Roache, J. D. & Zanca, N. A. 2001 Combining ondansetron and naltrexone treats biological alcoholics: corroboration of self-reported drinking by serum carbohydrate deficient transferrin, a biomarker. *Alcohol. Clin. Exp. Res.* **25**, 847–9. (doi:10. 1111/j. 1530–0277.2001.tb02289.x)

Altshuler, H. L., Phillips, P. A. & Feinhandler, D. A. 1980 Alteration of ethanol self-administration by naltrexone. *Life Sci.* **26**, 679–88. (doi:10.1016/0024–3205(80)90257–X)

Anthony, J. C., Warner, L. A. & Kessler, R. C. 1994 Comparative epidemiology of dependence on tobacco, alcohol, controlled substances, and inhalants: basic findings from the National Comorbidity Survey. *Exp. Clin. Psychopharmacol.* **2**, 244–68. (doi: 10.1037/1064–1297.2.3.244)

Anton, R. F., Oroszi, G., O'Malley, S., Couper, D., Swift, R., Pettinati, H. & Goldman, D. 2008 An evaluation of μ-opioid receptor (OPRM1) as a predictor of naltrexone response in the treatment of alcohol dependence: results from the combined pharmacotherapies and behavioral interventions for alcohol dependence (COMBINE) study. *Arch. Gen. Psychiatry* **65**, 135–44. (doi:10.1001/arch–psyc.65.2.135)

Bond, C. et al. 1998 Single-nucleotide polymorphism in the human mu opioid receptor gene alters β-endorphin binding and activity: possible implications for opiate addiction. *Proc. Natl Acad. Sci.* **95**, 9608–13. (doi:10.1073/pnas.95.16.9608)

Brodie, J. D., Figueroa, E., Laska, E. M. & Dewey, S. L. 2005 Safety and efficacy of γ-vinyl GABA (GVG) for the treatment of and/or cocaine addiction. *Synapse* **55**, 122–5. (doi:10.1002/syn.20097)

Brown, M. E., Anton, R. F., Malcolm, R. & Ballenger, J. C. 1988 Alcohol detoxification and withdrawal seizures: clinical support for a kindling hypothesis. *Biol. Psychiatry* **23**, 507–14. (doi:10.1016/0006–3223(88)90023–6)

Carroll, K. M., Fenton, L. R., Ball, S. A., Nich, C., Frankforter, T. L., Shi, J. & Rounsaville, B. J. 2004 Efficacy of disulfiram and cognitive behavior therapy in cocaine-dependent outpatients: a randomized placebo-controlled trial. *Arch. Gen. Psychiatry* **61**, 264–72. (doi:10.1001/archpsyc.61.3.264)

Childress, A. R., McLellan, A. T. & O'Brien, C. P. 1985 Behavioral therapies for substance abuse. *Int. J. Addict.* **20**, 947–69.

Childress, A. R., Mozley, P. D., McElgin, W., Fitzgerald, J., Reivich, M. & O'Brien, C. P. 1999 Limbic activation during cue-induced cocaine craving. *Am. J. Psychiatry* **156**, 11–18.

Childress, A. R. et al. 2008 Prelude to passion: limbic activation by "unseen" drug and sexual cues. *PLoS ONE* **3**, e1506. (doi:10.1371/journal.pone.0001506)

Comer, S. D., Sullivan, M. A., Yu, E., Rothenberg, J. L., Kleber, H. D., Kampman, K., Dackis, C. & O'Brien, C. P. 2006 Injectable, sustained-release naltrexone for the treatment of opioid dependence: a randomized, placebo-controlled trial. *Arch. Gen. Psychiatry* **63**, 210–18. (doi:10.1001/archpsyc.63.2.210)

Cornish, J. W., Metzger, D., Woody, G. E., Wilson, D., McLellan, A. T., Vandergrift, B. & O'Brien, C. P. 1997 Naltrexone pharmacotherapy for opioid dependent federal probationers. *J. Subst. Abuse Treat.* **14**, 529–34. (doi:10.1016/S0740–5472(97)00020–2)

Dackis, C. A. & O'Brien, C. 2003 The neurobiology of alcoholism. In *Handbook of psychiatric disorders* (eds S. Gershon & R. Soires), pp. 563–80. New York, NY: Marcel Dekker.

Dackis, C. A. & O'Brien, C. 2005 Neurobiology of addiction: treatment and public policy ramifications (commentary). *Nat. Neurosci.* **8**, 1431–6. (doi:10.1038/nn1105–1431)

Dackis, C. A. et al. 2003 Modafinil and cocaine: a double-blind, placebo-controlled drug interaction study. *Drug Alcohol Depend.* **70**, 29–37. (doi:10.1016/S0376–8716(02) 00335–6)

Dackis, C. A., Kampman, K. M., Lynch, K. G., Pettinati, H. M. & O'Brien, C. P. 2005 A double-blind, placebo-controlled trial of modafinil for cocaine dependence. *Neuropsychopharmacology* **30**, 205–11. (doi:10.1038/ sj.npp.1300600)

Deroche-Gamonet, V., Belin, D. & Piazza, P. V. 2004 Evidence for addiction-like behavior in the rat. *Science* **305**, 1014–17. (doi:10.1126/science.1099020)

Dole, V. P. & Nyswander, M. 1965 A medical treatment for diacetylmorphine (heroin) addiction: a clinical trial with methadone hydrochloride. *J. Am. Med. Assoc.* **193**, 80–4.

Ehrman, R., Robbins, S., Childress, A. R. & O'Brien, C. P. 1992 Conditioned responses to cocaine-related stimuli in cocaine abuse patients. *Psychopharmacology* **107**, 523–9. (doi:10.1007/BF02245266)

Ferry, L. 1994 Bupropion versus placebo for nicotine dependence. American Psychiatric Association, Annual Meeting Abstracts, New Research no. 544. Washington, DC: APA Press.

Foulds, J. 2006 The neurobiological basis for partial agonist treatment of nicotine dependence: varenicline. *Int. J. Clin. Pract.* **60**, 571–6. (doi:10.1111/j.1368–5031. 2006.00955.x)

Franklin, T R., Acton, P. D., Maldjian, J. A., Gray, J. D., Croft, J. R., Dackis, C. A., O'Brien, C. P. &
    Childress, A. R. 2002 Decreased gray matter concentration in the insular, orbitofrontal, cingulate,
    and temporal cortices of cocaine patients. *Biol. Psychiatry* **51**, 134–42. (doi:10.1016/S0006–3223
    (01)01269–0)

Fuller, R. K. et al. 1986 Disulfiram treatment of alcoholism. A Veterans Administration cooperative
    study. *J. Am. Med. Assoc.* **256**, 1449–55. (doi:10.1001/jama.256.11.1449)

Gelernter, J., Gueorguieva, R., Kranzler, H. R., Zhang, H., Cramer, J., Rosenheck, R. & Krystal, J. H.
    2007 Opioid receptor gene (*OPRM1, OPRK1,* and *OPRD1*) variants and response to naltrexone
    treatment for alcohol dependence: results from the VA Cooperative Study. *Alcohol Clin. Exp. Res.*
    31, 555–63.

Gerra, G., Zaimovic, A., Giusti, F., Di Gennaro, C., Zambelli, U., Gardini, S. & Delsignore, R. 2001
    Lofexidine versus clonidine in rapid opiate detoxification. *J. Subst. Abuse Treat.* **21**, 11–17.
    (doi:10.1016/S0740–5472(01)00178–7)

Gonzales, R. A. & Weiss, F. 1998 Suppression of ethanol-reinforced behavior by naltrexone is associ-
    ated with attenuation of the ethanol-induced increase in dialysate dopamine levels in the nucleus
    accumbens. *J. Neurosci.* **18**, 10 663–71.

Gorelick, D. A., Gardner, E. L. & Xi, Z. X. 2004 Agents in development for the management of
    cocaine abuse. *Drugs* **64**, 1547–73. (doi: 10.2165/00003495–200464 140–00004)

Haney, M., Hart, C. L., Vosburg, S. K., Nasser, J., Bennett, A., Zubaran, C. & Foltin, R. W. 2004
    Marijuana withdrawal in humans: effects of oral THC or divalproex. *Neuropsychopharmacology*
    29, 158–70. (doi:10.1038/ sj.npp.1300310)

Hart, C. L., Haney, M., Vosburg, S. K., Rubin, E. & Foltin, R. W. 2007 Smoked cocaine self-
    administration is decreased by modafinil. *Neuropsychopharmacology* **33**, 761–8. (doi:10.1038/sj.
    npp.1301472)

Johnson, B. A. et al. 1996 Ritanserin in the treatment of alcohol dependence—a multi-center clinical
    trial. *Psychopharmacology* **128**, 206–15. (doi:10.1007/s002130 050126)

Johnson, B. A., Roache, J. D., Javors, M. A., DiClemente, C. C., Cloninger, C. R., Prihoda, T. J.,
    Bordnick, P. S., Ait-Daoud, N. & Hensler, J. 2000 Ondansetron for reduction of drinking among
    biologically predisposed alcoholic patients: a randomized controlled trial [see comments]. *J. Am.
    Med. Assoc.* **284**, 963–71. (doi:10.1001/jama.284.8.963)

Jones, R. T., Benowitz, N. L. & Herning, R. I. 1981 Clinical review of cannabis tolerance and depen-
    dence. *J. Clin. Pharmacol.* **21**, 143S–52S. (doi:10.1007/BF00637515)

Jorenby, D. E., Hays, J. T., Rigotti, N. A., Azoulay, S., Watsky, E. J., Williams, K. E., Billing, C. B.,
    Gong, J. & Reeves, K. R. 2006 Efficacy of varenicline, an α4β2 nicotinic acetylcholine receptor
    partial agonist, vs placebo or sustained-release bupropion for smoking cessation: a randomized
    controlled trial. *J. Am. Med. Assoc.* **296**, 56–63. (doi:10.1001/jama.296.1.56)

Kampman, K. M. et al. 2001 Cocaine withdrawal symptoms and initial urine toxicology results
    predict treatment attrition in outpatient cocaine dependence treatment. *Psychol. Addict. Behav.* **15**,
    52–9. (doi:10.1037/0893–164X.15.1.52)

Kampman, K. M., Pettinati, H., Lynch, K. G., Dackis, C., Sparkman, T., Weigley, C. & O'Brien, C. P.
    2004 A pilot trial of topiramate for the treatment of cocaine dependence. *Drug Alcohol Depend.* **75**,
    233–40. (doi:10.1016/ j.drugalcdep.2004.03.008)

Kampman, K. M., Dackis, C., Lynch, K. G., Pettinati, H., Tirado, C., Gariti, P., Sparkman, T., Atzram, M.
    & O'Brien, C. P. 2006 A double-blind, placebo-controlled trial of amantadine, propranolol, and
    their combination for the treatment of cocaine dependence in patients with severe cocaine with-
    drawal symptoms. *Drug Alcohol Depend.* **85**, 129–37. (doi:10.1016/j.drugalcdep.2006.04.002)

Kantak, K. M., Collins, S. L., Lipman, E. G., Bond, J., Giovanoni, K. & Fox, B. S. 2000 Evaluation
    of anti-cocaine antibodies and a cocaine vaccine in a rat self-administration model.
    Psychopharmacology **148**, 251–62. (doi:10.1007/s002130050049)

Killian, A., Bonese, K., Rothberg, R., Wainer, B. & Schuster, C. 1978 Effects of passive immunization
    against morphine on heroin self-administration. *Pharmacol. Biochem. Behav.* **9**, 347–52.
    (doi:10.1016/0091–3057(78)90295–2)

Koob, G. F., Ahmed, S. H., Boutrel, B., Chen, S. A., Kenny, P. J., Markou, A., O'Dell, L. E., Parsons,
    L. H. & Sanna, P. P. 2004 Neurobiological mechanisms in the transition from drug use to drug
    dependence. *Neurosci. Biobehav. Rev.* **27**, 739–49. (doi:10.1016/j.neubiorev.2003.11.007)

Kranzler, H. R. & Gage, A. 2008 Acamprosate efficacy in alcohol-dependent patients: summary of results from three pivotal trials. *Am. J. Addict.* **17**, 70–6. (doi:10.1080/10550490701756120)

Kreek M. J. 1992 Rationale for maintenance pharmacotherapy of opiate dependence. In *Addictive states* (eds C. P. O'Brien & J. Jaffe), ch.13, pp. 205–30. New York, NY: Raven Press.

LeBlanc, A., Kalant, H., Gibbins, R. & Berman, N. 1969 Acquisition and loss of tolerance to ethanol by the rat. *J. Pharmacol. Exp. Ther.* **168**, 244–50.

Lerman, C., Roth, D., Kaufman, V., Audrain, J., Hawk, L., Liu, A., Niaura, R. & Epstein, L. 2002 Mediating mechanisms for the impact of bupropion in smoking cessation treatment. *Drug Alcohol Depend.* **67**, 219–23. (doi:10.1016/S0376–8716(02)00067–4)

Malcolm, R. et al. 2006 Modafinil and cocaine interactions. *Am. J. Drug Alcohol Abuse* **32**, 577–87. (doi:10.1080/ 00952990600920425)

Martell, B. A., Mitchell, E., Poling, J., Gonsai, K. & Kosten, T. R. 2005 Vaccine pharmacotherapy for the treatment of cocaine dependence. *Biol. Psychiatry* **58**, 158–64. (doi:10.1016/j.biopsych.2005.04.032)

McLellan, A. T., Lewis, D. C., O'Brien, C. P. & Kleber, H. D. 2000 Drug dependence, a chronic medical illness: implications for treatment, insurance, and outcomes evaluation. *J. Am. Med. Assoc.* **284**, 1689–95. (doi:10.1001/jama.284.13.1689)

McLellan, A. T., Weinstein, R. L., Shen, Q., Kendig, C. & Levine, M. 2005 Improving continuity of care in a public addiction treatment system with clinical case management. *Am. J. Addict.* **14**, 426–40. (doi:10.1080/105504 90500247099)

Mello, N. K. & Negus, S. S. 2007 Effects of d-amphetamine and buprenorphine combinations on speedball (cocaine + heroin) self-administration by rhesus monkeys. *Neuropsychopharmacology* **32**, 1985–94. (doi:10.1038/sj.npp.1301319)

Montoya, I. D. et al. 2004 Randomized trial of buprenorphine for treatment of concurrent opiate and cocaine dependence. *Clin. Pharmacol. Ther.* **75**, 34–48. (doi:10.1016/ j.clpt.2003.09.004)

NIDA 2007 Marijuana facts. NIDA. See http://www.nida. nih.gov/MarijBroch/parentpg17–18N. html#Addicted.

O'Brien, C. P. 2005 Anticraving medications for relapse prevention: a possible new class of psycho-active medications. *Am. J. Psychiatry* **162**, 1423–31. (doi:10.1176/ appi.ajp.162.8.1423)

O'Brien, C. P. 2006 Drug addiction and drug abuse. In *Goodman & Gilman's the pharmacological basis of therapeutics* (eds L. Brunton, J. Lazo & K. Parker), pp. 607–27, 11th. New York, NY: McGraw-Hill.

O'Brien, C. P. 2008 Prospects for a genomic approach to the treatment of alcoholism. *Arch. Gen. Psychiatry* **65**, 132–33. (doi:10.1001/archgenpsychiatry.2007.32)

O'Brien, C. P. & McLellan, A. T. 1996 Myths about the treatment of addiction. *Lancet* **347**, 237–40. (doi:10. 1016/S0140–6736(96)90409–2)

O'Brien, C. P., O'Brien, T. J., Mintz, J. & Brady, J. P. 1975 Conditioning of narcotic abstinence symptoms in human subjects. *Drug Alcohol Depend.* **1**, 115–23. (doi:10.1016/ 0376–8716(75)90013–7)

O'Malley, S. S., Krishnan-Sarin, S., Farren, C., Sinha, R. & Kreek, J. 2002 Naltrexone decreases craving and alcohol self-administration in alcohol-dependent subjects and activates the hypothalamo-pituitary-adrenocortical axis. *Psychopharmacology (Berl.)* **160**, 19–29. (doi:10.1007/ s002130100919)

Oslin, D. W., Berrettini, W., Kranzler, H. R., Pettinati, H., Gelernter, J., Volpicelli, J. R. & O'Brien, C. P. 2003 A functional polymorphism of the mu-opioid receptor gene is associated with naltrexone response in alcohol-dependent patients. *Neuropsychopharmacology* **28**, 1546–52. (doi:10.1038/ sj.npp.1300219)

Post, R. M., Weiss, S. R. B., Pert, A. & Uhde, T. W. 1987 Chronic cocaine administration: sensitization and kindling effects. In *Cocaine: clinical and biobehavioral aspects,* pp. 109–73. New York, NY: Oxford University Press.

Rawson, R., Huber, A., Brethen, P., Obert, J., Gulati, V., Shoptaw, S. & Ling, W. 2000 Methamphetamine and cocaine users: differences in characteristics and treatment retention. *J. Psychoactive Drugs* **32**, 233–8.

Ray, L. A. & Hutchison, K. E. 2004 A polymorphism of the mu-opioid receptor gene (*OPRM1*) and sensitivity to the effects of alcohol in humans. *Alcohol Clin. Exp. Res.* **28**, 1789–95. (doi:10.1097/01. ALC.0000148114. 34000.B9)

Ray, L. A. & Hutchison, K. E. 2007 Effects of naltrexone on alcohol sensitivity and genetic modera-
    tors of medication response: a double-blind placebo-controlled study. *Arch. Gen. Psychiatry* **64**,
    1069–77. (doi:10.1001/archpsyc.64.9.1069)
Roberts, D. C., Andrews, M. M. & Vickers, G. J. 1996 Baclofen attenuates the reinforcing effects of
    cocaine in rats. *Neuropsychopharmacology* **15**, 417–23. (doi:10.1016/ 0893–133X(96)00002–4)
Rocio, M., Carrera, A., Ashley, J. A., Parsons, L. H., Wirsching, P., Koob, G. F. & Janda, K. D. 1995
Suppression of psychoactive effects of cocaine by active immunization. *Nature* **378**, 727–30.
    (doi:10.1038/ 378727a0)
Rose, J. E., Behm, F. M. & Westman, E. C. 2001 Acute effects of nicotine and mecamylamine on
    tobacco withdrawal symptoms, cigarette reward and ad lib smoking. *Pharmacol. Biochem. Behav.*
    68, 187–97. (doi:10.1016/S0091–3057 (00)00465–2)
Satel, S. L. & Edell, W. S. 1991 Cocaine-induced paranoia and psychosis proneness. *Am. J. Psychiatry*
    148, 1708–11.
Shoptaw, S., Yang, X., Rotheram-Fuller, E. J., Hsieh, Y.C., Kintaudi, P. C., Charuvastra, V. C. & Ling,
    W. 2003 Randomized placebo-controlled trial of baclofen for cocaine dependence: preliminary
    effects for individuals with chronic patterns of cocaine use.J. *Clin. Psychiatry* **64**, 1440–8.
Sofuoglu, M. & Kosten, T. R. 2006 Emerging pharmacological strategies in the fight against cocaine
    addiction. *Expert Opin. Emerg. Drugs* **11**, 91–8. (doi:10.1517/ 14728214.11.1.91)
Stephens, R. S., Babor, T. F., Kadden, R. & Miller, M. 2002 The Marijuana Treatment Project:
    rationale, design and participant characteristics. *Addiction* 97(Suppl. 1), 109–24. (doi: 10.1046/j.
    1360–0443.97.s01.6.x)
Swan, G. E., McAfee, T. & Curry, S. J. 2003 Effectiveness of bupropion sustained release for smoking
    cessation in a health care setting: a randomized trial. *Arch. Intern. Med.* **163**, 2337–444. (doi:10.1001/
    archinte.163.19.2337)
Volpicelli, J. R., O'Brien, C. P., Alterman, A. I. & Hayashida, M. 1990 Naltrexone and the treatment
    of alcohol dependence: initial observations. In *Opioids, bulimia, alcohol abuse and alcoholism*
    (ed. L. B. Reid), pp. 195–214. New York, NY: Springer-Verlag.
Volpicelli, J. R., Alterman, A. I., Hayashida, M. & O'Brien, C. P. 1992 Naltrexone in the treatment of
    alcohol dependence. *Arch. Gen. Psychiatry* **49**, 876–80.
Weerts, E. M., Froestl, W., Kaminski, B. J. & Griffiths, R. R. 2007 Attenuation of cocaine-seeking
    by GABA B receptor agonists baclofen and CGP44532 but not the GABA reuptake inhibitor
    tiagabine in baboons. *Drug Alcohol Depend.* **89**, 206–13. (doi:10.1016/j.drugalcdep. 2006.12.023)
Wikler, A. 1973 Dynamics of drug dependence: implications of a conditioning theory for research and
    treatment. *Arch. Gen. Psychiatry* **28**, 611–16.

18

Concluding summary and discussion: New vistas

Trevor W. Robbins, Barry J. Everitt, and David J. Nutt

Royal Society Discussion meetings, as befits the name, are usually marked by the quality and range of discussion that occurs at them. This feature was encouraged in this meeting on the Neurobiology of Drug Addiction by arranging the talks around four main themes and having quite lengthy discussions, based on questions from the floor, after each presentation. This concluding chapter attempts to capture some of this discussion and controversy whilst also drawing out significant cross-cutting themes and points for debate, as gleaned in part from recordings of the lectures and the ensuing discussions.

Behavioural theories of addiction

The meeting opened with a series of talks describing key theoretical points that had emerged from recent scientific findings of relevance to addiction. They were dominated by descriptions of phenomena from basic research, which mainly used experimental animals in so-called models of addiction, such as that based on reinforcing effects of drugs as indicated by drug self-administration, whether by intravenous catheter or orally, in the case of alcohol. Self-administration is generally taken as the gold standard because the drug is administered in a way that is both predicted and regulated (to some extent) by the animal, which presumably removes obvious confounds such as stress induction that may detract from the reinforcing effects of drugs. However, Robinson did make the argument that some of the potentially important phenomena that accompany drug taking, such as the incremental responding observed following sensitization, are probably best observed when the drugs are administered in a controlled way, by the experimenter. This is a key issue, as the theory described by Everitt et al. does depend rather crucially on the fact that drug seeking and drug taking represent an integration of both elicited, Pavlovian responses, together with instrumental behaviour that makes contact with the goal (e.g. drug self-administration). What is crucial to all theories of addiction, and also has become embodied in many diagnostic descriptions, is why the behaviour becomes 'compulsive', i.e. loses its regulated nature with respect to drug intake and is performed 'out-of control' (see also the contribution of Koob and LeMoal). For Robinson and Berridge, this compulsive property comes from a dissociation between 'liking' and 'wanting' the effects of a drug, which is inferred mainly from the study of ingestive responses to food in the rat, in which so-called 'hedonic' reflexes sometimes appear intact when appetitive behaviour in general diminishes. The attraction of this hypothesis is that tolerance to 'hedonic' effects of drugs does occur, while addicts continue to seek (or 'want') drugs. This 'wanting' behaviour is held to be exacerbated by 'sensitization' to the effects of the drugs and environmental stimuli associated with them.

Another way of explaining this dissociation is to make use of a parallel dissociation that has emerged in learning theory for instrumental behaviour between action–outcome associations and stimulus–response (S–R) habits (Everitt et al.). The latter occur as the behaviour becomes increasingly divorced from the outcome or goal. Although this behaviour thus has the quality of becoming relatively 'automatic', it is important not to confuse it with procedural or skill learning, in which it is sensori-motor parameters that are practised to the point of producing invariant performance. Thus, drug seeking has more of the quality of occurring autonomously and outwith normal restraints on behaviour, than that of 'tying a shoelace' (c.f. Robinson and Berridge), which is of course, simply a highly practised motor programme.

However, there are important issues that remain; the extent to which Pavlovian behaviours influence the instrumental behaviour of drug seeking and taking, and the question of how habitual behaviour actually may become compulsive. These points are also bound almost inseparably with the important question of how this behaviour is controlled by the brain—the central point of the entire Discussion Meeting. There appears little doubt that Pavlovian conditioning mechanisms contribute to drug addiction; the evidence that cues paired with drug effects become important for subsequent drug-seeking behaviour, as occurs for example in relapse in experimental animals (Stewart; Crombag et al.) and humans (O'Brien) being overwhelming. However, the question of exactly how this happens is less clear; Pavlovian conditioned stimuli can become conditioned reinforcers for responding (i.e. they can act as 'sub-goals' in their own right), but such stimuli may directly energize responding through their incentive motivational qualities (Robinson & Berridge). But in the context of drug seeking and taking behaviour, it has proven difficult to detect the motivational effects of conditioned stimuli and much easier to demonstrate their role as conditioned reinforcers (Everitt et al.) or as attractants that capture attention and elicit approach (Robinson).

On the issue of how 'habits' may become compulsions, there are several possible notions. One is that this is achieved by drug-induced 'sensitization' (Robinson & Berridge). A key point that emerged from the Meeting is that psychostimulant sensitization can exaggerate a number of possible processes leading to addiction, including habit formation itself. Moreover, sensitization in rats is also expressed not in terms of drug-taking behaviour itself, but as increases in locomotor activity and stereotyped behaviour, which may arise in part from the influence of Pavlovian conditioning to the environment ('contexual' conditioning) by the unconditioned effects of stimulant drugs. Given that stereotyped behaviour itself is obviously an example of compulsive behaviour, occurring almost to the exclusion of other behaviour, it seems possible that psychostimulant sensitization could indeed turn 'habits' into 'compulsions'. A factor that then becomes significant is the situations in which sensitization is maximized; this does not necessarily occur as a function of massed conditioning trials, but rather more intermittently. Whether it is intermittency or massed trials in the form of 'bingeing', for example of cocaine, that is most relevant for human stimulant addiction remains open, as both patterns of intake can occur.

However, there are at least two other possible mechanisms that must be taken into account for the understanding of compulsive drug taking. The first of these was evident from the paper by Koob and LeMoal, whose focus is less on the type of addiction produced by stimulant drugs such as amphetamine and cocaine than more generally on other forms of drug addiction including to opiates and to alcohol. These authors place much more emphasis on the 'dark side' of addiction, viz., the negative emotional state induced by withdrawal, in providing a detailed account of the behavioural, neural, and neurochemical changes in withdrawal in temporal terms. This state can be understood in animal learning theory as a 'rebound' process that becomes increasingly marked during conditioning, as the initial positive affective, or 'a', process diminishes (e.g. through tolerance to the rewarding effects of drugs). The existence of the negative state then makes drug seeking and taking necessary for the curtailment or avoidance of the withdrawal state, a process termed negative reinforcement.

Important evidence for negative states included the fact that 'reward thresholds' appear to be elevated so that 'rewarding' brain stimulation becomes less effective in withdrawn animals.

Such changes were shown to occur during stimulant, nicotine, opiate, or alcohol withdrawal. This evidence makes it difficult to deny a possible negative reinforcing quality of drug seeking/taking behaviour, which promotes strong avoidance behaviour that is also well-known to be susceptible to habitual qualities. A possible criticism of the procedure that it reflects the abnormal 'rewarding' properties of brain stimulation, particularly in humans, was met by the assertion of motivational properties of such stimulation in many human subjects. A key question however remains whether this mechanism is sufficient to account for compulsive drug taking/seeking as opposed to being merely contributory. And are the changes that occur during withdrawal sufficiently long lasting to account for relapse months later? One possible answer to that objection lies in the long-lasting nature of conditioning processes themselves. A further question was whether agents that opposed withdrawal-induced relapse, such as CRF receptor antagonists, had intrinsic positive reinforcing properties? There was no evidence of this from place preference conditioning.

A final source of factors leading to compulsive behaviour may be neurological. Classically, drug addiction has been considered to arise from a failure of the 'will'. In modern terms, this might be construed in terms of failures of inhibitory control resulting from impaired 'top–down' influences from neural structures such as the prefrontal cortex. Theoretically, this could arise in drug addiction from neurotoxic effects of drugs impairing frontal lobe function, leading incidentally to a range of cognitive impairments including loss of inhibitory control. Typical evidence was presented in the contributions by Garavan et al. (for stimulants) and by Stephens and Duka (for alcohol), although Beveridge et al. showed clearly how cognitive functions other than those normally influenced by the frontal lobes were affected, including temporal-lobe-dependent memory processes. Evidence surveyed by Stewart and by Crombag et al. also made it clear that the prefrontal cortex played a major role in experimental models of relapse, presumably in terms of exerting 'top–down' control on behavioural tendencies mediated by sub-cortical substrates, particularly the striatum.

Relapse was considered to be a key target for both the understanding and treatment of addiction. Stewart mainly dealt with the reinstatement model of relapse in which drug seeking/taking is first extinguished and then 'reinstated' either by priming injections of the drug itself, or cues associated with it, or by exposure to stressors. By contrast, Crombag et al. focused on contextual conditioning of relapse in which the behaviour is conditioned by general environmental features rather than specific cues. Extinction itself is especially specific to contextual factors, and there was a good deal of evidence already that the extinction of contexual fear conditioning appeared to depend on similar neural structures (including parts of the prefrontal cortex). A prodigious amount of work by investigators such as Stewart and Shaham (at the meeting) and by others such as Kalivas and colleagues (e.g. Kalivas & McFarland 2003) had shown that the neural substrates for these three forms of relapse shared some common structures, suggesting that they were mediated in part by common underlying processes. Further details are discussed under the *Neural basis of addiction*. One factor that was discussed in some detail was whether extinction was an appropriate model for relapse in human drug addicts, where much of their behaviour depended instead upon spontaneous or enforced abstinence. It was, however, the case that many of the brain regions implicated in relapse in human drug addicts through functional brain imaging were also highlighted by the animal models of relapse based on reinstatement. Nevertheless, it seemed likely that abstinence would recruit a distinct neural network. Another issue is whether there was overlap in the neural substrates for stimulant dependence (for which much of the work had been done) with those for heroin, and indeed other drugs of abuse, including alcohol, or even food. The importance of treating early in addiction was also underlined in view of the fact that there may be relationship between the duration of drug exposure and the strength of the relapse tendency, although there was little evidence to date that the schedule of reinforcement exerted a major influence on the strength of relapse.

Other forms of addiction

Whilst there has been emphasis on the neurobehavioural mechanisms underlying stimulant addiction, including its dopaminergic mediation via structures such as the nucleus accumbens, several presentations, beginning with that of Koob and Le Moal, emphasized the problems posed by considering addiction to other drugs, such as alcohol (Stephens and Duka) and nicotine (Markou) as well as to other sources of reinforcement, such as food (obesity, Volkow) and money (Potenza, compulsive gambling). Markou provided convincing evidence for a withdrawal syndrome in nicotine addiction and focused on its neural basis, mainly in terms of cholinergic–gabaergic–dopaminergic changes in the midbrain ventral tegmental area. She emphasized the rapid pharmacokinetic properties of nicotine smoking as an important part of nicotine addiction. The role of the cognitive effects of nicotine, notably to enhance concentration, in addiction were still unknown, but were probably a powerful element of the drive to smoke (together perhaps with anxiety-reducing effects of nicotine). However, these aspects were relatively under-researched, although there were prominent research programmes designed to exploit the cognitive enhancing effects of nicotine in such disorders as schizophrenia and Alzheimer's disease. Another, perhaps unique, element of relapse to smoking came from the fact that part of the motivation for smoking was from body weight regulation. Consequently, those pharmaceutical agents that suppress weight gain, as well as smoking per se, will be advantageous in the treatment of smoking relapse.

The importance of repeated withdrawal for alcohol abuse following repeated bingeing was also highlighted by the Stephens and Duka contribution, which brought out the profound implications of such repeated withdrawal for emotional and cognitive sequelae of alcohol abuse, including progressive effects on anxiety, impulsivity, and impaired learning. However, it is less clear how these changes contribute to addiction to alcohol, presumably via the opponent processes defined by Koob and Le Moal. One possibility was of drinking to reduce the anxiety that was at least particularly induced by withdrawal from alcohol, another form of 'self-medication', but there were probably many different types of alcoholism, including for example alcoholism due to impulsivity and self-medication which only applied to a sub-set of alcoholic individuals. It was raised whether the syndrome produced by repeated alcohol withdrawal could conceivably have been present prior to alcohol exposure; however, the rodent models strongly suggested that the effects in humans were not due to underlying pre-dispositions. Another issue raised was whether the multiple withdrawals were confounded with overall exposure to alcohol; however, levels of exposure were matched in the rodent (although not of course in the human) experiments. Alcohol did not appear to remediate cognitive disturbances produced by bingeing; if anything, it led to further impairment. The point was raised that 95% of alcoholics in the USA also smoked nicotine cigarettes, and so there were possible interactions between smoking and nicotine consumption. However, smoking did not affect the prefrontal cognitive deficits, although the impact on anxiety induced by multiple withdrawals was not known.

The Meeting also discussed two forms of 'behavioural addictions': gambling and eating. The prevalence of 'pathological gambling' showed that this was indeed a serious social burden comparable to that of other more conventional drug addictions. Potenza emphasized that the criteria for drug dependence such as tolerance, withdrawal, relapse, and compulsive behaviour also applied to pathological gambling. Moreover, the progression to compulsive gambling did appear to proceed in an analogous manner to that observed for stimulant or alcohol addiction, including initial links with impulsivity. From the research that had been done so far, there were studies on neurochemical factors through pharmacological studies, which implicated the same systems as have been implicated in drug addiction, including the monoamines, especially dopamine, serotonin, and noradrenaline. To a more limited extent, they also include similar neural substrates as measured by human functional neuroimaging, including the nucleus accumbens, anterior cingulate cortex, and the orbitofrontal cortex. Thus, again there was considerable evidence of overlap in the key neural networks underling drug addiction and pathological gambling. This had also been revealed by the phenomenon of compulsive gambling in some patients with Parkinson's disease, as a consequence of their use of D2 receptor agonist medication. However, much of the research thus far had been on relatively small samples of male gamblers and so there was an important need to study females. The likely interactions of pathological gambling with substance use had also not been much studied, hitherto.

Overlapping circuits (and therefore underlying behavioural processes) in addiction and obesity was also an important theme of the presentation by Volkow. The argument was that both many addictive drugs and food exert their reinforcing effects via dopamine; moreover, in both conditions, a marked preference for one type of reinforcer relative to others is evident. A major difference with feeding is that it is controlled by many other multiple factors, including neuroendocrine as well as peripheral and central physiological factors; nevertheless, the rewarding effects of food were also identified as being crucial. The kinetic effects of food delivery in terms of messages to the brain had not been studied as much as for drugs, where such pharmacokinetic effects are clearly crucial. However, other factors, such as stress, conditioning and emotional reactivity had all been shown to be relevant. Some of the key evidence came from human brain imaging studies. In parallel with her seminal work on stimulant and alcohol abusers showing reduced striatal D2 receptors, Volkow described how morbidly obese human or rodent subjects also exhibited lower than normal D2 receptor availability, although the mechanisms for how this neural change led to over-eating were obscure. There have also been imaging studies of conditioned cue-induced food craving showing associations with amygdala, medial prefrontal cortex, and striatal activation, which also parallel studies of cue-induced drug craving.

Neural basis of addiction

Many of the talks at the Meeting endorsed a common circuitry for drug addiction that especially depended on the ventral striatum (including the nucleus accumbens) and was importantly modulated by dopamine pathways originating in the ventral tegmental area. The special role of this region was exemplified by Nestler's talk, which focused on the molecular sequelae of addiction as shown by the time-dependent nature of changes in genetic transcription factors such as delta *FosB* and *c-fos*, which might track and even underlie the addiction process. However, the possible role of other structures had not been studied in as much detail. It was acknowledged that the availability of a PET ligand, which could be used to image the changes in these key molecules in parallel with the hypothetically distinct stages of addiction, would be invaluable as an experimental tool, but was not yet feasible. The talks of Everitt et al., Stewart, and Crombag et al. all showed that different sub-regions within the nucleus accumbens may have distinct roles. For example, although the shell sub-region was implicated in context-induced relapse, it is the core that is commonly implicated in cue-induced relapse, perhaps reflecting the relative projections of the hippocampus and amygdala, respectively. On the other hand, Crombag et al. also summarized evidence for basolateral amygdala involvement in context-induced relapse. Indeed, the prefrontal cortex and limbic structures such as the amygdala and hippocampus were also much implicated in the addictive process. However, the precise details of the involvement of this neural network and how it is affected differentially by different drugs (or other forms of addiction) and the stage of the addictive process varied quite widely across the presentations.

For example, Everitt et al., as well as other investigators, drew attention to the fact that the dorsal striatum was increasingly implicated in the later phases of drug self-administration, as distinct from the generally accepted role of the dopamine-dependent ventral striatum (including the nucleus accumbens) in mediating the initial reinforcing effects of many drugs (though stimulants in particular). This theme was also evident in work in monkeys (Beveridge et al.), and the molecular analysis of delta *Fos*B provided by Nestler, which focused on the nucleus accumbens but also showed changes in the dorsal striatum. Delta *Fos*B appears to throw a molecular 'switch' from the induction of several short-lived Fos family proteins after acute drug exposure to the predominant accumulation of delta *Fos*B after chronic drug exposure. Moreover, Volkow also showed how cue-induced craving could activate dorsal striatal structures rather than the nucleus accumbens in human drug abusers. This devolution from ventral to dorsal striatum may underlie what Everitt et al. characterized as the shift from action–outcome to S–R habit-based processes controlling drug seeking and taking.

However, Koob and LeMoal also identified a different set of structures associated with the withdrawal state that included noradrenergic-modulated structures such as the bed nucleus of the stria terminalis. These structures were also shown to have a special role in the phenomenon of stress-induced reinstatement (Stewart). Moreover, certain neuropeptides that drive the stress response, such as corticotrophin releasing factor (CRF) were identified as being very important. This importance arises from its role not only in controlling the hypothalamic–pituitary axis via the paraventricular nucleus, and the sympathetic nervous system, but also the brain systems controlling anxiety that depend on structures such as the central nucleus of the amygdala. This CRF dominated system becomes profoundly activated during withdrawal states. The amygdala was also highlighted by Stephens and Duka as being a neural target of repeated withdrawals from alcohol, leading to anxiety and concomitant changes in associative plasticity. These data leave us with the issue of how drugs taken putatively as 'negative reinforcers', such as alcohol, opiates, and possibly nicotine, actually reduce the activity in these centres, possibly by affecting GABA-ergic mechanisms within the amygdala, as well as the ventral tegmental area (Markou).

The third main region implicated in addiction is the prefrontal cortex, which was mentioned by many of the speakers, although often in different contexts, perhaps reflecting the multi-faceted importance of this structure, and also with emphasis sometimes on different regions. The prefrontal cortex influences in particular the amygdala and striatal sectors via its top–down projections. The animal literature normally emphasizes the rat medial prefrontal cortex in studies of the neural basis of relapse (whether cue-, context-, drug-, or stress-induced; see Stewart & Crombag et al.). These regions contrast with the profound changes in metabolism reported in the orbitofrontal cortex by Volkow following chronic drug abuse. In contrast, it is apparent that the insular cortex plays an important role in humans suffering nicotine withdrawal (Naqvi et al. 2007), possibly because of its close association with the autonomic nervous system. However, both Beveridge's neuropsychological analysis and Garavan's review of functional imaging in the context of drug addiction emphasized those regions of the prefrontal cortex implicated in cognitive functions, in particular cognitive control and monitoring of performance. Several speakers and questions from the floor queried whether the involvement of the prefrontal cortex in the human studies could be linked to drug taking *per se*, or to pre-morbid personality characteristics or traits that may predispose to addiction. Such questions can best be addressed by animal studies and the metabolic mapping studies of Beveridge et al. showed that the first metabolic changes (generally decreases) that could be detected in rhesus monkeys self-administering cocaine were to be found in the cingulate and ventromedial prefrontal cortex (area 14), as well as the insula. There are also initial increases in the dorsolateral prefrontal cortex, a region associated with aspects of working memory. However, more chronic exposure led to more widespread changes throughout the cingulate and orbitofrontal cortex, as well as to reductions in the dorsolateral prefrontal cortex, associated with impaired working memory performance. Similar patterns were observed in chronic human cocaine abusers. It is evident that chronic cocaine exposure is associated with impaired cognitive functions, whether this is associated with effects of withdrawal, neurotoxicity, or perhaps additional effects of cocaine such as the disruption of sleep. Probably all of these factors contribute to the generally complex picture.

Garavan complemented these findings with observations in chronic cocaine abusers of reduced activation in those areas of lateral prefrontal cortex that are implicated in response inhibition and the control of impulsive behaviour. Remarkably, however, he was able to show that administering cocaine to abusers in the scanner actually *improved* behavioural performance in tests of inhibitory response control, as well as normalizing the BOLD responses in these individuals. These effects also extended to similar effects in the anterior cingulate cortex in an error-monitoring task. These data clearly suggest that some of the cognitive impairment resulting from cocaine exposure results from a dysmodulation of prefrontal cortical function rather than a permanent deficit. They also suggest a normal role for mono-aminergic modulation of error monitoring and cognitive control functions (although Garavan himself favoured a role for dopamine in these functions). Garavan noted in discussion an initial improvement in performance of delayed matching to sample in the rhesus monkeys treated with cocaine, as studied by Beveridge et al. Thus, analogous to the effects of nicotine, there may be some grounds for assuming that some initial stimulant use is associated with self-medication for enhancement of certain behavioural and cognitive functions, possibly analogous to the treatment of impulsivity by stimulant drugs in attention deficit/hyperactivity disorder.

Vulnerability and aetiology of drug addiction

A fourth major theme of the meeting centred around the predisposition towards drug addiction, including genetic and environmental factors. Both of the major reviews of genetic factors concentrated on the genetic basis of alcoholism, presumably because this has been most investigated, although its basis was likely polygenic. Crabbe reviewed the use of rodent (generally mouse) selective breeding studies (including inbred strains) and mutant strains for alcohol dependence. He advocated not a rodent 'model' of alcoholism but rather a focus on specific aspects of the disorder, such as the neuropharmacology of ethanol, including tolerance and withdrawal phenomena, as well as oral self-administration. Ideally, the use of the different techniques, including knock-out, transgenic, and quantitative gene expression, would lead to results converging on particular genes in one or other of these phenotypes.

One important result, which appeared to support the opponent motivational processing theory of Koob and Le Moal, was the existence of a negative genetic relationship between high drinking and low withdrawal phenotypes, a phenomenon often observed by alcoholism treatment clinicians. In terms of other measures of alcohol intake and preference, there was a strong correlation between home cage drinking and intravenous self-administration of alcohol but not with measures of conditioned place preference to alcohol. Other significant genetic relationships are between measures of alcohol dependence such as drinking and stress or opioid function. Moreover, work on selectively bred high-drinking ratlines has shown that they exhibit reductions in limbic 5-HT levels, although evidence for other neurotransmitter changes is either weak or lacking. Gene expression studies in high drinking rats were in their infancy but showed promise. The discussion focused around the suggestion that there were many paths to excessive drinking (as perhaps exist for excessive use of other addictive drugs) and the need to select for the most relevant phenotypes. However, these could be influenced by many factors that induce or unmask ethanol preference, including for example, taste factors that combat the bitter taste of alcohol and social factors (e.g. dominance–submissiveness relationships).

Crabbe's contribution was complemented by that of Wong, Clarke and Schumann, which focused on reducing phenotypic heterogeneity, epigenetic factors, and endophenotypes (i.e. measurable intermediate phenotypes), mainly for human studies. They advocated the use of functional neuroimaging and human electrophysiological indices (e.g. low amplitude P-300) in addition to behavioural measures in the definition of endophenotypes. Thus, for example, the potential biomarker of low P-300 is found in the unaffected offspring of alcoholic families, and in some sense may represent a risk factor for alcoholism. If such findings yield greater evidence of inheritance than traditional measures this might facilitate the search for relevant genetic factors. In terms of epigenetic factors, exposure to psychosocial stress had been shown to be a potent determinant of alcoholism and could be mediated by genetic regulation of CRF. Animal models had thrown up intriguing candidate genes that may merit further investigation—for example, the possible influence of genes controlling circadian rhythms were originally discovered through studies of *Drosophila*, and may have relevance to alcoholism, given its association with disruptions of circadian rhythmicity.

The possibility of endophenotypes contributing to the vulnerability to addiction was also highlighted by studies in rats (Everitt et al.) and rhesus monkeys (Nader et al.). Thus, Everitt et al. described how the screening for impulsivity in rats had produced a phenotype, which persistently self-administered cocaine when exposed to a long access, binge self-administration situation. These rats also exhibited impulsivity as defined by impulsive choice in a temporal discounting of reward situation, but were no worse at stop-signal inhibition, a commonly used test of motor response inhibition. Most strikingly, however, they exhibited reduced D2/D3 receptor binding in the ventral striatum, in some sense paralleling the reduced striatal D2/D3 binding of chronic human cocaine abusers. These findings suggest that this latter change in humans is not necessarily caused by cocaine exposure, but may be present premorbidly. Further data reviewed by Everitt et al. suggested that the high impulsive rats were exhibiting a trait that was quite distinct from that of sensation or novelty seeking previously associated with the altered initiation of stimulant self-administration (Piazza et al. 1989). Furthemore, the high impulsive rats also exhibited a tendency towards compulsive drug-seeking behaviour, as measured by the relative insensitivity of such behaviour to punishment.

These findings with rats had been preceded by previously published data described at this meeting by Nader et al. in rhesus monkeys. They too had found an inverse relationship between D2/3 receptor binding potential in the striatum and cocaine intake. Additionally, however, they found that striatal D2 availability was significantly reduced by further exposure to cocaine, showing that both prior disposition and the effect of the drug itself potentially contribute to the down-regulation of striatal D2/3 receptors show in humans (Volkow). The 'vulnerable' monkeys in the studies of Nader et al. tended to be those that had previously been exposed to psychosocial stress, for example, had been behaviourally subordinate in the social hierarchy of the colony. These observations have profound implications for behavioural therapy of cocaine dependence. Thus, for example, when a dominant monkey was introduced into a social colony, its sensitivity to the reinforcing effects of cocaine diminished in terms of dose-response (whereas the opposite was true of intruder submissive monkeys). Similar 'therapeutic' effects of introducing novel objects leading to environmental enrichment were also shown, suggesting that the vulnerability to cocaine reinforcement in these primates can be reduced by exposure to other preferred reinforcers. Clearly, there are profound implications here for the treatment of human stimulant abusers.

The other thread contributing to vulnerability came from quite frequent references to differential effects of drugs of abuse in early development. This was raised in the context of nicotine exposure, for example, and also with respect to reduced withdrawal symptoms observed in ethanol exposure. However, more systematic information was required concerning this important factor.

Implications for Treatment

The final theme running through many talks at the Meeting was that of the treatment of addiction, the paper by O'Brien being the only one that explicitly surveyed current clinical treatments. Several of the other talks, however, mentioned candidate therapies generally predicated on the experimental findings described. Thus, Koob and Le Moal mentioned animal studies that had shown efficacy of small molecule CRF-antagonists, kappa receptor antagonists, and Neuropetide-Y receptor agonists in their models of drug dependence and withdrawal, although none of these agents were yet available for human studies. Stewart referred to the possibility of effecting changes in glutamate-induced plasticity relevant to the treatment of relapse by using N-acetylcysteine to restore cytosine–glutamate exchange in the nucleus accumbens resulting perhaps from over-active prefrontal cortical glutamatergic inputs (Madayag et al. 2007). She also described possible remedial effects of a group II mGluR agonist on relapse when also infused into the nucleus accumbens. In an extensive experimental account, Markou had also shown that decreasing glutamate transmission or increasing GABA transmission by pharmacological means influenced the development of nicotine reinforcement and withdrawal in rodents, with implications for pharmacological therapy. She pointed out that $GABA_B$ receptor-positive allosteric modulators may decrease the rewarding effects of nicotine with a better side-effect profile than full $GABA_B$ receptor agonists.

In an horizon-scanning sense, the work of Nestler on molecular adaptations might also lead eventually to effective drugs in theory, for example, delta FosB antagonists. (The availability of such compounds would incidentally enable testing of the causal role of these molecular adaptations in addiction). However, the role of molecules such as delta FosB in other reward processes and also in certain situations, stress, means that any such drug is likely to have side–effects, which would have to be carefully considered before clinical application. Other future-looking contributions (Crombag et al.) chose to focus instead on refinements in possible behavioural treatments. Context-induced relapse suggests the need for future cue exposure therapy to arrange exposures to cues in diverse contexts to allow them to become more effective. They also mentioned the use of a richer variety of reinforcers along the lines being employed by Nader et al. in their environmental enrichment programmes. A very different type of treatment, although one with perhaps a neurobiological, as distinct from a psychological, basis was that of physical exercise that was raised by several of the questioners from the floor.

O'Brien finally reviewed in some detail the evidence base for addiction treatments, affirming the importance of both behavioural and pharmacological approaches and focusing on general principles. He made the point, not always appreciated from an animal approach, that there was enormous variation in response to drug treatments. He considered drug addiction as a chronic brain disorder with relapses and remissions in the long term. Drug detoxification was an initial step in treatment but could not be effective in itself without considering relapse, an unfortunate consideration in view of the fact that the focus of most drug-dependence treatments was on detoxification, usually attained by replacing the drug of dependence by another in the same pharmacological class in gradually decreasing doses. Buprenorphine, a partial mu-opiate receptor agonist, had recently been found to be a very effective treatment for opiate addiction and similar principles applied to nicotine substitutes (gum or patch or the alpha 4 beta 2 agonist varenicline), to alcohol (using benzodiazepines), stimulants (modafinil), and cannabis (dronabinol). However, most of these treatments were ineffective in treating craving or relapse except in the case of the opiates and nicotine treatments.

The use of opiate receptor antagonist treatments such as naloxone and naltrexone had not in general been as efficacious as agonists, but surprisingly naltrexone had been found to be useful in the treatment of alcoholism and may be augmented by pharmacogenomic evidence of individual responses to this treatment. (It was mentioned in discussion that naltrexone however did not block *conditioned* withdrawal responses, as monitored by fMRI). Other relatively novel treatments for addiction had arisen from animal models (in the case of vigabatrin, an inhibitor of GABA transaminase, and acamprosate), from clinical serendipity (bupropion) and from biological principles in the case of experimental vaccines, but the general dearth of treatments specifically for relapse was underlined, especially for stimulant drugs. Nevertheless, O'Brien was optimistic about the present state of addiction treatments, which often lead to improvements in occupational and functional status, though, as with other chronic relapsing disorders, when the treatment is discontinued, the symptoms usually recur. He pointed out that, in some sense, a future productive approach to the treatment of addiction would be to erase drug-associated memories if that was feasible without impairing normal memory.

References

Kalivas, P. W. & McFarland, K. (2003) Brain circuitry and the reinstatement of cocaine-seeking behavior. *Psychopharmacology*, **168**, 44–56.

Madayag, A., Lobner, D., Kau, K. S. et al. (2007) Repeated *N*-acetylcysteine administration alters plasticity-dependent effects of cocaine. *Journal of Neuroscience*, **27**, 13968–76

Naqvi, N. H., Rudrauf, D., Damasio, H., & Bechara, A. (2007) Damage to the insual disrupts addiction to cigarette smoking. *Science*, **315**, 531–4.

Piazza, P. V., Deminiere, J. M., Le Moal, M. & Simon, H. (1989) Factors that predict individual vulnerability to amphetamine self-administration. *Science* 245, 1511–13.

Index